HEART
TRANSPLANTATION

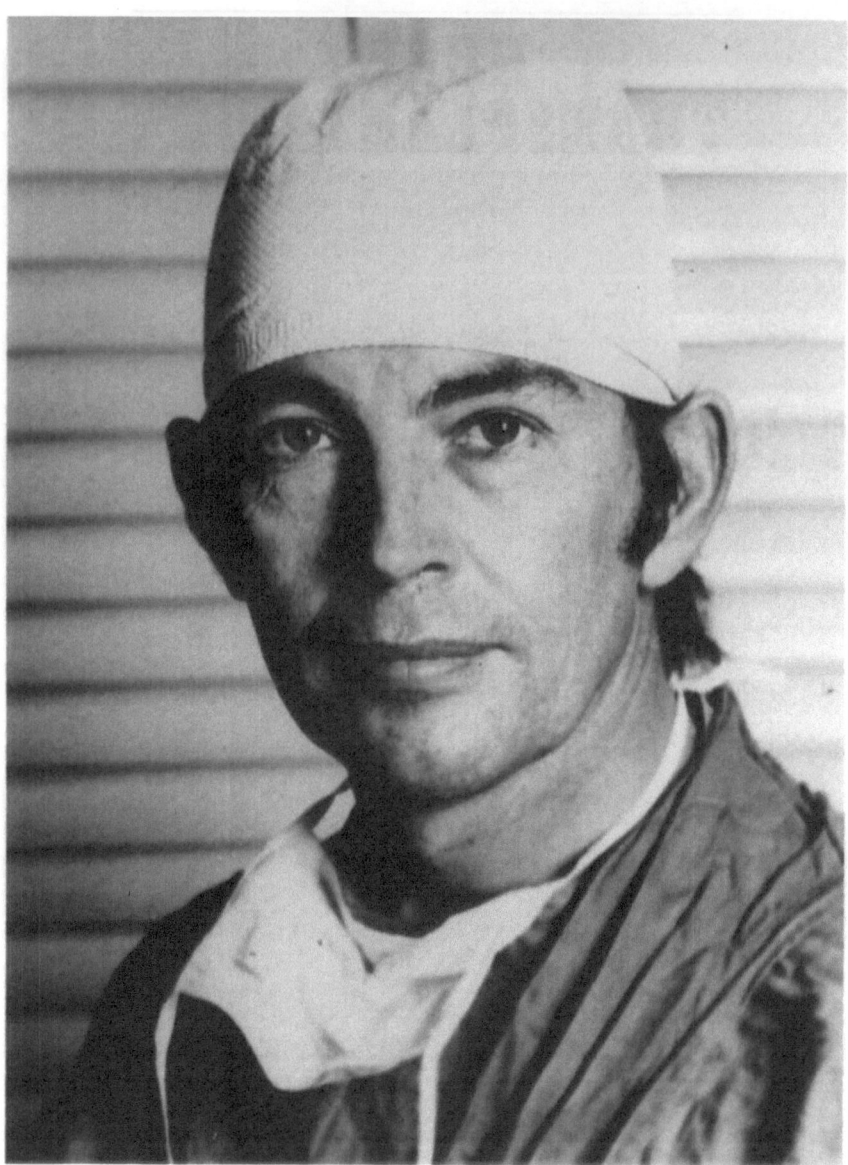

PROFESSOR CHRISTIAAN N. BARNARD, who was appointed to the specialist surgical staff of Groote Schuur Hospital and the University of Cape Town Medical School in 1958, became Head of the Department of Cardiac Surgery in 1961, Associate Professor of Surgery in 1962, and Professor of Surgical Science in 1972; he retired from these appointments at the end of 1983. To mark his retirement, the editors and authors offer this book as a tribute to his contributions to cardiac surgery and, in particular, to his pioneering work in the field of heart transplantation.

Photo: Don MacKenzie, Cape Town

HEART TRANSPLANTATION

THE PRESENT STATUS OF ORTHOTOPIC AND HETEROTOPIC HEART TRANSPLANTATION

EDITED BY

D. K. C. COOPER, MA, MB, BS, PhD, FRCS
Specialist in Cardiothoracic Surgery,
Groote Schuur Hospital and the
University of Cape Town Medical School, Cape Town, South Africa

and

R. P. LANZA, MD
Chris Barnard Fund Research Fellow,
Cardiac Surgical Research Unit,
Department of Cardiothoracic Surgery,
University of Cape Town Medical School, Cape Town, South Africa

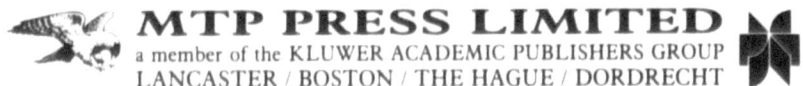

MTP PRESS LIMITED
a member of the KLUWER ACADEMIC PUBLISHERS GROUP
LANCASTER / BOSTON / THE HAGUE / DORDRECHT

Published in the UK and Europe by
MTP Press Limited
Falcon House
Lancaster, England

British Library Cataloguing in Publication Data

Heart transplantation
  1. Heart—Transplantation
  I. Cooper, D. K. C.   II. Lanza, R. P.
  617'.4120592   R9598

  ISBN-13: 978-94-011-7326-1   e-ISBN-13: 978-94-011-7324-7
  DOI: 10.1007/978-94-011-7324-7

Published in the USA by
MTP Press
A division of Kluwer Boston Inc.
190 Old Derby Street
Hingham, MA 02043, USA

Library of Congress Cataloging in Publication Data

Main entry under title:

Heart transplantation.

  Bibliography: p.
  Includes index.
  1. Heart—Transplantation.   I. Cooper, D. K. C.
(David K. C.), 1939– .   II. Lanza, R. P. (Robert
Paul), 1956– .   [DNLM: 1. Heart—transplantation.
2. Transplantation Immunology.   WG 169 H436]
RD598.H426   1984   617'.412   84-14319

ISBN-13: 978-94-011-7326-1

Mather Bros (Printers) Ltd, Preston

Contents

Foreword

It is a great pleasure for me to contribute a brief introduction to this volume, to which so many of my colleagues at Groote Schuur Hospital and the University of Cape Town Medical School have contributed.

Though considerable advances have been made in preventing or treating the complications of heart transplantation, even today a transplant programme remains a major undertaking for a hospital team. The acquisition of a sufficient number of donor hearts, the maintenance of viability of those hearts, and the prevention, diagnosis and treatment of acute and chronic rejection and infection remain major challenges to those caring for patients undergoing this operation. A transplant programme draws into it medical, surgical, nursing and paramedical staff from all quarters of the hospital and medical school, and requires sustained interest and dedication if patients are to be brought successfully through the procedure. If relevant experimental research is also to be carried out at such a centre, which in my opinion is essential, then an even greater number of highly skilled and creative people is required.

A few of the authors of this book have been involved with the Groote Schuur heart transplant programme since its inception in December 1967 with the operation on Louis Washkansky. I am sure that none of them (nor I) had any idea of the public interest this operation would attract. The other authors joined us subsequently and have made their own particular contributions to our work in both the clinical and experimental aspects of transplantation.

Over the years, very many others have, of course, been involved in this work in Cape Town. I remember, in particular, the great help I received from my brother, Marius, from immunologist Dr M. C. Botha, and from surgeons 'Bossie' Bosman, Rodney Hewitson, Jacques Losman, Alan Wolpowitz and Jannie Hassoulas. Our early explorations into the problems of heart transplantation were greatly encouraged and facilitated by that outstanding cardiologist, the late Professor Val Schrire, to whom I personally owe a debt of gratitude for his support throughout my early career at Groote Schuur.

The number of transplants performed at our own centre coud have been easily two or three times as large had we been able to acquire sufficient suitable donor hearts. This remains a major limiting factor, suggesting that, in South

Africa at least, the public and the medical profession have not yet fully accepted the donation of organs as a routine which should be considered in every brain-dead patient. A sustained effort in the education of the public will be required to correct the situation, not only in South Africa, but worldwide.

The contributors to this book and, in particular, the editors, David Cooper and Robert Lanza, are to be congratulated in bringing together such a wealth of information on this topic and presenting it in such a balanced and readable way. I believe this book will be essential reading for those considering initiating a heart transplant programme and, indeed, for any interested in progress in this field.

As this is the first year of my retirement from the staff of Groote Schuur Hospital and the University of Cape Town I can take this opportunity of wishing those who continue to work in the field of heart transplantation, not only in Cape Town, but worldwide, every success in their labours.

CHRISTIAAN N. BARNARD

April 1984

Preface

When Professor Christiaan Barnard and his surgical team performed the first human-to-human heart transplant at Groote Schuur Hospital in Cape Town on 2 December 1967, the event not only captured the public interest and imagination but also stimulated many other surgical centres to enter this demanding field of therapy. Interest soon died, however, since some of these groups were ill-prepared to deal with the many major complications of the procedure, and the results were poor.

A very small number of centres, including our own, persisted in their efforts to overcome the problems they faced. Recognition must be given, in particular, to the immense contribution made by the group at Stanford Medical Center, and to the groups at the Medical College of Virginia and La Pitié Hospital in Paris, who continued exploring this area of therapy whilst the enthusiasm of others waned. Now, some 16 years later, the number of centres actively engaged in this field has increased over fivefold, and heart transplantation has progressed from being a clinical research programme to a definitive form of surgical therapy.

It therefore seemed timely to review the present status of heart transplantation. In writing this book, though we have drawn greatly from our own experience at Groote Schuur Hospital and the University of Cape Town, we have endeavoured to review the experience of all of the major groups who have contributed to our knowledge in this area. Though we do not claim that our review has been totally comprehensive, we hope and believe that it provides an informative and balanced account of this form of therapy at the present time.

Professor Barnard retired from the staff of our hospital and medical school at the beginning of this year; this book marks the occasion of his retirement and is offered as a tribute to his pioneering work in the field of heart transplantation.

D. K. C. COOPER
R. P. LANZA
Department of Cardiothoracic Surgery
Groote Schuur Hospital and the
University of Cape Town Medical School

April 1984

List of Contributors

(All members of the staff of Groote Schuur Hospital and/or the University of Cape Town Medical School)

C. N. Barnard, MD, MMed, MS, PhD, FACS, FACC, DSc(HonCausa)
Formerly Professor of Surgical Science and Head
Department of Cardiac Surgery

E. D. Bateman, MB, ChB, DCH, MRCP
Senior Specialist
Respiratory Clinic
Department of Medicine

P. J. Commerford, MB, ChB, FCP(SA), FACC
Senior Specialist
Cardiac Clinic
Department of Medicine

D. K. C. Cooper, MA, MB, BS, PhD, FRCS
Specialist
Department of Cardiothoracic Surgery

J. C. de Villiers, MD, FRCS(Eng), FRCS(Edin)
Helen and Morris Mauerberger Professor and Head
Department of Neurosurgery

E. D. du Toit, MD
Head
Laboratory for Tissue Immunology
Cape Provincial Administration

A. A. Forder, MB, ChB, MMed(Path)
Wernher and Beit Professor and Head
Department of Medical Microbiology

A. R. Horak, MB, ChB, FCP(SA)
Specialist
Cardiac Clinic
Department of Medicine

R. P. Lanza, MD
Chris Barnard Fund Research Fellow
Cardiac Surgical Research Unit
Department of Cardiothoracic Surgery

E. S. Nash, MB, ChB, FRCP, DPM, FFPsych(SA)
Senior Specialist
Department of Psychiatry

D. Novitzky, MD, FCS(SA)
Specialist
Department of Cardiothoracic Surgery

J. Ozinsky, MB, ChB, DA, FFARCS
Chief Specialist
Department of Anaesthetics

A. G. Rose, MB, ChB, MMed(Path), MRCPath, FACC
Associate Professor
Department of Pathology

L. S. Smith, MB, BCh, DPH, DBact, FRCPath
Professor and Head
Department of Forensic Medicine and Toxicology

C. J. Uys, MD, DClin Path, FRCPath
Wernher and Beit Professor and Head
Department of Pathology

J. van Heerden
Chief Technologist
Department of Cardiothoracic Surgery

W. N. Wicomb, PhD
Chris Barnard Fund Research Fellow
Cardiac Surgical Research Unit
Department of Cardiothoracic Surgery

Acknowledgements

We wish to express our appreciation to the contributing authors, who have expertly presented their information in a clear and concise manner. Our surgical colleague, Dimitri Novitzky, reviewed several of the chapters and gave us the benefit of his expertise and experience; his comments proved most helpful. Other colleagues—Jack Jacobson, Machteld Oudshoorn, Gwen Sayers and John Stevens—also read and commented on several chapters at various stages of their preparation. We thank all of them.

Mrs Desirée Fray proved untiring in producing a carefully typed manuscript and is deserving of our sincere gratitude; her contribution greatly facilitated the preparation of this book. Her secretarial colleagues, Mrs Doreen Lambie and Mrs Doris Walker, gave her valuable support.

The excellent illustrations are the work of Miss Jenny Bosman, medical artist in the Department of Clinical Photography at Groote Schuur Hospital. We are most grateful to her and to her departmental colleagues for the photographic work which appears in the book.

We gratefully acknowledge permission to reproduce tables and illustrations previously published in the following journals: Figure 5.1 from *Transplantation*, **34**, 247, 1982; Figure 5.2 from *S. Afr. Med. J.*, **60**, 246, 1981; Figure 6.1 from *Heart Transplant.*, **3**, 89, 1983; Figures 6.2 and 6.3 op. cit. p. 90; Figures 8.10 and 8.11 from *Ann. Thoracic Surg.*, **36**, 477, 1983; Figures 8.12 and 8.13 op. cit. p. 478; Figure 8.20 op. cit. p. 481; Figure 8.22 from *Br. J. Clin. Pract.*, **36**, 340, 1982; Figure 11.15 from *Arch. Path. Lab. Med.*, **107**, 368, 1983; Figure 17.3 from *Heart Transplant.*, **3**, 258, 1984; Figures 19.7 and 19.8 from *Heart Transplant.*, **3**, 88, 1983; Figure 20.1 from *Ann. Thoracic Surg.*, **37**, 246, 1984; Figure 20.2 from *Br. J. Clin. Pract.*, **36**, 331, 1982; Table 13.2 from *Thorax*, **38**, 823, 1983; Table 13.3 op. cit. p. 825; Table 14.2 from *J. Am. Med. Assoc.*, **249**, 1747, 1983; Tables 19.2 and 19.3 from *Heart Transplant.*, **3**, 89, 1983; Table 19.4 from *Heart Transplant.*, **3**, 249, 1984.

One of us (R.P.L.) is indebted to Dr Eliot Stellar and the University Scholars' Program of the University of Pennsylvania, and to Scott Randall, and Barbara and Eugene O'Donnell for their valuable support.

Since the inception of the heart transplant programme in 1967 many members of the medical, nursing and paramedical staff of Groote Schuur

Hospital and the University of Cape Town Medical School have contributed towards the care of our patients and to our research activities; to all of them we give our thanks. We also take this opportunity of expressing our gratitude to the generous and continuing support given to our research programmes by the Cape Provincial Administration, the University of Cape Town, and the Chris Barnard Fund.

Finally, we wish to record our gratitude to Dr H-Reeve Sanders, the present Chief Medical Superintendent of Groote Schuur Hospital, for the support and encouragement she has given to both the clinical and experimental work on heart transplantation in our department.

D. K. C. COOPER
R. P. LANZA
Groote Schuur Hospital and the
University of Cape Town Medical School

April 1984

1
Experimental Development and Early Clinical Experience

INTRODUCTION

Clinical heart transplantation was made possible by the considerable experimental work carried out earlier this century which embraced mainly the technical, physiological and immunological aspects of the procedure. This chapter endeavours to review briefly the evolution and results of experimental surgical techniques utilized by cardiac transplant research workers; a comprehensive review appears elsewhere[1].

Experimental work on cardiac transplantation evolved through several overlapping phases. In the earliest experiments animals were given a second, often parasitic, heart which enabled certain physiological, pharmacological and pathological studies to be made. Initially the neck was chosen as the locus, though the abdomen and inguinal regions were occasionally used. The subsequent evolution of surgical techniques permitted the insertion of the donor heart into the chest as an auxiliary pump in circuit with the recipient organ. With the advent of hypothermia and the pump oxygenator, total excision and replacement of the recipient heart became more feasible. Finally, after technical and physiological problems had been studied and minimized, efforts were made to combat the immune response with immunosuppressive agents.

TRANSPLANTATION OF AN ACCESSORY HEART

The first reported attempts at experimental heart transplantation were by Carrel and Guthrie in 1905[2,3]. The principal technique they used is inadequately described as 'anastomosing the cut ends of the jugular vein and the carotid artery to the aorta, the pulmonary artery, one of the vena cava and a pulmonary vein'. This procedure took approximately 75 minutes. Although contractions of the donor atria appeared immediately after the operation, effective contractions of the ventricles did not begin for approximately 1 hour. The operation was performed without aseptic technique; the experiment was interrupted after a further 2 hours when coagulation occurred in the cavities of the heart. Carrel also attempted transplantation of the heart and both lungs into the neck of a cat, but the lungs became oedematous with subsequent distension of the right chambers of the heart[3].

The crucial factor of donor coronary perfusion (viviperfusion) was simplified in 1933 when Mann and his colleagues developed a technique of cervical transplantation[4] (Figure 1.1). The donor coronary system was perfused by anastomosing the recipient common carotid artery to the donor aorta. Coronary sinus blood returned to the recipient jugular vein via the right atrium, right ventricle and pulmonary artery. Immediately after the coronary circulation was established the heart usually began to contract at a heart rate of approximately 100–130 beats per minute. This rate increased further if the animal

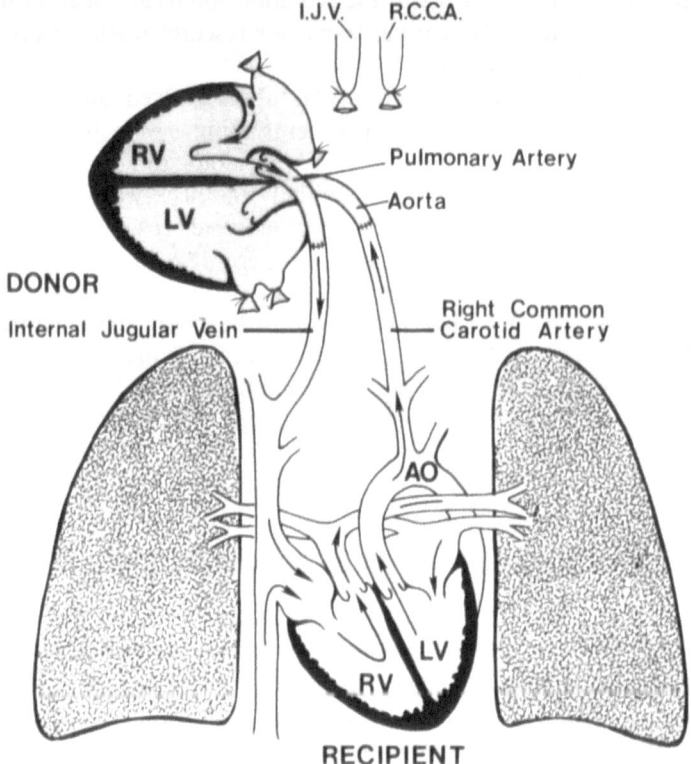

Figure 1.1   Technique of experimental heterotopic heart transplantation in the neck (Mann et al., 1933)[4]. I.J.V. = Internal jugular vein; R.C.C.A. = Right common carotid artery

Figure 1.1   Technique of experimental heterotopic heart transplantation in the neck (Mann et al., 1933)[4]. I.J.V. = Internal jugular vein; R.C.C.A. = Right common carotid artery

Electrocardiographic (ECG) tracings were 'surprisingly normal'. Numerous investigators have subsequently used modifications of the Mann technique to study problems of heart transplantation and the response of the denervated heart to pharmacological agents and physiological stresses[1]. One such modification remains a standard model in many laboratories, including our own, for experimental animal studies on acute rejection and immunosuppression (Figure 1.2).

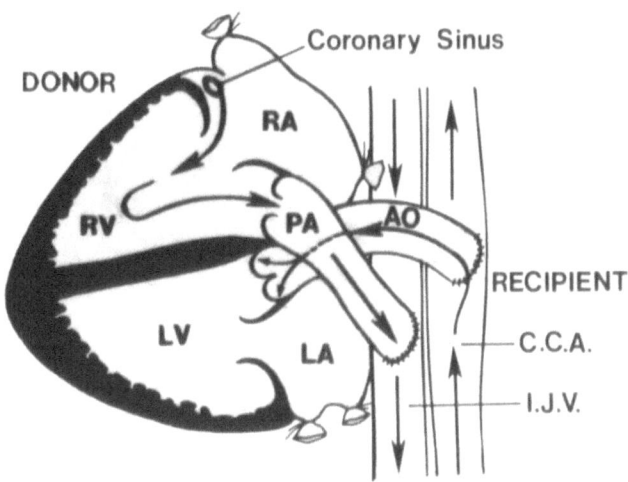

Figure 1.2 Modification of the Mann experimental cervical heterotopic heart transplantation technique as used in our own laboratory

Mann and his colleagues reported irregularities in the pulse rate of the transplanted heart after an average of 4 days; these were soon followed by fibrillation or absence of pulsation. When the heart was excised just prior to becoming quiescent, the left atrium was found to be filled with clot, both the right atrium and ventricle were distended, the surface of the heart was mottled, and the myocardium friable on section. Histologically, the heart was completely infiltrated with lymphocytes, large mononuclear cells, and polymorphonuclear leukocytes. From these results the investigators concluded that a functioning cardiac allograft was no less 'resistant' than a renal allograft, the graft failing to survive due to the same 'biologic factor' which also prevented survival of other homotransplanted tissues and organs.

With regard to short experiments performed within 24 hours of transplantation, the same research team had no hesitation, however, in concluding that the transplanted heart should be a valuable test object for the investigation of various physiological problems. For example, they investigated the effect of the intravenous administration of thyroxine to the host animal. Although the pulse rate of the transplanted organ increased significantly within 18 hours, the rate of the host's heart remained unchanged. This experiment demonstrated that thyroxine-induced tachycardia was independent of the central nervous system (CNS), and that the denervated heart was more sensitive to the accelerating influence of the drug since CNS influence was inhibitory.

In more recent years, techniques for transplanting the auxiliary donor heart into the abdomen of the recipient have been described (Figure 1.3). Anastomoses are made between the recipient abdominal aorta and the donor ascending aorta to allow perfusion of the myocardium through the coronary arteries.

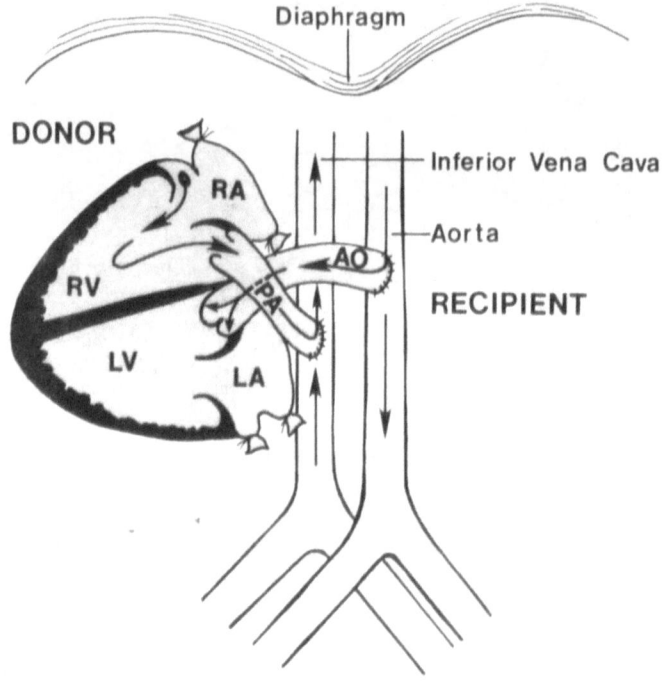

Figure 1.3 Technique of experimental heterotopic heart transplantation in the abdomen (Abbott *et al.*, 1964)

Coronary venous return drains through the right heart and pulmonary artery to the recipient inferior vena cava. This technique has also been used principally for the study of the immune response and its modification by therapeutic agents, particularly using microsurgical techniques in rats[5,6] where it remains an important model.

THE TRANSPLANTED HEART AS AN AUXILIARY INTRATHORACIC PUMP

In 1946, Demikhov began extensive studies on transplantation of the heart into the thorax. These involved the addition of a second heart (occasionally with an attached lobe of a lung) as an auxiliary pump, as well as orthotopic transplantation of the heart with and without both lungs[7]. The ambitious nature of Demikhov's attempts can be appreciated best when it is remembered that supportive techniques, such as hypothermia and cardiopulmonary bypass, had not yet been developed.

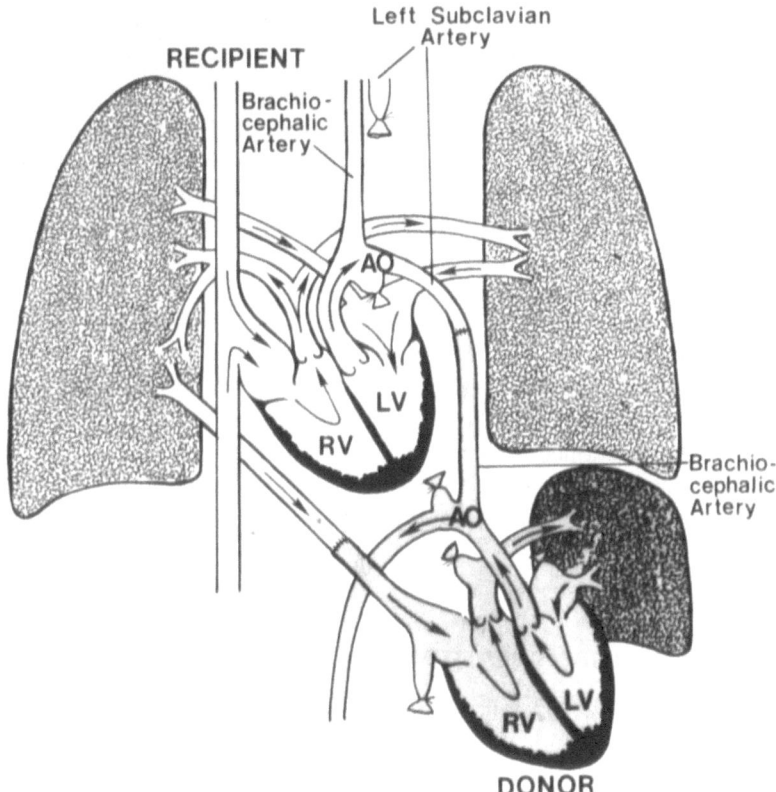

Figure 1.4 Technique of insertion of the heterotopic heart in the chest as an auxiliary pump (Demikhov, 1962)[7]

In all, Demikhov described 24 variants of his technique to place an additional heart within the thorax. He performed 250 operations on dogs utilizing most of the major vessels within the chest cavity; 43 animals died on the operating table, 87 during the first 2 days, 110 between the 2nd and 19th day, and one on day 32. Most of the early deaths were associated with technical problems. The best results with regard to functional activity of the transplanted heart and preservation of its structure were obtained after operations using the technique illustrated in Figure 1.4.

Physiologically the transplanted heart was distinguished by the comparative constancy of its rhythm and by its greater resistance to the action of toxic doses of various cardiac glycosides. Marked bradycardia of the dog's own heart occurred after injection of large doses of strophanthin, although no changes took place in the rhythm of the transplanted heart. When lethal doses of cardiac glycosides were administered, the transplanted heart continued to function for 10–15 minutes after the animal's own heart had arrested. It was also observed that when a dog died from haemorrhage or peritonitis the coordinated activity of the animal's own heart ceased long before that of the transplanted heart. The physiological and pharmacological responses of the denervated, transplanted heart are discussed more fully in Chapter 10.

Several years later, Reemtsma[8] described a method of inserting an additional intrathoracic heart as an auxiliary pump, which was similar in principle to that later developed and used clinically in our own heterotopic heart transplant programme in Cape Town[9, 10]. The donor inferior vena cava was anastomosed to the recipient's right atrial appendage, followed by anastomosis of the two left atrial appendages, and end-to-side anastomoses of the two pulmonary arteries and aorta. Function as an auxiliary pump was maintained for a maximum period of 72 hours.

Sen and his colleagues described a further technique in which the transplanted heart supported only the systemic circulation of the recipient[11]. This auxiliary heart functioned in one animal for 48 hours, when it was surgically excised and the animal supported solely by its own heart once again, thus demonstrating the heterotopic heart transplant as a temporary left ventricular assist device.

ORTHOTOPIC TRANSPLANTATION OF THE HEART

Between 1946 and 1955, Demikhov used an ingenious method in 67 attempts to transplant the heart and both lungs in dogs, with survival up to the 6th day[7] (Chapter 21). Deaths resulted primarily from thrombosis at the sites of blood vessel anastomosis, or from bronchopneumonia in the lower lobes.

On 25 December 1951—a date which surely tells us a great deal about this surgeon—Demikhov made the first recorded attempt to replace the heart alone. Without the availability of hypothermia or pump oxygenator support the technique was necessarily complicated. The procedure consisted of end-to-side anastomoses between the corresponding thoracic aortae, superior and inferior venae cavae, and pulmonary arteries. The two inferior pulmonary veins of the donor were joined together and connected to the recipient's left atrial appendage. After these anastomoses, the ascending parts of the recipient's thoracic aorta and pulmonary artery were ligated, and the recipient's left atrium was indrawn at its border with the ventricle by means of a purse-string suture. The entire segment of the recipient's heart thus excluded from the circulation was then excised.

Demikhov performed this procedure on 22 occasions, and in 1955 was successful in obtaining good cardiac function in two cases for periods of $11\frac{1}{2}$ and $15\frac{1}{2}$ hours respectively. In the former case, death was due to thrombosis at the superior vena caval anastomosis, whereas in all other cases death resulted from technical problems. These were amongst the first reported experiments, however, where animals survived for a few hours solely on the activity of the transplanted heart.

ADVENT OF SUPPORTIVE TECHNIQUES

With the advent of methods of supporting the recipient during the operative procedure, workers in this field became more ambitious. Neptune and his colleagues used hypothermia in three attempts at transplantation of the heart and both lungs, with survival for up to 6 hours[12]. Webb and Howard performed cardiopulmonary replacement on an animal maintained on mechanical pump-oxygenator support, with survival to 22 hours[13, 14]; they studied cardiac and unilateral pulmonary transplants, autotransplants of the heart and lungs and of the heart alone.

In 1958, Goldberg and Berman used a technique which differed from that of Webb in that a left atrial cuff was preserved in the recipient, thus nullifying the need to anastomose the pulmonary veins. They reported three experiments, with survival for only 21, 117 and 86 minutes; in two of these cases pacemakers had to be inserted to maintain an adequate heart rate[15, 16].

Cass and Brock reported six attempts at autotransplantation and homotransplantation using a modification of Goldberg's technique, where both atria were left intact in the recipient, thus simplifying the procedure even further[17]. Anastomoses of the atria, aorta and pulmonary artery were now all that were required. This procedure was described again 1 year later at Stanford Medical School by Lower and Shumway, who obtained the first consistently successful results[18]. With a further modification made by Barnard[19], the technique is now used in the clinical operation of orthotopic heart transplantation and is described in detail in Chapter 8.

It was, therefore, not until 1960 that the major experimental advance was made, when Lower and Shumway reported that five out of eight consecutive dogs undergoing transplantation had lived for 6–21 days[18]. During convalescence the dogs ate and exercised normally, the pulse rate was variable and increased moderately with exercise, and only a few hours before death the ECG remained virtually normal, showing no evidence of arrhythmia or conduction defects. The terminal course was usually rapid, occurring within approximately 24 hours, during which time the animal became lethargic and progressively tachypnoeic. Postmortem examination of the heart showed it to be ecchymotic and oedematous with a fibrinoid pericarditis and generalized dilatation. Microscopical examination of sections demonstrated severe myocarditis, with massive round-cell infiltration, patchy necrosis, interstitial haemorrhage, and oedema. The authors concluded that in all likelihood the graft would have continued to function for the normal life span of the animal if the immunologic mechanisms of the host had been suppressed.

In the following year, Lower et al. reported complete homograft replacement of the heart and both lungs, with survival of up to 5 days; deaths were from respiratory insufficiency, which was apparently secondary to infiltration of mononuclear cells into the lung parenchyma[20].

These investigators and their colleagues subsequently confined their studies to autotransplantation[21,22] and allotransplantation[23-25] of the heart alone, achieving long-term survival, and contributing extensively to our knowledge of this subject[26-28]. In the experimental animal the transplanted heart was found to have the capacity to increase cardiac output, primarily by increasing stroke volume, under a variety of physiological stresses, including hypoxia and exercise; a normal cardiac output was demonstrated 1 year after allotransplantation and $5\frac{1}{2}$ years after autotransplantation; evidence of autonomic reinnervation of the heart after autotransplantation was obtained.

In 1962, Willman and his colleagues produced the first of several papers on the subject of myocardial structure and function following autotransplantation of the heart[29]. Their technique differed from those of previous workers in being a piecemeal division and resuture in turn of each of the vessels connecting the heart to the rest of the body. Twenty-seven out of 40 animals died within 2 days, primarily from technical causes; 13 survived longer than 2 days. All survivors appeared critically ill during the first week, though a few long-term survivors were obtained. They concluded that there was a specific adverse effect of severing the heart from the body and suggested that this resulted from severance of the extrinsic innervation and/or the lymphatic drainage. The specific mechanism of adaptation by which long-term survival was achieved remained unclear. Shumway's group later disputed these pessimistic findings, having obtained autotransplants in dogs which survived for over 18 months[21]. The disparity between these results has never been explained. Willman and his associates subsequently used their technique to carry out extensive studies of the physiology[30-33], histology[34,35], metabolism[36-38], and pharmacology[39] of the autografted heart, including autotransplantation in the primate[40].

USE OF PROFOUND HYPOTHERMIA

Kondo and his colleagues performed orthotopic transplantation in puppies under profound hypothermia rather than with a pump oxygenator[41]. Total body cooling by iced water immersion of both recipient (to 16–17 °C rectally) and donor (to 27–29 °C) was carried out, allowing complete circulatory arrest of the recipient for the 45 ± 5 minute operation. Heart massage was begun immediately after the anastomoses were completed. After being warmed to 26–28 °C by body immersion and flushing of the chest cavity with warm saline the heart was electrically defibrillated, and rewarming continued until the temperature returned to normal. In their first reported series of 40 experiments the group obtained 24 1-day survivors, 13 7-day survivors, and one which remained alive and well 112 days after operation. Although none was given immunosuppressive therapy, histological and other signs of rejection occurred much later than in previously reported series. The surprisingly long survival of some of their animals was attributed to accidental histocompatibility, though the fact that 3-month-old puppies were used for these experiments was thought to be a significant factor in the relative mildness of the immune response.

In preparation for human heart transplantation in our institution, M. S. Barnard performed orthotopic cardiac allografting in dogs with pump-oxygenator support, though the donor was cooled by immersion in ice as described by Kondo. The donor heart supported a satisfactory circulation in 90% of cases[42].

PROLONGATION OF GRAFT SURVIVAL BY IMMUNOSUPPRESSION

When many of the technical and physiological problems had been overcome, investigators turned their attention to the problem of combating the immune response by chemotherapy. Reemtsma and his colleagues used Mann's cervical transplantation technique to study the effect of methotrexate, a folic acid antagonist[43]. In a control series of untreated dogs, cardiac activity continued for a maximum of only 10 days, whereas in the methotrexate-treated group maximal survival extended to 27 days. When the recipient was given azathioprine, the maximal survival was 32 days[8]. In both drug groups approximately 40% of the transplanted hearts functioned for more than the maximum 10 days of the control animals. Drug toxicity was less severe in the azathioprine-treated group. Blumenstock and his colleagues, using methotrexate in dogs with orthotopic transplants, obtained five dogs that survived from 12 to 42 days[44].

The Stanford group reported its experience with a combination of steroids (hydrocortisone or methylprednisolone) and azathioprine or mercaptopurine, achieving a mean survival of 17 days, in comparison to 7 days in control dogs[25]. Three dogs survived for more than a month, dying from infection and drug toxicity. The complications which arose as a result of the daily administration of these drugs were numerous and clearly prohibitive. Six dogs were therefore given immunosuppressant drugs only during threatened rejection, as determined by diminution of the R-wave voltage in all leads of the ECG, which had previously been found to accompany immune disease of the cardiac allograft. Five of the six dogs survived for over a month, and three for over 3 months.

CARDIAC TRANSPLANTATION IN MAN—FIRST ATTEMPT USING A XENOGRAFT

By the mid-1960s a considerable fund of knowledge had been acquired. The increasing success of experimental cardiac transplantation led Hardy and his colleagues to consider heart transplantation in man. This group had considerable experience of cardiac and lung transplantation in animals and had carried out lung transplantation in man on one occasion[45].

In 1964 they reported their attempt to transplant the heart of a large chimpanzee into the chest of a 68-year-old man with hypertensive cardiovascular disease, widespread atheroma, and evidence of previous myocardial infarction[46]. Before operation the patient deteriorated suddenly and passed into terminal shock. He was taken to the operating room, and supported by a pump-oxygenator just as effective heart action ceased. Subsequent dissection of his heart revealed gross atherosclerosis with about 90% occlusion of the coronary arteries. As no human donor was available, and as some of the members of the group had been impressed by the early results of kidney xenografts from chimpanzees to man reported by Reemtsma et al.[47], the heart of a 96 lb (43.6 kg) chimpanzee was excised and its viability maintained by retrograde hypothermic perfusion of the coronary sinus. Orthotopic transplantation was performed, and the donor heart beat regularly and forcefully after defibrillation at a rate of about 80 beats per minute. It soon became apparent that the rather small heart would not be able to support the circulation unless its rate were increased. The heart was paced at 100 per minute to maintain a systolic blood pressure of 60–90 mmHg. About 1 hour after the removal of the bypass catheters, however, the heart was judged incapable of accepting the large venous return without intermittent decompression by manual massage. Further support was abandoned.

THE FIRST HUMAN-TO-HUMAN HEART TRANSPLANT

After nearly 4 years and much further experimental work another attempt was reported. Barnard and his colleagues performed the first human-to-human heart transplantation on a 57-year-old man with ischaemic heart disease at our own institution in December 1967[48]. The operative procedure was successful and the patient's orthotopically transplanted heart functioned satisfactorily throughout the early postoperative course. Like many patients who followed, however, he developed pneumonia, and died on the 18th postoperative day. At autopsy his transplanted heart showed features of mild to moderate acute rejection[49].

The first patient who could realistically be acclaimed a 'long-term' survivor was operated on in Cape Town 1 month later. This 60-year-old patient lived an active and full life for over $1\frac{1}{2}$ years until he died from the hitherto undescribed complication of chronic rejection[50] (see Appendix).

EARLY CLINICAL PROGRESS

The initial enthusiasm for heart transplantation waned as the problems of acute rejection and infection became apparent to those who had embarked upon a transplant programme without a full understanding of the complications which might be involved. Four centres, those of Stanford University[51] and the Medical College of Virginia[52] in the USA, the La Pitié Hospital in Paris[53], and our own group in Cape Town[54], continued with planned programmes of heart transplantation. With improved patient selection based on experience, and improved postoperative care, in particular with regard to the administration of immunosuppressive drugs and the prevention, diagnosis and treatment of infectious complications, the results in these centres slowly improved. The introduction of the technique of percutaneous transvenous endomyocardial biopsy to diagnose acute rejection by Caves and his colleagues in 1973[55, 56] contributed much to the successful management of patients with cardiac allografts, allowing timely increased immunosuppression or, of equal importance, the avoidance of over-immunosuppression.

The introduction of the operation of heterotopic heart transplantation by Barnard and Losman in 1975[10] added a further surgical technique, with some advantages and some disadvantages over orthotopic transplantation, which could be used by those treating patients with terminal myocardial disease.

During the late 1970s cardiac transplantation came to be accepted as a definitive form of therapy rather than as a clinical research programme. As a result, in the late '70s and early '80s several other groups in North America and Europe initiated clinical heart transplant programmes, and the number of active centres involved in this work has increased by at least fivefold. The introduction during this period of the immunosuppressive drug, cyclosporin A[57], has brought about a further significant improvement in the results of this procedure, and has further stimulated other major cardiac surgical centres to become involved clinically in this field of therapy.

References

1. Cooper, D. K. C. (1968). Experimental development of cardiac transplantation. *Br. Med. J.*, **4**, 174
2. Carrel, A. and Guthrie, C. C. (1905). The transplantation of veins and organs. *Am. Med. (Philadelphia)*, **10**, 1101
3. Carrel, A. (1907). The surgery of blood vessels. *Bull. Johns Hopkins Hosp.*, **18**, 18
4. Mann, F. C., Priestley, J. T., Markowitz, J. and Yater, W. M. (1933). Transplantation of the intact mammalian heart. *Arch. Surg.*, **26**, 219
5. Abbott, C. P., Lindsey, E. S., Creech, O. Jr. and De Witt, C. W. (1964). A technique for heart transplantation in the rat. *Arch. Surg.*, **89**, 645
6. Abbott, C. P., De Witt, C. W. and Creech, O. Jr. (1965). The transplanted rat heart: histologic and electrocardiographic changes. *Transplantation*, **3**, 432
7. Demikhov, V. P. (1962). *Experimental Transplantation of Vital Organs*. Authorized translation from the Russian by Haigh, B. (New York: Consultants Bureau)
8. Reemtsma, K. (1964). The heart as a test organ in transplantation studies. *Ann. NY Acad. Sci.*, **120**, 778
9. Losman, J. G. and Barnard, C. N. (1977). Hemodynamic evaluation of left ventricular bypass with a homologous cardiac graft. *J. Thorac. Cardiovasc. Surg.*, **74**, 695
10. Barnard, C. N. and Losman, J. G. (1975). Left ventricular bypass. *S. Afr. Med. J.*, **49**, 303
11. Sen, P. K., Parulkar, G. B., Paruday, S. R. and Kinare, S. G. (1965). Homologous canine heart transplantation: a preliminary report of 100 experiments. *Indian J. Med. Res.*, **53**, 674
12. Neptune, W. B., Cookson, B. A., Bailey, C. P., Appler, R. and Rajkowski, F. (1953). Complete homologous heart transplantation. *Arch. Surg.*, **66**, 174
13. Webb, W. R. and Howard, H. S. (1957). Cardiopulmonary transplantation. *Surg. Forum*, **8**, 313
14. Webb, W. R., Howard, H. S. and Neely, W. A. (1959). Practical methods of homologous cardiac transplantation. *J. Thorac. Surg.*, **37**, 361
15. Goldberg, M., Berman, E. F. and Akman, L. C. (1958). Homologous transplantation of the canine heart. *J. Int. Coll. Surg.*, **30**, 575
16. Berman, E. F., Goldberg, M. and Akman, L. (1958). Experimental replacement of the heart in the dog. *Transplant. Bull.*, **5**, 10
17. Cass, M. H. and Brock, R. (1959). Heart excision and replacement. *Guy's Hosp. Rep.*, **108**, 285
18. Lower, R. R. and Shumway, N. E. (1960). Studies on orthotopic homotransplantation of the canine heart. *Surg. Forum*, **11**, 18
19. Barnard, C. N. (1968). What we have learned about heart transplants. *J. Thorac. Cardiovasc. Surg.*, **56**, 457
20. Lower, R. R., Stofer, R. C., Hurley, E. J. and Shumway, N. E. (1961). Complete homograft replacement of the heart and both lungs. *Surgery*, **50**, 842
21. Hurley, E. J., Dong, E. Jr., Stofer, R. C. and Shumway, N. E. (1962). Isotopic replacement of the totally excised canine heart. *J. Surg. Res.*, **2**, 90
22. Dong, E. Jr., Hurley, E. J., Lower, R. R. and Shumway, N. E. (1964). Performance of heart two years after autotransplantation. *Surgery*, **56**, 270
23. Lower, R. R., Stofer, R. C. and Shumway, N. E. (1961). Homovital transplantation of the heart. *J. Thorac. Cardiovasc. Surg.*, **41**, 196
24. Lower, R. R., Stofer, R. C., Hurley, E. J., Dong, E. Jr., Cohn, R. B. and Shumway, N. E. (1962). Successful homotransplantation of the canine heart after anoxic preservation for seven hours. *Am. J. Surg.*, **104**, 302
25. Lower, R. R., Dong, E. Jr. and Shumway, N. E. (1965). Long-term survival of cardiac homografts. *Surgery*, **58**, 110
26. Shumway, N. E. and Lower, R. R. (1964). Special problems in transplantation of the heart. *Ann. NY Acad. Sci.*, **120**, 773

27. Lower, R. R., Dong, E. Jr. and Glazener, F. S. (1966). Electrocardiograms of dogs with heart homografts. *Circulation*, **33**, 455

28. Angell, W. W., Dong, E. Jr. and Shumway, N. E. (1967). Four-day storage of the canine cadaver heart. *Surg. Forum*, **18**, 223

29. Willman, V. L., Cooper, T., Cian, L. G. and Hanlon, C. R. (1962). Autotransplantation of the canine heart. *Surg. Gynecol. Obstet.*, **115**, 299

30. Willman, V. L., Cooper, T., Cian, L. G. and Hanlon, C. R. (1962). Mechanism of cardiac failure after excision and reimplantation of the canine heart. *Surg. Forum*, **13**, 93

31. Willman, V. L., Cooper, T. and Hanlon, C. R. (1964). Return of neural responses after autotransplantation of the heart. *Am. J. Physiol.*, **207**, 187

32. Willman, V. L., Cooper, T. and Hanlon, C. R. (1966). Coronary blood flow in dogs after cardiac transplantation. *J. Am. Med. Assoc.*, **195**, 206

33. Willman, V. L., Merjavy, J. P., Pennell, R. and Hanlon, C. R. (1967). Response of the autotransplanted heart to blood volume expansion. *Ann. Surg.*, **166**, 513

34. Napolitano, L., Cooper, T., Willman, V. L. and Hanlon, C. R. (1964). Fine structure of the heart after transplantation with special reference to the neural elements. *Circulation*, **29–30** (Suppl.), 81

35. Cooper, T., Hirsch, E. F., Willman, V. L. and Hanlon, C. R. (1964). Transplantation of the heart. *Arch. Surg.*, **89**, 915

36. Cooper, T., Willman, V. L., Jellinek, M. and Hanlon, C. R. (1962). Heart autotransplantation: effect on myocardial catecholamine and histamine. *Science*, **138**, 40

37. Willman, V. L., Jellinek, M., Cooper, T., Tsunekawa, T., Kaiser, G. C. and Hanlon, C. R. (1964). Metabolism of the transplanted heart: effect of excision and reimplantation on myocardial glycogen, hexokinase, and acetylcholine esterase. *Surgery*, **56**, 266

38. Potter, L. T., Cooper, T., Willman, V. L. and Wolfe, D. E. (1965). Synthesis, binding, release and metabolism of norepinephrine in normal and transplanted dog hearts. *Circ. Res.*, **16**, 468

39. Cooper, T., Willman, V. L. and Hanlon, C. R. (1964). Drug responses of the transplanted heart. *Dis. Chest*, **45**, 284

40. Willman, V. L., Cooper, T., Kaiser, G. C. and Hanlon, C. R. (1965). Cardiovascular response after cardiac autotransplant in primate. *Arch. Surg.*, **91**, 805

41. Kondo, Y., Grädel, F. and Kantrowitz, A. (1965). Heart homotransplantation in puppies. *Circulation*, **31–31** (Suppl.), 181

42. Barnard, M. S. (1967). Heart transplantation: an experimental review and preliminary research. *S. Afr. Med. J.*, **41**, 1260

43. Reemtsma, K., Williamson, W. R. Jr., Iglesias, F., Pena, E., Sayegh, S. F. and Creech, O. Jr. (1962). Studies in homologous canine heart transplantation: prolongation of survival with a folic acid antagonist. *Surgery*, **52**, 127

44. Blumenstock, D. A., Hechtman, H. B., Jaretzki, A., Hosbein, J. D., Zingg, W. and Powers, J. H. (1963). Prolonged survival of orthotopic homotransplants of the heart in animals treated with methotrexate. *J. Thorac. Cardiovasc. Surg.*, **46**, 616

45. Hardy, J. D., Webb, W. R., Dalton, M. L. Jr. and Walker, G. R. Jr. (1963). Lung homotransplantation in man: report of the initial case. *J. Am. Med. Assoc.*, **186**, 1065

46. Hardy, J. D., Chavez, C. M., Kurrus, F. E., Neely, W. A., Webb, W. R., Eraslan, S., Turner, M. D., Fabian, L. W. and Labecki, J. D. (1964). Heart transplantation in man: developmental studies and report of a case. *J. Am. Med. Assoc.*, **188**, 1132

47. Reemtsma, K., McCracken, B. H., Schlegel, J. U., Pearl, M. A., De Witt, C. W. and Creech, O. Jr. (1964). Reversal of early graft rejection after renal heterotransplantation in man. *J. Am. Med. Assoc.*, **187**, 691

48. Barnard, C. N. (1967). A human cardiac transplant: an interim report of a successful operation performed at Groote Schuur Hospital, Cape Town. *S. Afr. Med. J.*, **41**, 1271

49. Thomson, J. G. (1968). Heart transplantation in man—necropsy findings. *Br. Med. J.*, **2**, 511

50. Thomson, J. G. (1969). Production of severe atheroma in a transplanted human heart. *Lancet*, **2**, 1088

51. Baumgartner, W. A., Reitz, B. A., Oyer, P. E., Stinson, E. B. and Shumway, N. E. (1979). Cardiac homotransplantation. *Curr. Probl. Surg.*, **61**, 1

52. Lower, R. R., Szentpetery, S., Thomas, F. T. and Kemp, V. E. (1976). Clinical observations on cardiac transplantation. *Transplant. Proc.*, **8**, 9

53. Cabrol, C., Gandjbakhch, I., Guiraudon, G., Pavie, A., Villemot, J. P., Viars, P., Gabrol, A., Mattei, M. F. and Rottembourg, J. (1982). Cardiac transplantation: our experience at La Pitié Hospital in Paris. *Heart Transplant.*, **1**, 116

54. Barnard, C. N., Barnard, M. S., Cooper, D. K. C., Curcio, C. A., Hassoulas, J., Novitzky, D. and Wolpowitz, A. (1981). The present status of heterotopic cardiac transplantation. *J. Thorac. Cardiovasc. Surg.*, **81**, 433

55. Caves, P. K., Stinson, E. B., Graham, A. F., Billingham, M. E., Grehl, T. M. and Shumway, N. E. (1973). Percutaneous transvenous endomyocardial biopsy. *J. Am. Med. Assoc.*, **225**, 228

56. Caves, P. K., Billingham, M. E., Stinson, E. B. and Shumway, N. E. (1974). Serial transvenous biopsy of the transplanted human heart—improved management of acute rejection episodes. *Lancet*, **1**, 821

57. Jamieson, S. W., Oyer, P. E., Bieber, C. P., Hunt, S. A., Billingham, M., Miller, J., Gamberg, P., Stinson, E. B. and Shumway, N. E. (1983). Cardiac transplantation at Stanford. *Heart Transplant.*, **2**, 243

2
Selection and Management of the Recipient

INTRODUCTION

Cardiac transplantation offers an attractive alternative form of therapy for the physician caring for a patient with intractable heart failure in whom symptoms are poorly controlled. The option of referring patients for cardiac transplantation presents the physician with several difficult questions:

(1) Should cardiac transplantation be performed at all?
(2) Considering the variable and unpredictable natural history of congestive heart failure, when is the optimum time for the procedure to be performed in the individual patient?
(3) Which patients will benefit from transplantation and who should be referred?
(4) How best may the recipient be maintained prior to surgery?

SHOULD PHYSICIANS REFER PATIENTS FOR CARDIAC TRANSPLANTATION?

A heart transplant programme has a major impact on patient care. It commits scarce and costly resources to a procedure that, at best, will benefit only a very small number of patients. The argument that they should be kept available for the benefit of many is strong. A heart transplant programme further loads the already overburdened intensive care facilities, not only with postoperative patients, but with potential transplant recipients, some of whom will die while awaiting a donor heart[1,2].

Thus the questions of cost and potential benefit arise. It is not an accurate economic and social analysis of the cost of end-stage cardiac disease to simply compute the cost of providing medical and surgical treatment for such patients. The emphasis should be on the cost of treating end-stage cardiac disease by conventional medical and surgical therapy versus heart transplantation[3]. Some authors have concluded that both methods are in the same range of cost to society[4]. The true cost of heart transplantation, however, is not simply what appears on the bottom line when all the bills come in; it must also include the value of what must be sacrificed to make room for transplantation[5]. This value, of course, is subjective and inevitably controversial.

It is difficult to separate society's interest in a fair distribution of resources from the individual patient's right to treatment. Most physicians are uncomfortable when called on to withhold treatment from an individual patient on the grounds that prescribing such therapy may jeopardize the treatment of others. In an ideal world such decisions obviously would not be necessary. With the improving results of heart transplantation[6,7], and the dramatic improvement in the quality of life offered by the procedure in suitable recipients, physicians will continue to refer patients for transplantation as long as the procedure is available.

Having taken the decision to refer a patient for transplantation, the procedure must be explained to the patient and informed consent must be obtained. Patients who have undergone an acute cardiac catastrophe, such as acute myocardial infarction, or who have end-stage chronic congestive heart failure, are usually placed in intensive care units, treated with drugs that may impair judgement, surrounded by formidable-looking equipment, and subjected to the psychological stress of their diminished state of health. Under these conditions, truly informed consent is difficult, if not impossible, to obtain[8]. The physician has a responsibility to ensure that the patient understands the nature of the treatment offered, the potential benefits, as well as the necessity of prolonged postoperative hospitalization, follow-up, and the hazards associated with immunosuppression.

WHEN SHOULD THE PROCEDURE BE PERFORMED?

The prognosis of patients in severe left ventricular failure is variable, and prediction of life expectancy is extremely difficult. Most experienced consultants indicate that they often misjudge the duration of survival of patients with chronic congestive heart failure[8]. This renders the timing of the intervention difficult. Selection of the optimum time for surgery is, however, extremely important. Although one does not wish to subject patients who still have a reasonable prognosis to an operation that carries a significant postoperative mortality, it is equally important not to delay the operation until permanent, non-cardiac organ damage has occurred. As the patient reaches the terminal stages of his cardiac disease, other organs, particularly the kidneys, lungs and liver, may deteriorate. If transplantation is delayed until death is imminent, the patient may not survive, regardless of how successful the transplant operation is. While the availability of donor hearts will always be the final factor determining the time of transplantation, it is important that patients be referred for consideration for transplantation before irreversible organ damage has occurred.

A recent prognostic study of patients in severe New York Heart Association (NYHA) functional class 3 or 4 heart failure, who were treated optimally with vasodilators and antiarrhythmics, showed overall 1 and 2 years' survival of 52% and 32% respectively for the whole group[9]; patients in NYHA class 4 had an even lower 1-year survival. The annual mortality rate was lower (20%) in those patients with 'stable' heart failure, and considerably higher (approximately 50%) in those with progressively worsening heart failure. These findings have been confirmed by other groups[10]. Resting haemodynamic measurements, echocardiographic left ventricular dimensions, and electrocardiographic monitoring do not add useful prognostic information over and above that obtained from careful clinical evaluation and determination of effort tolerance.

Patients in class 4 heart failure are potential candidates for assessment for transplantation, as are patients in class 3 with progression of symptoms over the preceding weeks or months.

WHICH PATIENT WILL BENEFIT FROM HEART TRANSPLANTATION?

The substantial improvement in survival that has recently occurred following transplantation is the result, primarily, of improvement in survival during the first 3 postoperative months[6]. This reflects improvement not only in management but also in patient selection. Retrospective analysis has aided recognition of recipient-related factors that influence survival after transplantation[11].

There are a number of absolute and relative contraindications to cardiac transplantation (Table 2.1)[1,11-14].

Patients with active infection must be excluded because of the risk of exacerbation by postoperative immunosuppression. Insulin-requiring diabetes

Table 2.1 Absolute and relative contraindications to cardiac transplantation

Absolute	Relative
Active infection	Age >45 years
Insulin-dependent diabetes mellitus	Unresolved pulmonary infarction
Malignancy	Active peptic ulcer disease
Fixed pulmonary vascular resistance >8 Wood units (orthotopic)	Significant peripheral vascular or cerebrovascular disease
	Significant irreversible dysfunction of any other major organ (e.g. kidney, liver or lungs)
	Drug addiction, alcoholism, active mental illness, or psychological instability

mellitus is a contraindication as the administration of the corticosteroids necessary for immunosuppression makes control of diabetes difficult and increases the already high risk of infection in this group of patients. Even patients without preoperative abnormality of glucose homoeostasis may develop postoperative diabetes mellitus[12]. Pre-existing malignancy will almost certainly progress rapidly in the immunocompromised patient.

In the early days of cardiac transplantation it became obvious that an elevated pulmonary vascular resistance was a contraindication to orthotopic transplantation; the procedure of heterotopic transplantation was introduced in part to deal with this problem. A fixed high pulmonary vascular resistance of above 8 Wood units is therefore an absolute contraindication only to orthotopic transplantation. In heterotopic transplantation the recipient's right ventricle remains functional and, unless right-sided failure has occurred, has adapted to the pressure overload, and will continue to support the pulmonary circulation. A high pulmonary vascular resistance in patients with advanced myocardial disease may be, at least, partly reversible, and a significant fall in resistance may be observed after transplantation[15]. The degree of reversibility can frequently be predicted before transplantation by recording the pulmonary vascular resistance both before and during the administration of 100% oxygen or of tolazoline or sodium nitroprusside, all of which may bring about a marked fall in resistance in patients with a large reactive component.

The first transplants performed were in older patients. It is now clear, however, that the best results are seen in patients under 35–40 years of age. Using conventional immunosuppressive therapy with azathioprine and methylprednisolone, our local experience has been that mortality rises over the age of 40 and no recipient aged 50 or over at the time of transplantation has survived beyond his second year[11]. This age criterion in selection of recipients has been questioned[16], but the authors' assertion that equally good results are obtained in the elderly is not supported by other published evidence[17]. The impact of age on survival possibly reflects the increased prevalence of undetected noncardiac disease in older patients prior to transplantation, as well as their inability to tolerate the side-effects of the high level of immunosuppression required by cardiac allograft recipients.

Patients with recent unresolved pulmonary infarction must be excluded because of the risk of cavitation and secondary infection. Because of the risk of exacerbation by steroid therapy, patients with active peptic ulcer disease must be excluded, unless healing of the ulceration can be obtained prior to transplantation. The presence of significant peripheral or cerebrovascular disease will prevent the patient obtaining maximum benefit from the procedure and/or increase the short-term risks.

It is always difficult to determine whether dysfunction of other major organs will be reversible once myocardial function has returned to normal. Correction of the underlying circulatory state often results in a surprising degree of recovery of organ dysfunction. In the patient with chronic congestive cardiac failure, therefore, every effort must be made to demonstrate whether renal or hepatic insufficiency is reversible or not. Significant chronic obstructive pulmonary disease, resulting from chronic bronchitis and emphysema, must be differentiated from the features of left ventricular failure, but, if clearly demonstrated, will contraindicate cardiac transplantation; active chronic bronchitis and emphysema predispose to postoperative pulmonary infection. The recently introduced immunosuppressive agent cyclosporin A (CYA) induces significant nephrotoxicity and alters hepatic excretion of bilirubin; its use, therefore, means that great care must be taken to ensure that irreversible renal and hepatic dysfunction are not already present.

Many of the above contraindications are particularly related to the postoperative use of high-dose corticosteroids. It is, as yet, too early to know whether the long-term use of CYA and lower doses of corticosteroid will be associated with a more favourable outlook for cardiac recipients, and allow liberalization of some of the criteria for selection.

Patients addicted to drugs or who consume excessive amounts of alcohol or who are otherwise emotionally unstable or suffer from acute mental illness are not suitable candidates for cardiac transplantation. The addicted or alcoholic patient is unlikely to comply during the postoperative period, when compliance with a complex drug regimen and regular attendance for follow-up visits are important.

As with all major cardiac surgical procedures, the success of the operation depends on the patient's ability to understand fully the life-long treatment and follow-up programme that is an essential part of this management. A strong supportive family is of great value in seeing the patient through the difficult postoperative period[18,19].

Perhaps the most important practical difficulty is to ensure that the patient has sufficient financial resources to pay for those expenses not covered by the State, insurance, or a medical aid agency. Whilst the State or other organization may bear the cost of the operation and postoperative care, the facilities available to maintain the recipient awaiting transplantation and his family may be inadequate. In planning transplantation, great care is needed to ensure that patients and their families do not incur unnecessary expense by needlessly travelling great distances in the hope of a life-saving procedure, only to die whilst awaiting a donor.

In summary, the ideal transplant recipient should be younger than 40 years and have severe cardiac failure untreatable by conventional surgery or medical therapy. He should be free of any condition likely to predispose to the complications of immunosuppression, be psychologically stable, and have sufficient resources to support himself and his family through the perioperative period prior to full rehabilitation.

Further assessment

Screening of the recipient begins with a full history and physical examination, including a chest radiograph and electrocardiogram; at this stage any major contraindications should become evident. Many patients will be rejected at this early, informal evaluation, as they are seen to be completely unsuitable. Usually this is on the grounds of age, coexistent disease in other organ systems, or an unsuitable social or psychological background.

Once having passed this informal assessment, candidates undergo systematic and extensive medical screening. This includes cardiac catheterization, haemodynamic evaluation, and angiography, if recent results are not available. Once the patient is judged to be a candidate for transplantation on the basis of clinical status and cardiac catheterization, then further screening is performed to ensure that major contraindications to the use of immunosuppression are not present. This screening process is obviously guided by clinical judgement, but includes a full blood count, biochemical screening of blood and urine, a glucose tolerance test, respiratory function tests, dental examination and radiography, and bacteriological screening where indicated. Barium studies and intravenous pyelography are performed where appropriate. Based on the results of these investigations, specific therapy may be indicated, or the patient may be deemed unsuitable for transplantation. If no contraindication is detected, then the patient becomes a candidate and awaits a suitable donor.

MAINTENANCE OF THE SELECTED RECIPIENT

These patients are all seriously ill, and have a very short life expectancy, usually measured in weeks. The mean survival of patients accepted as recipients, but who died whilst awaiting a donor at our own institution, was 26 days[1]; similar observations have been reported by other groups[12,16]. Maintenance of these patients prior to transplantation poses a formidable problem. The management of chronic congestive heart failure in the transplant recipient is no different from that in other patients, and has been reviewed recently[20].

A few points, however, deserve emphasis. Most patients are receiving very large doses of diuretics at the time of referral, which are usually unnecessary and can often be reduced following the introduction of vasodilators or a converting enzyme-inhibitor such as captopril. These changes often result in considerable improvement of renal function and electrolyte balance, and are best carried out in an intensive care unit with appropriate monitoring of left ventricular filling pressure by means of a Swan–Ganz catheter. Every effort must be made to avoid the introduction of infection or the complication of pulmonary infarction[1].

Some patients will temporarily require aggressive management with inotropic agents such as dopamine or dobutamine, and a few will become dependent on intravenous inotropes. In the absence of an adequate supply of donor hearts this is an unfortunate situation, since few patients dependent on intravenous inotropes will survive until operation, and those that do will have such severe non-cardiac organ dysfunction (renal, hepatic) that, in our experience, a successful outcome from transplantation is unlikely.

Reports of transplantation in patients dependent on the intraaortic balloon pump suggest that, unless donor hearts are freely available, patients with end-stage heart failure should not be submitted to this procedure[21]. Similarly, when only a limited number of balloon pumps are available, they should not be committed to pump-dependent patients, with a poor prognosis, for a period of time which cannot be determined in advance.

The availability of heart transplantation has provided physicians with a novel form of therapy for heart failure. At the same time, however, it has posed difficult questions related to allocation of resources, selection of patients for therapy, and maintenance of the dying patient.

References

1. Cooper, D. K. C., Charles, R. G., Beck, W. and Barnard, C. N. (1982). The assessment and selection of patients for heterotopic heart transplantation. *S. Afr. Med. J.*, **61**, 575
2. Leaf, A. (1980). The MGH trustees say no to heart transplants. *N. Engl. J. Med.*, **302**, 1087
3. Evans, R. W. (1982). Economic and social costs of heart transplantation. *Heart Transplant.*, **1**, 243
4. Thomas, F. T. and Lower, R. R. (1978). Heart transplantation—1978. *Surg. Clin. North Am.*, **58**, 335
5. Centerwall, B. S. (1981). Cost-benefit analysis and heart transplantation. *N. Engl. J. Med.*, **304**, 901
6. Jamieson, S. W., Oyer, P. E., Bieber, C. P., Hunt, S. A., Billingham, M., Miller, J., Gamberg, P., Stinson, E. B. and Shumway, N. E. (1983). Cardiac transplantation at Stanford. *Heart Transplant.*, **2**, 243
7. Losman, J. G., Levine, H., Campbell, C. D., Replogle, R. L., Hassoulas, J., Novitzky, D., Cooper, D. K. C. and Barnard, C. N. (1982). Changes in indications for heart transplantation. *J. Thorac. Cardiovasc. Surg.*, **84**, 716
8. Woolley, F. R. (1984). Ethical issues in the implantation of the total artificial heart. *N. Engl. J. Med.*, **310**, 292
9. Wilson, J. R., Schwartz, S., St John Sutton, M., Ferraro, N., Horowitz, L. N., Reichek, N. and Josephson, M. E. (1983). Prognosis in severe heart failure: relation to hemodynamic measurements and ventricular ectopic activity. *J. Am. Coll. Cardiol.*, **2**, 403
10. Massie, B., Ports, T., Chatterjee, K., Parmley, W., Ostland, J., O'Young, J. and Haughom, F. (1981). Long-term vasodilator therapy for heart failure: clinical response and its relationship to hemodynamic measurements. *Circulation*, **63**, 269
11. Cooper, D. K. C., Lanza, R. P., Boyd, S. T. and Barnard, C. N. (1983). Factors influencing survival following heart transplantation. *Heart Transplant.*, **3**, 86
12. Thompson, M. E. (1983). Selection of candidates for cardiac transplantation. *Heart Transplant.*, **3**, 65

13. Oyer, P. E., Stinson, E. B., Bieber, C. P. and Shumway, N. E. (1982). Cardiac transplantation. In Chatterjee, S. N. (ed.) *Organ Transplantation*. p. 347. (Bristol and Littleton, Mass.: Wright)

14. Lower, R. R., Szentpetery, S., Quinn, J. and Thomas, F. T. (1979). Selection of patients for cardiac transplantation. *Transplant. Proc.*, **11**, 293

15. Pucillo, A. L., Reison, D. S., Rose, E. A., Drusin, R. E., Reemtsma, K. and Powers, E. R. (1983). Reversibility of elevated pulmonary vascular resistance after cardiac transplantation. (Abstract) *J. Am. Coll. Cardiol.*, **1**, 72

16. Fuller, J. K. and Copeland, J. G. (1983). The age criterion and recipient selection. Presented at Third Annual Scientific Session, International Society for Heart Transplantation, March 1983. *Heart Transplant.* (Suppl.), p. 30. (Abstract)

17. Baumgartner, W. A., Reitz, B. A., Oyer, P. E., Stinson, E. B. and Shumway, N. E. (1979). Cardiac homotransplantation. *Curr. Probl. Surg.*, **16**, 1

18. Lunde, D. T. (1969). Psychiatric complications of heart transplants. *Am. J. Psychiatry*, **126**, 369

19. Cooper, D. K. C., Lanza, R. P., Nash, E. S. and Barnard, C. N. (1984). Non-compliance in heart transplant recipients: the Cape Town experience. *Heart Transplant.*, **3**, 248

20. Packer, M. (1983). Vasodilator and inotropic therapy for severe chronic heart failure: passion and scepticism. *J. Am. Coll. Cardiol.*, **2**, 841

21. Bregman, D., Drusin, R., Lamb, J., Reemtsma, K. and Rose, E. (1982). Heart transplantation in patients requiring mechanical circulatory support. *Heart Transplant.*, **1**, 154

3
Selection and Management of the Donor

INTRODUCTION

The concept of brain death or coma dépassé, as opposed to clinical death, which is the absence of all vital signs, was first formulated by Mollaret and Goulon in 1959[1]. As could be expected, this new concept of death evoked considerable controversy in both medical and lay circles. It is, however, not an academic or philosophical question but one of very real practical importance, with wide ethical, legal and economic implications.

The present-day availability of efficient resuscitation facilities after injury or acute organ failure has created a situation where patients may be mechanically ventilated and the circulation artificially maintained without any possibility of recovery of cerebral function. This state has come to be known as cerebral death. It is now virtually universally accepted in the Western world that cerebral death means death of the individual, but there are a few countries where this is not so[2]. The high cost of maintaining such patients in intensive care units has led to financial evaluation of this care by those who have to foot the bill for health care—individuals, insurance companies and the State. Other treatable patients may be precluded from curative care by such 'brain dead' patients. The additional work-load for nursing and medical staff, the emotional toll taken of the relatives and distress caused to nursing staff are also very real considerations. The care of these patients has also acquired medico-legal and ethical significance since they may be potential donors of essential organs such as kidneys, heart and liver[3]. It is not the task of the neurosurgeon or any other medical practitioner to provide organs for donation, but neither can any doctor deny patients in need of transplant surgery the chance of a cure on insufficient evidence or mere prejudice.

CLINICAL DEATH

The classical features of clinical death have been accepted for centuries and can be simply stated as the absence of spontaneous heart beat and respiration. In most countries legislators have steered clear of any definition of death, for very understandable reasons; in the Republic of South Africa, a patient is regarded as dead when he is certified to be so by a qualified medical practitioner.

BRAIN DEATH

It is universally accepted that irreversible loss of function of the brain must inevitably lead to progressive deterioration in function and death of the rest of the body. The next step, that is to equate brain stem death with brain death, came later, but few would question this concept today[4]. The practical problem that arose in the beginning was the need for a system of diagnosing brain stem death with such certainty that there could be no reasonable doubt that this diagnosis was unquestionably correct, and that further resuscitative or sustaining activities were pointless and could be terminated. This has, however, been overcome, and the diagnosis is now an acceptable clinical exercise[5].

PATHOPHYSIOLOGY OF IRREVERSIBLE BRAIN STEM DAMAGE

In order to produce coma, pathological processes must either affect the brain diffusely or directly encroach upon its deep central structures[6]. Three major groups of lesions can be differentiated:

(1) Supratentorial lesions, such as subdural, subarachnoid or intracerebral haematoma, or cerebral infarction, tumour or abscess.
(2) Infratentorial masses or destructive lesions that directly damage the brain stem, e.g. brain stem/cerebellar haemorrhage, abscess, brain stem infarction or tumour.
(3) Metabolic disorders which widely depress or interrupt brain stem function, including anoxia, ischaemia, infections such as meningitis or encephalitis, exogenous toxins, and deficiencies.

The end result of major trauma, whether physical or chemical, which leads to progressive brain swelling, is progressive herniation of the parahippocampal gyri with lateral compression and downward displacement of the brain stem, eventually resulting in loss of brain stem function. Unless relieved in time, any expanding lesion will increase intracranial pressure until it is equal to systemic arterial pressure, at which point there will be complete arrest of cerebral circulation. Cerebral circulatory arrest can therefore be confidently used as a criterion of irreversible cerebral injury.

Functional disintegration, following on the conditions mentioned, leads to cessation of spontaneous respiration, which in turn results in hypoxic cardiac arrest. If gaseous exchange is maintained artificially, the heart, kidneys and liver may continue to function for some hours or days, although progressive circulatory collapse will occur unless adequate support is given.

DIAGNOSIS OF BRAIN DEATH

Before a patient can be considered as being in a state of brain stem death, a positive diagnosis of the structural alteration in the brain that has caused this damage must have been made. All investigations necessary to make this diagnosis, and efforts to reverse this process, if it is at all reversible, should be instituted. In the early phases of declining brain stem function, the clinician should be concerned with diagnostic and resuscitative measures and not with speculations about irreversible coma. Three questions therefore have to be answered:

(1) What is the cause of the deterioration?
(2) Can it be reversed?
(3) Can this state be simulated by any other condition?

The diagnosis of brain stem death is a clinical one with no need for any additional investigative procedures. Once it has been established that there is irreversible structural damage of the brain, other conditions that may simulate brain stem death have to be excluded, such as depressant drugs, hypothermia, or metabolic or endocrine disturbances (e.g. hypo- or hyper-glycaemia, acid-base or electrolyte disturbances), although the last three may have resulted from extensive brain damage or from the patient's subsequent management.

Clinical features of brain stem death

1. *Level of consciousness*

A patient can only be considered cerebrally dead if he is in absolutely non-responsive coma, with bilaterally fixed, non-reacting pupils, and makes no spontaneous respiratory effort; these conditions must be due to an irremediable cause. This has also been called coma stage 4. To consider any patient with a level of activity higher than this as having a dead brain stem reveals a complete lack of understanding of the condition and may lead to serious errors.

The patient with a supratentorial space-demanding lesion may show progressive rostro-caudal disintegration of brain stem function during which he descends irretrievably from a high level of consciousness to the stage of irreversible coma. In the established case there is little diagnostic difficulty;

the patient is totally unresponsive as far as brain stem reactivity is concerned, and is artificially respired because spontaneous respiration had become inadequate during the clinical decline. After 24 hours, the patient is often hypothermic and may have diabetes insipidus.

The real problem is to know how soon this diagnosis can be established with absolute, incontrovertible certainty. If this step has to be taken for the sake of organ transplantation as well as for the other reasons mentioned, the sooner the better.

2. Respiratory function

A patient may have all the signs of severe cerebral and upper brain stem injury, but as long as he breathes spontaneously he may still recover[7]. Obvious as this may seem, it does bear repetition and, if this is remembered, the embarrassing situation of the patient who has been considered for organ donation recovering consciousness will not occur.

The reason for maintaining the patient on a mechanical ventilator must be that spontaneous respiration has previously become inadequate or has ceased altogether[7]. Neuromuscular blocking agents as a cause of respiratory inadequacy must be excluded. The necessity for artificial ventilation may be determined when the patient is seen to make no respiratory effort throughout a 5-minute period of observation (off the ventilator). The arterial carbon dioxide partial pressure (P_aCO_2) should be within the normal range 5.3–6.1 kPa) at the beginning of the period of observation, and must be allowed to rise above the threshold for stimulating respiration (6.7 kPa). In order to prevent hypoxaemia, oxygen is delivered at 6 l/min via an endotracheal catheter throughout the test period.

If blood gas analysis is not available to measure the P_aCO_2, an alternative procedure is to supply the ventilator with pure oxygen for 10 minutes (preoxygenation), then with 5% carbon dioxide in oxygen for 5 minutes to avoid hypocarbia, and to disconnect the ventilator for 10 minutes, while delivering oxygen at 6 l/min by endotracheal catheter. This establishes diffusion oxygenation and ensures that hypoxia will not occur during the 10 minutes of respiratory arrest.

3. Brain stem reflexes

Because of the anatomical position of the brain stem nuclei and their well-known connections, their integrity can be tested systematically, level by level, utilizing standard clinical reflex responses for this purpose. All brain stem reflexes must be absent if brain death is to be diagnosed.

(1) *Pupillary response* (second/third nerve interaction). For an effective test of pupillary function, the room should be darkened and the pupil

observed through a magnifying glass. If a diagnosis of coma dépassé is to be made, the pupil must be fixed on testing reaction to a strong light. The pupils are nearly always dilated. Depending on the cause of the cerebral damage, there may, of course, be pupillary inequality, one pupil having enlarged first and the other later. On the other hand, with massive downward central herniation of the brain stem, both pupils are small initially and may dilate later. The pupils are not only fixed to light, but obviously also do not react to painful stimulation either locally or distantly. In some patients there is no pupillary dilatation, the pupils being small or mid-sized and, in these instances, it is presumed that there is associated central damage to the sympathetic system with inability to effect mydriasis.

(2) *Corneal reflex* (fifth/seventh nerve interaction). A firm contact with the cornea should be made with a soft object, such as a tuft of cotton wool; light touch with a wisp of cotton wool is not enough. If this evokes a blink in addition to upward movement of the eyes (Bell's phenomenon), it indicates integrity of the third/seventh nerve connections. A corneo-mandibular reflex (deviation of the jaw to the opposite side) is seen in upper brain stem injury, particularly in the early stages of rostro-caudal disintegration.

(3) *Grimace response* (fifth/seventh nerve interaction). Painful stimulation or irritation in the field of the fifth nerve will evoke a grimace response in the normal individual. In the deeply unconscious patient, supraorbital stimulation is used, but a more sensitive test is irritation of the nasal mucosa with a vibration fork, tickling, or *light* pinprick. This response disappears in brain stem death. Lower brain stem responses such as coughing or gagging on stimulation of the throat will usually have been noted by the nursing staff during suctioning, but should be tested by the physician himself.

(4) *Oculo-cephalic reflex*. In a normal alert person, turning the head from side to side is followed by virtual instantaneous adjustment of the resting eye position to that of the head[6]. This cortical response diminishes with progressive loss of cortical control in the presence of an intact brain stem. In this situation, the eyes lag behind the eye movement and then rapidly adjust their position again. When the brain stem centres that integrate the vestibulo-cervical input with ocular position have been completely destroyed, these responses are lost, and there is no movement of the eye independently from that of the head. This test should not be performed when there is suspicion of a cervical spinal injury.

(5) *Vestibulo-ocular reflexes* (cold caloric tests). This response involves pathways almost identical to those subserving the oculo-cephalic response,

but disappears later because a stronger stimulus is needed to evoke it. In an awake person lying supine, irrigation of the external auditory meatus with 20 ml of iced water will elicit slight deviation of the eyes towards the irrigated side, followed by nystagmus with the coarse beat to the contralateral side.

In the unconscious patient with an intact brain stem and loss of cortical control, the eyes will deviate towards the irrigated ear and remain immobile for 2–3 minutes before they gradually return to their initial resting position. With progressive decline in consciousness, the sequence of response is as follows:

(i) Conjugate ocular deviation with nystagmus
(ii) Conjugate ocular deviation without nystagmus
(iii) Dysconjugate ocular deviation or possibly response only from the ipsilateral eye
(iv) Loss of caloric response in the presence of coma stage 4

It must be stressed that cold caloric responses are also lost completely in patients in deep barbiturate coma; accordingly, this test is of decisive importance only in the determination of brain stem death in patients who have suffered structural cerebral lesions.

Spinal segmental reflexes

These are mentioned because they can be a cause of confusion. They may be retained for a long period of time after all evidence of cerebral activity has ceased, or they may even reappear after the initial loss of all neural activity. Reflexes which may remain present for a long time are the superficial abdominal, the cremasteric, and plantar withdrawal responses, as well as an isolated knee or ankle jerk. The persistent plantar response is usually a very slow flexion withdrawal reaction. The upper limb may display a slow extension/ internal rotation movement elicited from a limited skin area on the arm and chest[8]. It is a localized response and indicates a transection above C8.

These reflexes are subserved by local arcs through the spinal cord and occur independently of suprasegmental influences from the brain[9]. Similarly, the spinal sympathetic outflow may remain intact for a considerable time. Fluctuations in intensity of these responses are probably dependent on fluctuations in spinal cord perfusion. Physiologically, one is looking at a peculiar form of acute transection with spinal shock, which is modified by the fact that previous destruction of the brain stem has occurred. It must be emphasized that persistent spinal cord function has nothing to do with irreversible loss of cerebral or brain stem function, and need not interfere with the diagnosis of brain stem death. Indeed, spinal cord areflexia is uncommon after central cerebral circulatory arrest[9].

It bears repetition that the clinical diagnosis of the loss of brain stem function is the mainstay in establishing brain stem death. If reversible causes of brain stem dysfunction have been excluded, and the basic criteria of functional loss have been satisfied, this clinical conclusion is as valid as any other absolute clinical observation. Before a final diagnosis can be made, one further question must be answered. Could this state be simulated by other conditions such as drugs, hypothermia, metabolic or endocrine disturbance, or electrical injury? The latter is particularly important in a country (such as South Africa) where lightning injury is common and can cause cessation of respiration and fixed dilated pupils that can be reversed after prolonged resuscitation[10]. All these causes are theoretically reversible and should be considered from the outset; if not, it is worth while to ask the question at this stage because patients should not have been considered as brain stem dead if there was earlier evidence of any one of these conditions[11].

Ancillary tests

1. *Electroencephalography*

Historically, when the concept of brain death first arose, great importance was attached to electroencephalography (EEG), which was thought to be essential for making this diagnosis. The reason for this was probably the search for an 'objective' and absolute non-clinical mode of diagnosis.

Despite a great interest in the electroencephalographic features of brain death, and extensive research into methods of recording and safeguards to be observed, this investigation rapidly fell into disuse. In 1969, a year after the publication of the Harvard criteria[12], it was recommended that the EEG was not essential for the diagnosis of irreversible coma[13]. For a complete and balanced review of the argument about the EEG, the writings of Pallis should be consulted[14].

The practical fact is that the EEG has been dropped from the criteria for determining brain stem death; unavailability of this facility does not debar anyone from making the diagnosis clinically with complete confidence.

2. *Carotid and vertebral angiography*

Often these studies would have been done as part of the initial diagnostic procedure (for example, in suspected subarachnoid haemorrhage), and where computerized axial tomography is not available it will probably be the first method of investigation of a patient with a severe head injury. In the patient with an expanding intracranial lesion, the rising intracranial pressure will eventually be equal to systemic arterial pressure; complete circulatory arrest will be shown on the arteriogram, a feature which can confidently be used as a criterion of irreversible cerebral injury[16]. Cerebral circulatory arrest has also been demonstrated with isotope angiography, which may serve to show this state effectively[16].

3. *Cerebral evoked responses*

Brain stem auditory evoked responses recorded after clickstimuli, and short-latency, somatic evoked responses recorded after median nerve stimulation, have been used in patients in deep coma showing evidence of brain death, and can serve to test various levels of brain stem integrity. There is, however, no absolute agreement between various experts on the value of this method, and it must remain in abeyance for the time being until contradictory findings have been clarified[6].

Repetition of clinical examination

In the final analysis, therefore, one must return to the clinical examination for one's final conclusion in this diagnosis. The only question that remains after one has made the diagnosis of brain stem death is at what time interval one has to repeat the examination. Only by allowing time to pass can one have absolute proof of irreversibility and of further progression. The clinician's judgement is important because the rapidity of decline in neurological status may vary from patient to patient, depending on the basic pathology and on how the patient has progressed until the time of the first testing. When one has fulfilled all the criteria above and the patient has already deteriorated for a period of 6 or more hours prior to testing, there would be little point in waiting for longer than 3 hours before the tests are repeated. To wait for 24 hours would be pointless.

CERTIFICATION OF BRAIN DEATH

In order to facilitate and clarify the examination of patients on whom the diagnosis of brain death is being considered, a simple form based on that of Searle and Collins[17] (*see* Appendix 3.1), abbreviating the above points, is provided at our own institution for completion by the examining doctor. Legally (in South Africa), two registered doctors must certify the fact of death, and it would seem wise for each one to examine the patient independently and draw his or her own conclusions, thus minimizing the risk of mutual influence and observer error. In situations where the observers disagree, repeated examination after a few hours becomes imperative. No further investigative procedure is necessary to make a confident diagnosis of brain death, and the patient may be declared dead if the above criteria have been met, safeguards observed and an adequate examination performed. Mechanical ventilation may be discontinued at this point.

If the viability of certain organs is to be maintained for possible subsequent transplantation, mechanical ventilation can be continued and the circulation supported artificially, but with a clear understanding that these measures are not therapeutic but are continued in order to maintain a cadaver in a perfused condition. A member of the transplantation team is informed of the patient's condition. In the Cape Town area, if the referring physician so requests, all subsequent medical and administrative care of the potential donor will be carried out by the transplant team.

SELECTION OF DONOR HEARTS

Hearts are probably of insufficient size to support the circulation of an adult recipient, even after heterotopic transplantation, if taken from children under the age of approximately 10–14 years. In South Africa, white and coloured (mixed race) patients are rarely considered as heart donors if over the age of 40 (male) or 45 (female) years because of the high incidence of coronary atheroma in these ethnic groups; coronary arteriography and left ventriculography may be indicated in potential donors older than 35 (male) or 40 (female) years. Black patients of both sexes, having a significantly lower incidence of coronary atheroma, are considered suitable up to the age of approximately 50 years.

Those with transferable disease, such as a malignant lesion (other than primary tumours of the central nervous system) or serious infection, are excluded. Mild bronchial infection of recent onset resulting from aspiration is not a contraindication to organ donation. The presence of pyrexia in the hours or days before death may be related to the brain injury itself and may not necessarily indicate serious infection, although every effort must be made to exclude this possibility; once brain death has occurred, body temperature usually falls to subnormal levels over the course of a few hours. The length of time that the patient has been ventilated mechanically is equated with an unavoidable degree of infection, overt or otherwise. Not more than 3 days is desirable, and longer than 7 days is usually unacceptable.

Patients with pre-existing cardiac disease are obviously unsuitable for heart donation, and diabetes mellitus and hypertension may also preclude donation. The presence of cardiac disorders can be excluded by taking, whenever possible, a clinical history from the patient's relatives or his/her own medical practitioner, by clinical examination, by study of a chest radiograph of adequate quality, and a 12-lead ECG. If murmurs or added sounds are not to be missed, it is essential that the clinical examination be performed when a normal arterial pressure is present. Intracranial damage itself may cause ST and T wave changes on the ECG[18,19], and hypothermia leads to bradycardia and/or the presence of J waves, which are of no pathological significance but can be confused with electrocardiographic changes suggestive of ischaemia

(Figure 3.1). Rarely, cardiac catheterization and angiography may be indicated to exclude suspected cardiac disease.

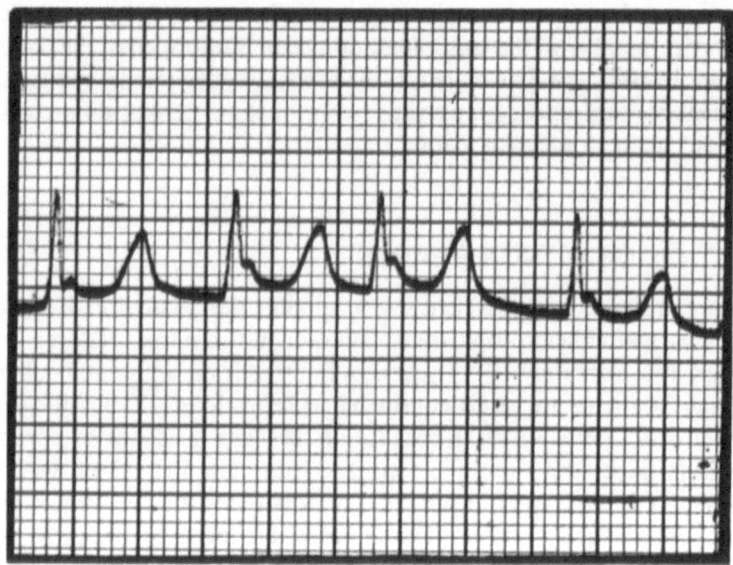

Figure 3.1   Electrocardiogram of a hypothermic potential organ donor showing typical J waves

Ideally, there should have been no episodes of severe hypotension or cardiac arrest at any time[20]. Recovery from such episodes, however, with return of an adequate blood pressure and diuresis, suggests that myocardial function remains satisfactory.

Blood specimens are taken for bacterial culture and serological tests for syphilis and hepatitis B (Australia) antigen. Although the results may not be available before the organ is transplanted, they may, if positive, be of considerable importance in the subsequent care of the recipient. When the presence of hepatitis B antigen is strongly suspected, the result of the serological investigation must be awaited; it remains our policy not to transplant organs taken from patients in whom a positive result is obtained.

OBTAINING CONSENT FOR DONATION FROM THE RELATIVES

The doctor who takes care of the patient from the time of admission clearly has a responsibility to the relatives who are passing through an extremely anxious time. For the layman it is still a macabre concept that the heart can be beating when doctors speak of death. They may not be able to grasp this concept, and this possibility should be respected, particularly when such understanding has to occur across cultural dividing lines. Continued small 'progress' reports to the relatives as the doctor works with the patient, informing them of the patient's deterioration, help to prepare them for the inevitable blow which must follow.

Medical and nursing staff who cared for the potential donor when alive are naturally concerned that an approach to the relatives of the deceased, requesting donation, may add to their distress. On a number of occasions, however, relatives derive solace and comfort from the knowledge that from their own loss someone else may benefit. When an autopsy is legally inevitable, the relatives may feel more inclined to consent to organ donation.

Although occasionally the attending doctor may prefer to approach the next-of-kin personally to request donation, in our experience the request comes best from the transplant team, and not from those who treated the primary pathology.

THE BRAIN-DEAD DONOR

The major source of donor hearts has been, and would appear to continue to be, from persons dying of head injury or spontaneous intracranial haemorrhage. The adverse effect of brain dysfunction on the heart has been demonstrated[21-25]. Electrocardiographic changes have been reported clinically in association with subarachnoid haemorrhage, intracranial infections, and cerebral tumours. Subendocardial haemorrhage and even myocardial necrosis have been reported in association with intracranial lesions. Electrocardiographic changes can be produced in animals by midbrain stimulation, and chronic stimulation produces myocardial necrosis; excessive sympathetic discharge may be aetiologically responsible.

Griepp and his colleagues[20], however, found no evidence of central nervous system mediated cardiac damage in a series of 22 patients evaluated as potential cardiac donors, but stressed that continuing consideration of this possibility was necessary. In the selection of donor hearts, the presence and severity of 'neurogenic heart lesions' should be assessed as far as possible. Such occult cardiac damage may conceivably contribute to the failure of some transplants and obscure or complicate the histological manifestations of rejection or ischaemia in others.

Studies in our own experimental laboratory in baboons have shown that myocardial damage, depletion of myocardial energy stores, and a reduction in circulating levels of various hormones result from sudden brain stem infarction (Novitzky et al., unpublished data). Heart function as judged by numerous haemodynamic observations is frequently considerably subnormal immediately following brain stem infarction and remains so, despite full supportive measures.

MANAGEMENT OF THE DONOR

Care of the donor can be a time-consuming activity; if the patient is to be maintained in an ideal state for organ donation as much care has to be taken over his management as would be given to any patient in an intensive care unit. Mechanical ventilation will already be employed and blood gases are maintained within the normal range. A urinary catheter may already be *in situ*; if not, one is inserted. A central venous pressure (CVP) monitoring catheter is essential if the volaemic state of the patient is to be well controlled. An arterial pressure line is an advantage but is not essential if monitoring by sphygmomanometer cuff is satisfactory; its presence, however, facilitates the frequent estimation of arterial blood gases. At least one and preferably two other peripheral venous infusions are set up for fluid and drug administration. Care is taken to introduce all vascular and urinary catheters under sterile conditions.

Brain-dead patients frequently pass large quantities of urine and rapidly become hypovolaemic and hypotensive if fluid is not replaced. Fluid, preferably warmed to help prevent hypothermia, is administered in the form of electrolyte solution or colloid. If the patient has bled significantly, e.g. from a head or other injury, whole blood is given to maintain the haemoglobin level above 8 g/dl. The serum sodium may rise to high levels in patients with impairment of production of antidiuretic hormone, and the administration of sodium chloride as a replacement fluid is therefore avoided. Potassium is lost in the urine and may require replacement on a large scale. 30 mmol potassium chloride are added to each litre of intravenous fluid given; supplements of 15 mmol/l administered in 30–50 ml of intravenous fluid over periods of 15–20 minutes may be necessary to maintain the serum potassium level above 3.5 mmol/l.

Until recently, it was our policy to maintain a mean arterial pressure (MAP) of approximately 80 mmHg until the heart was ready for excision. This was achieved by maintaining the CVP at between 5 and 10 cmH$_2$O and by adding a continuous infusion of inotropic agent when necessary. If these measures failed to maintain the MAP at the required level, vasopressin was administered either as an intravenous infusion or in small increments by intramuscular injection. Recent experimental work in our laboratory suggests, however, that excessive fluid administration and cardiotonic support may be neither necessary nor even desirable, and that maintenance of a lower MAP of between 40 and 60 mmHg may be preferable (Wicomb *et al.*, unpublished data).

Very high left atrial pressures can occur in brain-dead animals in which fluids are given to maintain the CVP at 5–10 cmH$_2$O and there is evidence to suggest that the left ventricle may undergo deterioration if a high preload is maintained, thus forcing the left ventricle to increase its cardiac output. A systemic MAP of between 40 and 60 mmHg would appear sufficient to provide an adequate coronary flow. Such a pressure may be best obtained by a combination of fluids to maintain a moderate preload and small increments of intramuscular vasopressin to increase the afterload. Excessive increases in either preload or afterload may be damaging to the myocardium. Maintenance of an MAP in excess of 60 mmHg would appear to be unnecessary. If the kidneys are also to be excised for the purposes of transplantation, as is usually the case, an MAP of much below 60 mmHg may, however, prove inadequate.

When inotropic support is given, dopamine is preferably avoided, as there is evidence that it depletes myocardial catecholamine reserves[26].

If urinary output is extreme, making adequate fluid replacement difficult, vasopressin given intravenously or intramuscularly is of value in reducing this loss. Since vasopressin acts by peripheral (including renal) vasoconstriction, great care is required in its administration if the kidneys are to remain suitable for donation. (Similarly, phenylephrine is contraindicated, although neither of these agents is harmful if the heart alone is to be donated.) We have found the intramuscular administration of vasopressin to be particularly effective, only small doses being required (0.1–0.25 U/kg). For intravenous infusion, vasopressin (20 U/200 ml electrolyte solution, administered initially at 10–20 microdrops/min) may suffice, although the solution strength may have to be doubled or even quadrupled if an increase in the rate of administration does not result in the desired decrease in urine flow and/or increase in blood pressure.

Brain-dead patients lose thermoregulation and rapidly cool to low temperatures if not actively warmed with an electric warming blanket. Although a mild degree of hypothermia may, in fact, be beneficial to the preservation of organs in a satisfactory condition, ventricular fibrillation can occur at temperatures below 30 °C. Our policy has been to maintain the central temperature at approximately 35 °C.

If the P_aO_2 and P_aCO_2 are maintained within normal limits by mechanical ventilation, and if the central venous and arterial pressures are also maintained within the desired range, acid-base balance will frequently remain within normal limits. If acidosis occurs, which is often a result of peripheral vasoconstriction associated with hypothermia, sodium bicarbonate should be administered to correct the base deficit (base deficit × body weight (kg) × 0.3/2 = ml 8.4% sodium bicarbonate).

There is some evidence that the administration of steroids leads to improved kidney[27] and heart[28] protection against ischaemic injury. However, doses of 30 mg/kg are necessary to achieve this effect, and administration must be carried out at least 2 hours before excision of the donor organ.

Studies in our experimental laboratory have conclusively shown that the circulating levels of various hormones such as insulin, glucagon, thyroxine and cortisol are significantly diminished following brain death (Novitzky et al., unpublished data). We are presently investigating the possibility that replenishment of these hormones is beneficial, and that their presence at normal levels may contribute to haemodynamic stability.

A suitable wide-spectrum, non-nephrotoxic antibiotic (e.g. chloramphenicol or cefamandole nafate) is initially administered at a dose of 3 g intravenously, and at 1 g 6-hourly thereafter until the donor is taken to the operating theatre for organ excision.

By the measures outlined above, the hearts of most brain-dead donors can be maintained in a viable state for several hours, occasionally up to 24 hours. In our experience, however, increasing instability of the circulation is the rule, and every effort should be made to organize the transplant operation as soon as possible.

References

1. Mollaret, P. and Goulon, M. (1959). Le coma dépassé (Mémoire préliminaire). *Rev. Neurol.*, **101**, 3
2. Stuart, F. P., Veith, F. J. and Cranford, R. E. (1981). Brain death laws and patterns of consent to remove organs for transplantation from cadavers in the United States and 28 other countries. *Transplantation*, **31**, 238
3. Jennett, B. (1975). The donor doctor's dilemma: observation on the recognition and management of brain death. *J. Med. Ethics*, **1**, 63
4. Conference of Medical Royal Colleges and their Faculties in the United Kingdom (1976). Diagnosis of death. *Br. Med. J.*, **2**, 1187
5. Black, P. McL. (1978). Brain death. *N. Engl. J. Med.*, **299**, 338
6. Plum, F. and Posner, J. B. (1980). *The Diagnosis of Stupor and Coma.* 4th Edn. (Philadelphia: F. A. Davis)
7. Brendler, S. J. and Selverstone, B. (1970). Recovery from decerebration. *Brain*, **93**, 381
8. Ivan, L. P. (1973). Spinal reflexes in cerebral death. *Neurology*, **23**, 650
9. Jörgensen, E. O. (1973). Spinal man after brain death. *Acta Neurochirurg.*, **28**, 259
10. Hanson, G. C. and McIlwraith, G. R. (1973). Lightning injury: two case histories and a review of management. *Br. Med. J.*, **2**, 271
11. Pallis, C. (1982). A B C of brain stem death. Pitfalls and safeguards. *Br. Med. J.*, **285**, 1720
12. Report of the *ad hoc* committee of Harvard Medical School to examine the definition of brain death: 'Definition of irreversible coma'. 1968. *J. Am. Med. Assoc.*, **205**, 337
13. Beecher, H. K. (1969). After the 'definition of irreversible coma'. (Editorial). *N. Engl. J. Med.*, **281**, 1070
14. Pallis, C. (1983). A B C of brain stem death. The arguments about the EEG. *Br. Med. J.*, **286**, 284
15. Korein, J., Brunstein, P. and George, A. (1977). Brain death. I. Angiographic correlation with the radioisotopic technique for evaluation of critical deficit of cerebral flow. *Ann. Neurol.*, **2**, 195
16. Goodman, J. M., Mishkin, F. S. and Dyken, M. (1969). Determination of brain death by isotope angiography. *J. Am. Med. Assoc.*, **209**, 1869
17. Searle, J. and Collins, C. (1980). A brain death protocol. *Lancet*, **1**, 641
18. Fentz, V. and Gormsen, J. (1962). Electrocardiographic patterns in patients with cerebrovascular accidents. *Circulation*, **25**, 22
19. Cooper, D. K. C. (1976). The donor heart: the present position with regard to resuscitation, storage, and assessment of viability. *J. Surg. Res.*, **21**, 363
20. Griepp, R. B., Stinson, E. B., Clark, D. A., Dong, E. Jr. and Shumway, N. E. (1971). The cardiac donor. *Surg. Gynecol. Obstet.*, **133**, 792
21. Burch, G. E., Meyer, R. and Abildskov, J. (1954). A new electrocardiographic pattern observed in cerebrovascular accidents. *Circulation*, **9**, 719

22. De Pasquale, N. P. and Burch, C. E. (1969). How normal is the donor heart? *Am. Heart J.*, **77**, 719

23. Greenhoot, A. H. and Reichenbach, D. D. (1969). Cardiac injury and subarachnoid haemorrhage. *J. Neurosurg.*, **30**, 521

24. Heggtveit, H. A. (1970). The donor heart: brain death and pathological changes in the heart. *Laval Med.*, **41**, 178

25. Smith, R. P. and Tomlinson, B. E. (1954). Subendocardial haemorrhages associated with intracranial lesions. *J. Pathol. Bacteriol.*, **68**, 327

26. Goldberg, L. I. (1974). Dopamine—clinical use of an endogenous catecholamine. *N. Engl. J. Med.*, **291**, 707

27. Miller, H. C. and Alexander, J. W. (1973). Protective effect of methylprednisolone against ischaemic injury to the kidney. *Transplantation*, **16**, 57

28. Toledo-Pereyra, L. H. and Jara, F. M. (1979). Myocardial protection with methylprednisolone. *J. Thorac. Cardiovasc. Surg.*, **77**, 619

APPENDIX 3.1

MINIMUM CRITERIA FOR A DIAGNOSIS OF BRAIN DEATH

THE DIAGNOSIS OF BRAIN DEATH CAN ONLY BE MADE IF THE ANSWER TO <u>ALL</u> THE QUESTIONS IS <u>NO</u>.

1. *RESPIRATION**
(a) Is there spontaneous ventilation within 5 minutes of disconnecting the ventilator (with P_aCO_2 normal before the ventilator was disconnected)?

OR

(b) Is there any spontaneous ventilation within 10 minutes of disconnecting the ventilator?

2. *BRAIN STEM REFLEXES*
(a) Do the pupils react to light?
    Do the pupils react to painful stimulation?
(b) Are doll's eye movements present?
(c) Does nystagmus occur when each ear is in turn irrigated with ice-cold water for 1 minute?
(d) Is there any movement in the head and neck, either spontaneously or in response to stimulation?
(e) Is there a gag or a reflex response following bronchial stimulation by a suction catheter passed down the trachea?

3. *BODY TEMPERATURE*
Is the rectal temperature below 35°C?

4. *DRUGS*
Have any drugs which may affect ventilation or the level of consciousness been administered during the past 12 hours?

5. *CEREBRAL STATE*
Have you any doubt that this patient's cerebral state is due to an irreversible cause?

DATE_____ DOCTOR_____

_____

*Details of testing for spontaneous respiration are given on the reverse of this form.

4
Medico-legal Aspects

INTRODUCTION

Although the specific laws relating to organ donation vary from country to country, in broad terms the statutory requirements have much in common.

Prior to 1952 there was no *statutory* provision in most countries for the removal of tissues from bodies of deceased or living persons for the purpose of transplantation. With advances in surgical techniques it was inevitable that representations would be made by the various organizations seeking statutory sanctions for their activities. For example, this process was initiated in the Republic of South Africa (RSA) by the National Council for the Blind, who were in urgent need of corneas for transplantation. They were largely instrumental in initiating the passage of legislation that provided for postmortem examinations for purposes other than medico-legal, as well as for the removal of tissue for therapeutic and scientific purposes, and for the preservation and use of such tissues. This far-sighted legislation lawfully entitled a doctor to remove tissue of a recipient and replace it with tissue removed from a donor. At that time this represented a state of affairs considerably in advance of many other countries in which transplantation operations were being contemplated.

The first human-to-human heart transplant in 1967 inevitably precipitated discussion about the legality and ethics of such operations, despite the legislation enacted some 15 years earlier. This legislation, of course, facilitated the performance of the operation, since surgical skill and medical knowledge are not sufficient if the operation itself is unlawful[1-5].

Problems of interpretation of this 1952 South African legislation (amended in 1962) arose as a result of the first heart transplant, which necessitated further legislation to provide more adequately for the donation of human bodies and tissue for therapeutic and scientific purposes, as well as for the removal, preservation and use of such tissues in living persons. In 1970, legislation was enacted to overtly encourage anatomical donations by facilitating the acquisition and use of human tissue where necessary, yet ensuring that the public and individual interests were adequately safeguarded[6, 7].

The need for not infrequent changes in transplantation legislation has become necessary as 'advances in science and medicine have their less positive side and may pose increasingly different moral, ethical, clinical and legal difficulties for all concerned. The law, as always, lags some way behind, fearful of new changes which may prove worse than the uneasy *status quo* of the common law, which has itself evolved gradually over the years to take account of the changing face of society'[8]. Understandably, thus during 1983 the Human Tissues Act was consented to by the State President, representing a consolidation of relevant legislation in South Africa, i.e. Anatomy Act, Blood Transfusion Regulations, and the 1970 'transplantation' Act.

In this chapter attention will be directed to the statutory requirements relating to heart transplantation in South Africa for comparison with the relevant laws in a number of other countries. Professional ethical codes and issues relating to civil litigation are not discussed. The following legislative areas are briefly considered: (1) certification of the fact of death, (2) donation, (3) the purpose of donation, (4) donees, (5) authority for removal of donated tissue, (6) confidentiality, and (7) certain related administrative matters.

1. CERTIFICATION OF THE FACT OF DEATH

In the RSA the *fact* of death must be certified by two registered medical practitioners, who may not be members of the transplant team, one of whom must have been practising for at least 5 years since registration. What constitutes 'death' is left to the discretion of the two doctors concerned. The grounds for so certifying would have to be justified by these doctors should this become an issue of litigation. The 1961 British Human Tissues Act allows removal of tissue once a registered medical practitioner has satisfied himself by personal examination of the body that life is extinct.

The words 'death' and 'life is extinct' make the issue more one of semantics than science. There has generally been opposition to making provision in the RSA law that would define the moment of death 'because the *moment* of death cannot be defined. . . . The solution to this problem will seem to be to define those who should be qualified to determine death, for, in the final analysis, it is the opinion of the physician that determines the time of death, regardless of what instruments or methods he uses to assess the condition'[9].

The 22nd World Medical Assembly, at the meeting in Sydney, Australia, in 1963, issued a statement that 'the determination of death should be based on clinical judgement supplemented if necessary by a number of diagnostic aids, of which electroencephalography is currently most helpful'. In the case of those persons kept alive by artificial means of resuscitation (in use or contemplated), or in which the transplantation of an organ is being considered, it emphasized that the moment of irreversibility of the processes leading to death must be determined rather than the moment of death. This latter part defies definition as it varies from cell to cell, tissue to tissue, and organ to organ, so it may be impossible by known means to determine when a body is extinct. This declaration further states that, while the electroencephalograph is the most useful diagnostic aid, 'no single technological criterion is entirely satisfactory in the present state of medicine, nor can any one technological procedure be substituted by the overall judgement of the physician'[9].

Unquestionably, the moment of death may be of vital concern to the civil and criminal law when issues of liability for alleged murder or culpable homicide or succession must be solved. Questions may arise as to whose act was the true cause of the deceased's death? Was the deceased still alive when a second assailant joined in the 'assault', in which case the latter may be shown to be guilty of murder[10]?

'While many may recoil from the suggestion of removal of organs from a body whilst the heart is still beating, it is clear that there is substantial support for the view that cerebral death is an acceptable criterion. The difficulty, however, is that absolute unanimity as to what constitutes irreversible cerebral death has so far not been achieved'[11].

Any acceptable definition of the moment of death in terms of heart transplantation would by necessity be only applicable where facilities are available to fulfil the prescriptions of international concepts of death. Obviously these criteria will not be applicable beyond the hospital situation, where the process of dying and death eventually present unmistakable evidence that the tripod of life—respiration, cardiac action and cerebral function—has ceased permanently[12].

By 1979, 25 states in the USA had recognized brain death as a basis for declaring the fact of death. The 1978 Uniform Brain Death Act specifies that: 'For legal and medical purposes, an individual who has sustained irreversible cessation of all functioning of the brain, including the brain stem, is dead. A determination under this section must be made in accordance with reasonable medical standards'. The law is, however, silent on the actual criteria to be used for determining death. The time of death is determined by the physician who attends the death, or, if none, by the physician who certifies the death. By this law too, this physician may not participate in the procedures for removing or transplanting a part of the deceased's body[13].

In contrast, most other countries, including South Africa, have no specific laws relating to brain death as evidence of the fact of death, and generally rely on acceptable medical criteria. A Working Party on behalf of the Health Departments of Great Britain and Northern Ireland has prepared a quasi-legal Code of Practice intended for hospital staff and medical administrators relating to 'Cadaveric Organs for Transplantation' (1983)[14]. In the section dealing with brain death, it states: 'There is no legal definition of death. Death has traditionally been diagnosed by the irreversible cessation of respiration and heart beat. This Working Party accepts the view held by the Conferences of Royal Colleges that death can also be diagnosed by the irreversible cessation of brain-stem function—"brain death". In diagnosing brain death, the criteria laid down by the Colleges[15] should be followed'.

In an attempt to seek clarity in regard to 'reasonable medical standards' a US report was issued by 'The Medical Consultants on the Diagnosis of Death to the President's Commission for the Study of Ethical Problems in Medicine and Biomedical Behavioral Research', entitled 'Guidelines for the Determination of Death'[16]. In this report, attention is directed towards: (a) eliminating errors in classifying a living individual as dead, (b) minimizing errors in classifying a dead body as alive, (c) allowing a determination of death to be made without unreasonable delay, and making the guidelines (d) adaptable to a variety of clinical situations, and (e) explicit and accessible to verification. These guidelines are advisory, in the authors' words 'representing a distillation of current practice tending to be too inflexible to be mandatory'.

Subsequently, the American Bar Association, the American Medical Association, and the National Conference of Commissions of Uniform State Laws, together with the aforementioned Commission, proposed a model statute, to replace the Uniform Brain Death Act by a Uniform Determination of Death Act[16]. The relevant section reads: 'An individual who has sustained either (1) irreversible cessation of circulatory and respiratory functions, or (2) irreversible cessation of all functions of the entire brain, including the brain stem, is dead. A determination of death must be made in accordance with accepted medical standards'. The changed emphasis is underlined and tends to give legal standing to a decision made in terms of 'good medical practice', i.e. accepted standards, rather than reasonable medical standards.

Although recommendations and codes of practice regarding the criteria for death certification are generally not statutory prescriptions, they carry such evidential weight as to be read almost as a rider to what the laws would generally consider to constitute 'good medical practice'. The main differences, which are substantial, between the approach to brain death in the UK and the USA are summarized by Pallis[17] (Table 4.1). (The clinical diagnosis of brain death is discussed in detail in Chapter 3.)

The certification of the *fact* of death must not be confused with other legal requirements where the doctor attending the patient is required to certify

Table 4.1 Comparison of features considered essential for the diagnosis of brain death in the UK and USA (after Pallis[17])

	Death the sum of the following:	
	UK	USA
Comatose patient on ventilator with known diagnosis	+	−
Irremediable structural brain damage	+	−
Necessary exclusions	+	−
Loss of brain stem reflexes (apnoeic)	+	+
Other tests (electroencephalography, etc.)	−	+

forthwith the *cause* of death (or his inability to do so where death is not solely and exclusively due to natural causes). In the issuing of such a death (cause) certificate, the purpose is the registration of the death and the disposal of the body by burial or cremation. In the case of an organ donation, both certifications are required to be completed.

2. DONATIONS AND THE ACQUISITION OF TISSUE

In South Africa—there is similar legislation in several other countries—the donation of a human heart may be made in one of three ways, as described below.

(a) Any individual prior to death

Any person may make such a donation to be implemented after his death: (i) in his will, if he is competent to make such a will, (ii) in any document attested to by two competent witnesses, (iii) by an oral statement made by the deceased during life in the presence of two persons of at least 18 years of age, (iv) by wearing a prescribed identity tag issued by an institution approved by the Minister of Health and Welfare. Any such donation may be revoked prior to death by the donor.

In the USA the Uniform Anatomical Gift Act of 1968, which remains the last statute in the USA relating to transplantation, allows any individual of sound mind who is over 18 years of age to make a gift during his life by will (to be effective immediately upon death without waiting for probate), or by a card or other document. If the donor is incapable of signing for any reason, including sickness, then the document can be signed on his behalf, if validated by two witnesses.

The system of donor cards has the merit of simplicity and portability. A typical example is the Uniform Card developed in the USA following the Uniform Anatomical Gift Act. This card, which can be carried easily in a pocket or wallet, states in simple words the donor's desire to make an anatomical gift to take effect upon death. On the reverse side the card contains provisions for signature, witnessing and personal details. Similar cards are available in several other countries, including Australia, Canada and Britain. In Britain, under the Human Tissues Act, 1961, a patient may carry a signed donor card or record his wishes 'in writing at any time or orally in the presence of two or more witnesses during his last illness'.

(b) A relative of the deceased

In the absence of a donation made by the individual himself whilst alive (as above), certain *specified* relatives of the deceased, i.e. the spouse, any major child, any parent or any major brother or sister of the deceased may make a donation, provided the deceased donor had not forbidden such a donation. Any donation by a relative may be revoked by the relative who made it. In this context, in the RSA a major child refers to a person over the age of 21 years.

In the USA, relatives of a deceased may also legally donate by document, telegraph, recorded telephone or other recorded message; in order of legal priority are the spouse, adult children, parents and adult siblings.

In many countries 'relative' is not defined.

(c) An authority empowered to donate

The acquisition of hearts in the absence of a donation as in (a) or (b) above is still possible. If a relative authorized in law to consent to a donation cannot be traced, the law in many countries allows for a designated official to authorize under certain prescriptions the removal of tissue from a deceased person for purposes of a donation. In South Africa this is the District Surgeon, and in England and Wales the Coroner. In the USA, however, the law makes no actual reference to the deposition in use of an unclaimed cadaver. A few states allow transplantation of certain organs (such as corneas) if a reasonable effort has been made to trace the relatives; authorization must be given by the Medical Examiner. This official can only authorize removal of organs if he has satisfied himself on certain points.

For example, in South Africa the District Surgeon must be clear that: (i) the deceased did not give a contrary direction prior to his death, (ii) two doctors have stated in writing that in their opinion the use of the tissue in the body of another person is immediately necessary to save the life of the envisaged recipient, and (iii) all reasonable steps have been taken to trace the relatives of the deceased. This third provision is difficult to implement, and District Surgeons are loath to give such consent where the identity of the deceased is not known, as it is argued, if this be the case, that it is impossible for any meaningful effort to have been made to trace the relatives of such a deceased.

Where the body is to become the subject of a medico-legal examination, in many countries certain authorities are empowered under certain circumstances to remove tissue (e.g. a heart) and donate such tissue to an authorized institution. Such removal or donation is not subject to the consent of the relatives. The medical practitioner who gives this authority must, however, satisfy himself that removal of the organ will in no way affect the outcome of the autopsy.

In South Africa this particular provision was introduced primarily to facilitate the acquisition of pituitary glands for the purposes of extracting pituitary growth hormone. The Minister is empowered, however, to prescribe any tissue on application from an institution. Hearts, *inter alia*, have been included as prescribed tissue for certain institutions. This has proved to be an ideal and major source of hearts for purposes of transplantation by the very nature of the victims being the subject of violent death. These provisions could best be equated with the 'presumed consent' referred to in the legislation of a number of countries.

Despite this provision it has nevertheless been internal hospital policy in the RSA to seek the consent of the family to such removal and use. On the very infrequent occasions where the relatives cannot be traced, and the deceased has not indicated his opposition to tissue donation in a statement or document made before death, or by virtue of his particular religious background, or where there would not appear to be a contrary sentiment, the removal, donation and the acquisition is proceeded with.

In the USA, the State is given an overriding power to conduct legally required autopsies, and the exercise of this power cancels out the 'anatomical gift' (i.e. the donation for purposes of transplantation). When death occurs under suspicious, violent or unusual circumstances, the Medical Examiner or Coroner assumes jurisdiction and control of the body immediately; he may, however, give permission for transplantation.

Stuart and his colleagues[13] analysed patterns of consent to remove cadaveric organs for transplantation in 29 different countries (Table 4.2). Their findings were based on their own experience and the USA and on a mailed questionnaire sent to renal transplant programmes in 40 countries; replies were forthcoming from 28. A system of donor card/disc, prepared before death, was used in 19 countries; in 16 consent to remove organs had to be obtained from the donor or a family member, whilst 13 countries used 'presumed consent' as a basis for removal of organs for transplantation, though in 6 of the 13 the family was approached before proceeding with organ salvage. Some countries provided for both card donations and presumed consent. In the USA, in no state is consent presumed.

3. PURPOSE OF DONATION

As in most countries, in South Africa each donation or 'removal' must be for purposes of medical and dental education, research, therapy (including use in any other living person) or for any other scientific purpose; such purpose need not be specifically expressed.

4. THE DONEE

In the RSA a donee may be any hospital, medical practitioner, dentist, medical or dental school, authorized institution or any person. The donee may upon delivery of the tissue have exclusive right over it subject to the prohibition of the sale of the tissue. Except in the case of a donation of a whole body, the donee has 24 hours after death of a donor to have the tissue removed, since the relatives may claim the body for burial or cremation 24 hours after death.

Table 4.2 Donation consent procedures in various countries in the 1980s (after Stuart et al.[13])

Country	Donor cards/disc	Presumed consent	Presumed consent, but family agreement sought
Argentina	+	−	−
Australia	−	−	−
Austria	−	+	−
Belgium	+	−	−
Canada	+	−	−
Czechoslovakia	−	+	−
Denmark	+	+	−
Finland	+	+	+
France	+	+	−
Germany	+	−	−
Great Britain	+	−	−
Greece	+	+	+
India	−	−	−
Ireland	+	−	−
Israel	−	+	−
Italy	+	+	+
Japan	+	−	−
Netherlands	−	−	−
New Zealand	−	−	−
Norway	+	+	+
Poland	−	+	−
Puerto Rico	+	−	−
South Africa	+	−*	−
South Korea	+	−	−
Spain	−	+	+
Sweden	−	+	+
Switzerland	+	+	−
Thailand	+	−	−
USA	+	−	−

+ = Yes.
− = No.
*Under certain circumstances.

In the USA, state statutes vary with regard to permissible recipients of donated tissue but, in general, licensed hospitals, teaching institutions, colleges, medical schools, universities, storage banks, state public health and anatomy boards, and institutes approved by the State Department of Health, may be donees. Unless the donee has been previously indicated during life by the deceased, the attending physician becomes the donee. If he so desires, he can transfer his ownership to another person. Although he is not permitted to participate personally in removing and transplanting organs or parts, he is allowed to communicate with other relevant donees or transplant teams.

5. AUTHORIZATION FOR THE REMOVAL OF ORGANS

Once a donation has been made in the RSA, a donee specified, and the fact of death certified, the transplant surgeon or a member of the team must request authority from the appropriate medical practitioner (for example, the medical superintendent of the hospital in which the donor is being cared for, or his authorized medical deputy) to remove the donated organ, which removal may only be undertaken by or on the authority of a medical practitioner or dentist. The person authorizing removal must satisfy himself that the body is not required for examination in terms of other legislation which has a higher ranking claim on the body, e.g. the Inquest Act.

Authority to remove a valid donation in the United Kingdom is not essentially different from the above provisions, with the noticeable exception that the person lawfully in possession of the body of a deceased may so authorize, after practicable enquiries, providing that the deceased had not expressed objection to his body being so dealt with, or the surviving spouse or any relative of the deceased expressed objection. Normally the 'person' lawfully in possession of a dead body is a National Health Service hospital until such time as the body is claimed by the person with the right to possession, that is the Coroner, executor, or the next of kin[14].

6. CONFIDENTIALITY

Disclosure to any other person of any fact whereby the identity of the deceased donor or donee may be established is prohibited by statute in South Africa, unless consented to in writing by the deceased prior to his death, by one of the specified relatives, or by the District Surgeon who authorized the removal of tissue.

In the United Kingdom, confidentiality is not prescribed, but the staff of hospitals and organ exchange organizations 'must respect the wishes of the donor, the recipient, and the families with respect to anonymity'[14]. There appear to be no statutory laws regarding confidentiality in the USA.

In common law the privacy of the individual may not normally be intruded upon. The ethical obligation of a medical practitioner to treat patient information as confidential appears to be based on contract[18]. Experience has shown that breaches in confidentiality in regard to heart transplantation have generally had their origin beyond the profession. A general clause, as provided by South African law, would seem desirable, though this is viewed by some as an 'overkill' in the light of common law requirements.

7. ADMINISTRATIVE AND GENERAL PROVISIONS

Importation/exportation of tissue

In South Africa the importation or exportation of tissues is subject to permission being obtained from the Director General, Health and Welfare.

Sale of tissue

An authorized institution or the importer of tissue may receive payment for providing tissue to any person for therapeutic or scientific purposes. If any other person receives payment for such tissue, he shall refund such payment to the person who made it.

The object of this and the aforementioned provision is to prohibit trading in tissue, which ethically and scientifically is unacceptable. This prohibition, however, does not prevent a medical practitioner from being paid for his services in the collecting or use of such tissue as a part of therapy.

In the USA, the Uniform Anatomical Gift Act is believed to exclude all sales from dead bodies. Although there is no express restriction on the sale of body parts from *living* persons, the subject is treated under the general principles of law.

CONCLUSION

Jeddeloh[19], in a review, of legal aspects of transplantation, emphasizes that the law today is for the purpose of *inter alia* protecting individual rights in a complex technological society which has the capability to transplant tissue from one person to another as a form of medical treatment. This poses new, ever-changing challenges with regard to the rights and obligations of, and relationships between, the donor, whether living or dead, and the donee of human body tissue. 'Presently these issues have not been fully settled. While the law recognizes that the transplantation of human body tissue is an important, and in many cases, highly successful means of treatment which should be encouraged, it also seeks vigorously to protect potential donors from exploitation in all forms. In most recent decisions and cases, courts have struggled to balance socictal nccds and rights of individual donois. The law is only beginning to consider matters such as facile procurement and easy distribution of various body parts, right of minor and incompetent donors, proper standards of informed consent for giving a human body part, liability for injury caused to a donee by the transplantation procedure itself, the time at which a necessary human body part may be removed from a deceased donor, the legitimate scope of protection which ought to be afforded the transplant surgeon, and other questions'[19].

References

1. Shapiro, H. A. (1968). Organ grafting in man. *J. For. Med.*, **15**, 1
2. Shapiro, H. A. (1968). Brain death and organ transplantation. *J. For. Med.*, **15**, 89
3. Shapiro, H. A. (1969). Criteria for determining that death has occurred. *J. For. Med.*, **16**, 1
4. Shapiro, H. A. (1969). Organ transplantation and the law. *J. For. Med.*, **16**, 77
5. Shapiro, H. A. (1968). The Cape Town human heart transplants. *J. For. Med.*, **14**, 1
6. Smith, L. S. (1967). The acquisition of human tissue for transplantation purposes: legal requirements in South Africa. *S. Afr. Med. J.*, **41**, 1274
7. Cooper, D. K. C., De Villiers, J. C., Smith, L. S., Crombie, Y., Boyd, S. T., Jacobson, J. E. and Barnard, C. N. (1982). Medical, legal, and administrative aspects of cadaveric organ donation in the RSA. *S. Afr. Med. J.*, **62**, 933
8. Brahams, D. (1983). The problems posed by the advance of science. *Medico-Legal J.*, **51**, 191 (Editorial)
9. Report: Select Committee (1968). *The Anatomical Donations and Post Mortem Examinations Bill.* (Government Printer, Republic of South Africa)
10. Strauss, S. A. (1980). *Doctor, Patient and the Law.* p. 295. (Pretoria: Van Schaik)
11. Strauss, S. A. (1980). *Doctor, Patient and the Law.* p. 125. (Pretoria: Van Schaik)
12. Strauss, S. A. (1980). *Doctor, Patient and the Law.* p. 299. (Pretoria: Van Schaik)
13. Stuart, F. P., Veith, F. J. and Crawford, R. E. (1981). Brain death laws and patterns of consent to remove organs for transplantation from cadavers in the United States and 28 other countries. *Transplantation*, **31**, 238
14. Working Party of the Health Departments of Great Britain and Northern Ireland. (1983). *Cadaveric Organs for Transplantation.* (London: HMSO)
15. Conference of Medical Royal Colleges and their Faculties in the United Kingdom. (1976). *Br. Med. J.*, **2**, 1178
16. Report of the Medical Consultants on the Diagnosis of Death to the President's Commission for the Study of Ethical Problems in Medicine and Biomedical Behavioural Research. Guidelines for the determination of death. (1981). *J. Am. Med. Assoc.*, **246**, 2184
17. Pallis, C. (1983). A B C of brain stem death. The position in the USA and elsewhere. *Br. Med. J.*, **286**, 209
18. Masters, N. C. and Shapiro, H. A. (1966). *Medical Secrecy.* p. 6. (Cape Town: Balkema)
19. Jeddeloh, N. P. (1980). Legal aspects of transplantation. In Chatterjee, S. N. (ed.) *Renal Transplantation—A Multi-disciplinary Approach.* (New York: Raven Press)

5
Donor Heart Storage

INTRODUCTION

The development of successful methods of myocardial protection during open heart operations has been one of the major advances in cardiac surgery in recent years[1]. At present, cardioplegic arrest followed by simple storage in ice-cold saline provides good protection of the myocardium against ischaemic damage for up to 3–4 hours[2]. This allows for transport of a donor heart from one hospital to another over distances of up to approximately 1500 km (940 miles), but necessitates highly organized and expensive forms of communication and transportation between these centres[3].

Methods of storage of the heart for periods longer than 3–4 hours are still in their infancy. Improved techniques of preservation must be devised, however, if cardiac transplantation is to develop fully as a routine therapeutic procedure.

The essential gain from storing the isolated heart is, of course, time. This includes time to transport the donor heart to the recipient, time to tissue type the donor and perform donor–recipient lymphocytotoxic cross-matching, time to do an elective operation, and time, possibly, to resuscitate a heart too damaged by ante-mortem changes to transplant immediately.

At our own institution the need for a larger donor pool is acute. Geographically, Cape Town is relatively isolated from the other major cities in Southern Africa, and the distances are too great for donor hearts preserved by cardioplegic arrest and storage in ice to be transported to Cape Town. Where this simple method of storage has been utilized elsewhere over relatively long distances, privately chartered jet aircraft have been available[3]; the expense is obviously considerable and beyond the resources of many centres, including our own. It is therefore particularly important for our own institution to be involved in the development of a system of storage which will allow less expensive long distance transportation.

Today, in most countries involved in cardiac transplantation, the law allows the patient to be certified dead once the brain has undergone total and irreversible death. This enables the heart to be excised whilst still beating

51

within the donor, which therefore gives some indication of its viability. The effects of brain death on subsequent myocardial function have already been mentioned briefly (Chapter 3). Unprotected anoxic or ischaemic arrest of the heart leads to significant damage of the organ[4], and no group involved in cardiac transplantation is at present attempting to resuscitate and transplant hearts which have already ceased functioning under less than ideal cardioplegic conditions. The effects of anoxia or ischaemia on the myocardium, and experimental experience in resuscitating cadaveric hearts, therefore, need not concern us here, though they have been reviewed briefly elsewhere[5].

MYOCARDIAL CELL METABOLISM

The myocardium is composed of highly specialized cells, which function satisfactorily only within the narrow limits of a defined, regulated, biochemical environment. The cells of both the vascular and cellular compartments of the myocardium require specific osmotic pressures, pH and inorganic ions to function adequately, and metabolic substrates for their energy requirements. A change in any one or more of these factors results in a change in energy production. The pathways involved in the conversion of chemical energy from nutrient substrates into a form which can be utilized by the myocardium for useful work, that is, the normal metabolic pathways, are fully described in standard biochemical texts[6].

In outline, under normothermic conditions, four major pathways are operative in the myocardial cell in the oxidation of glucose: (1) glycolysis, (2) the hexosemonophosphate shunt, (3) the Krebs cycle, and (4) the electron transport chain. The former two can operate under aerobic or anaerobic conditions and are functional in the cytoplasm of the cell, whereas the latter two take place in the mitochondria only under aerobic conditions. The metabolic activity of these four pathways is interrelated. This unity will be disturbed if the supply of any essential factors, such as oxygen or glucose, is inadequate. In the absence of an adequate oxygen supply, there is significant depression of the Krebs cycle and of electron transport, and myocardial energy is derived from the anaerobic glycolytic pathway. Anaerobic glycolysis is a much less efficient system of energy supply compared with the oxidation of glucose under aerobic conditions; the efficiency of energy conservation in anaerobic glycolysis is only 3%, whereas that of aerobic metabolism is 50%[7].

The stability of myocardial metabolic activity is interrupted as soon as a period of *in situ* or *in vitro* preservation intervenes, whether it be by pharmacological arrest, simple ice storage, or by one of the various forms of normothermic or hypothermic preservation methods discussed later. Satisfactory myocardial preservation will only be achieved if compensation is made for the altered myocardial environment, either by efficient metabolic inhibition or by metabolic support.

DONOR PRETREATMENT

Studies on the rat kidney have shown that if the donor animal is treated variously with methylprednisolone, phenoxybenzamine, chlorpromazine or heparin before the organ is removed, subsequent function after a period of warm ischaemia can approximate that in control experiments[8]. The steroid, α-receptor blocker and phenothiazine are believed to function by 'stabilizing membranes', by which it is inferred that the cell and intracellular organelle membranes retain a greater degree of control over the exchange of ions across them, particularly the intracellular compartments; the α-blocker and chlorpromazine reduce agonal vascular spasm, and heparin prevents intravascular clotting. In addition, phenoxybenzamine maintains both the intracellular concentrations of adenosine triphosphate (ATP) and the electron microscopic structure of the organ. There is also evidence that donor pretreatment with methylprednisolone improves subsequent myocardial function if a period of preservation intervenes[9, 10].

In the clinical situation, most donors receive heparin (and some, a corticosteroid) immediately before cardiectomy. We do not know of any group which routinely administers other agents, other than antibiotics, to the donor.

METHODS OF ORGAN STORAGE

Organ preservation can therefore be achieved in two fundamental ways: (1) by reducing the metabolic demands of the tissues, increasing the organ's resistance to injury, and (2) by increasing the supply of vital substances such as oxygen and nutrients to the organ. Several techniques combine a method of increasing resistance to injury with maintenance of a supply of vital substances to the organ.

Whatever method is employed, most research workers in this field have felt that it is desirable to prevent intravascular thrombosis in the coronary vessels by heparinizing the donor before excision of the heart. Our own experimental and clinical observations would suggest, however, that, though desirable, this is not absolutely essential[11].

Preservation methods can be divided into two basic groups—those which utilize some form of perfusion system and those which do not (Table 5.1).

Table 5.1   Major methods of storage of the heart which have been investigated experimentally

Non-perfusion methods	Perfusion methods
Simple ice storage	Total body perfusion using a pump-oxygenator
Hypothermia and hyperbaric oxygenation	Autoperfusion (biological oxygenation)
Supercooling	Intermediate host perfusion (parabiosis)
Freezing	Extracorporeal normothermic perfusion
	Extracorporeal hypothermic perfusion

Non-perfusion methods

1. Hypothermia

The simplest method of preservation is hypothermia, which has been used in renal transplantation since 1956[12]. Much of the early work on preservation of the heart by simple hypothermia resulted from studies devoted to arrest of the heart during intracardiac surgical procedures[13, 14]. Myocardial protection by cooling remains of great interest to both the cardiac surgeon and the transplanter, though the latter seeks longer periods of protection.

Webb and Howard[15] were the first to study preservation by refrigeration, and demonstrated that the heart could be maintained viable and functional for periods of at least 8 hours.

Local myocardial hypothermia induced by surface cooling with isotonic saline has been used by the Stanford group to maintain viability of the cardiac transplant graft in both experimental and clinical situations[16]. In 1962 this group was the first to report successful orthotopic transplantation of the dog heart after 7 hours of preservation in cold saline[17].

The physiological basis for the efficiency of hypothermia as a cell protectant during ischaemia is its effect on reducing the metabolic demands of the organ[18]. Cooling of cells reduces the number of molecules available for physiological processes. This, in turn, reduces the metabolic demands of the cell and protects against ischaemic injury. The metabolic rate of the cell can be gauged by the Arrhenius plot (or the Q_{10}). This is the ratio of the reaction rates at two temperatures separated by $10\,°C$. Decreasing the temperature by $10\,°C$ decreases the metabolic rate by a factor of 2–3. Metabolic activity still continues at temperatures of $-60\,°C$ and, as a result, tissue stored at $0\,°C$ by simple ice storage is still subject to the relatively fast onset of ischaemic damage. During hypothermic storage, oxygen depletion, increased lactate production, and acid-base imbalance all occur. Unless these three features are continually corrected during the preservation period, tissue damage will occur following reperfusion (reperfusion injury), and, in the case of the heart, result in arrhythmia, gross oedema formation and inadequate function. Similar damage will follow any inadequate storage technique.

Continuing metabolic activity in an ischaemic organ will result in exhaustion of its oxygen supply and glycogen reserves, during which time the organ resorts to anaerobic glycolysis as its major energy contributor. The pH progressively decreases, predominantly from ATP hydrolysis[19]. The low pH inhibits the glycolytic regulatory enzyme phosphofructokinase (PFK)[20], and energy production by glycolysis is thereafter reduced. The low oxygen tension that develops results in a decreased formation of calcium chelating agents (ATP and citrate) predisposing the myocardium to inadequate calcium homeostasis. It is also likely that leakage from the sarcoplasmic reticulum and the extracellular space results in a net increase in cytoplasmic ionized calcium[21]. This may result in an increased resting myocardial tension, which increases the metabolic demands of the cell. The ultimate effect of an increase in intracellular calcium will be a stone heart. Tissue lactate has already reached high levels, though a further rise may be somewhat inhibited by the continuing fall in pH.

In the case of the myocardium, the reversibility of injury is limited to a maximum ice storage period of approximately 12 hours at 4°C. The injury occurs during storage, but it is only during the phase of reperfusion that the effects of the injury become evident, when normothermia increases the metabolic rate of the organ. The replenishment of oxygen, of which the organ was starved, has a paradoxical effect, because ionized calcium is now rapidly taken up by the mitochondria[22]. This is followed by explosive cell swelling, mitochondrial and myofibrillar damage, and the appearance of contraction bands and intramitochondrial calcium phosphate deposits[23].

Unless metabolism can be effectively arrested during the period of hypothermic storage, such that the need for oxygen is eliminated, extended periods of hypothermic organ storage will prove unsuccessful.

2. *Pharmacological inhibition*

During the early years of open heart surgery, surgeons experimented with various methods of inducing cardiac arrest; of the chemical agents tested, potassium citrate is perhaps the best known[24]. Electron microscopic studies revealed, however, that, although the cardiac arrest induced with potassium citrate led to a ·stabilization of the ultrastructure, after reanimation heart muscle necrosis with dilatation of the heart occurred[25]. This early phase of potassium arrest was almost certainly related to the high concentrations of potassium used. In the correct doses, however, potassium is a safe, reversible agent, and today is a constituent of many cardioplegic solutions.

The metabolic inhibition achieved by magnesium sulphate, used singly or in combination with chlorpromazine, has been shown to maintain the anoxic normothermic heart at virtually its ante-mortem functional state for at least 3 hours[26].

A large number of other pharmacological agents has been shown to have some metabolic inhibitory effect on the myocardium. Phenothiazines have a general inhibitory effect on the leakage of lysosomal enzymes[27], cellular metabolism[28] and mitochondrial swelling[29]. They also conserve purine nucleotides by inhibiting the membrane-bound 5 nucleotidase[30], preventing catecholamine depletion by inhibiting adenyl cyclase[31], and may have the additional function of α-adrenergic blockade, preventing vasospasm.

Phenoxybenzamine has vasodilator properties and a lysosomal membrane stabilizing effect[32, 33]. Other effects include inhibition of catecholamine uptake and degradation[34], and inhibition of serotonin and histamine activity resulting in vasodilatation[32]. A cardioplegic effect is produced by procaine hydrochloride in high concentrations by prolongation of the asystolic period through counteracting the return of electromechanical activity. Procaine also has membrane stabilization and vasodilator properties[35, 36]. Combinations of various agents in perfusion solutions were tested at normothermia by Hearse et al.[37].

3. Combined hypothermia and pharmacological inhibition

The combination of some pharmacological cardioplegic agents with hypo-thermia appears to be synergistic. The combination of magnesium sulphate and hypothermia extends more than two-fold the effects of either alone in the preservation of the isolated rat heart[38]. Coronary perfusion with hypothermic solutions or solutions containing high concentrations of potassium induces arrest without depleting ATP or creatine phosphate[39]. It appears important to maintain these myocardial high energy phosphates during arrest. Dypirid-amole has also been shown to increase tissue levels of ATP in the heart[40], and is successful in prolonging anoxic storage times when added to a cold flushing perfusate before storage of the rat heart[41].

Hearts have been stored at 4°C in intracellular-like solutions containing a high potassium content for periods of 18–26 hours without oxygen or per-fusion[42]. Subsequent orthotopic transplantation was successful in 14 of 21 cases with survival for 8 hours–4.5 days, with four dogs surviving to rejection. To date, 26 hours is the longest reported period of anoxic arrest which has been followed by indubitably viable heart function. High potassium solutions act as metabolic inhibitors by depolarizing cell membranes; intracellular-based solutions attempt to abolish all ionic gradients across the cell mem-brane, further reducing metabolic requirements and maintaining cellular integrity.

The addition of phenoxybenzamine, chlorpromazine, lignocaine or insulin to a flushing solution significantly increased the survival of rat hearts pre-served at 5°C[43]. Magnesium in high concentrations has a cardioplegic effect and at reduced temperatures it protects against membrane phase transitions (membrane stabilization), increasing cold tolerance[44].

4. Hypothermia and hyperbaric oxygenation

Manax and Lillehei, in 1964, first used hyperbaric oxygenation as a method for tissue preservation[45]. In this method the tissue can be protected under varying oxygen atmosphere (atm) pressures at 4°C in either a perfused or non-perfused state. Having too high an oxygen tension may, however, have an adverse effect on cellular integrity[46].

Bloch and his colleagues[47] were the first to report some success in preserving the heart with a combination of hypothermia and hyperbaria. Thirty hearts preserved at 3.3 atm pressure (99% O_2 : 1% CO_2) at 0–4°C for 24 h resumed a coordinated ventricular beat after revascularization. Prolonged storage for

72 h with subsequent defibrillation was possible by increasing the hyperbaria to 15 atm pressure at 2 °C[48]. The authors concluded that hypothermia and hyperbaria acted synergistically to improve preservation, rather than by addition of individual effects.

Reacting to this work, Shumway and his colleagues[49] transplanted numerous heart grafts orthotopically after storage under hyperbaric oxygenation and hypothermia for 24–48 hours. Although such hearts would defibrillate and maintain a coordinated beat, regular maintenance of the circulation could not be assured.

Lacombe and his colleagues[50] also orthotopically transplanted puppy hearts after various periods of 4 atm pressure at 4 °C. The longest period of storage compatible with survival of the recipient animal was 4 hours 10 minutes. A few attempts were made to preserve hearts at pressures up to 10 atm, but no improvement in the results was obtained. The same group has stressed that progressive decompression after periods of hyperbaric preservation causes less myocardial damage than abrupt, stepwise decompression, though histological examination revealed that even the progressively decompressed hearts were severely damaged[51].

From the results reported to date, it must remain doubtful whether the addition of hyperbaric oxygen produces more successful preservation of the heart than hypothermia alone.

5. *Supercooling*

The low molecular weight solutes of the majority of cells depress the freezing point to -0.6 °C. In practice, most cells do not freeze internally, however, unless they are cooled below -10 °C[52]. A cell which remains unfrozen below its theoretical freezing point (-0.6 °C) is by definition 'supercooled', and therefore not in thermodynamic equilibrium with ice. Supercooling is a theoretically attractive mechanism for prolonging organ preservation beyond that attainable at 0 °C, by further suppressing metabolism. Cells in this state, particularly in the absence of a cryoprotectant agent, are unstable, and at risk from damage resulting from spontaneous freezing[53]. As a result, there may be uncertainty as to what extent any tissue damage which occurs may be attributed to ice formation as distinct from the effect of supercooling alone[54, 55]. Published data indicate that no perfect method of preservation by supercooling has yet been achieved.

Personal work (performed by one of us in collaboration with Professor G. Collins of San Diego) provided clear evidence of a damaging effect on renal function resulting from 1 hour of supercooling at -4 °C[56]. Although the precise biochemical nature of this injury was not defined by these experiments, it can nevertheless be concluded that it was not due to freezing nor to rapid cooling (thermal shock). The latter is known to be dependent more on the rate of cooling than on the absolute temperature achieved. In these experiments cooling was approximately 20 times faster in the range 37°C–0°C, when no injury was evident, than between 0°C and −4°C. Ice formation could be excluded as the damaging agent since the thermal history of all kidneys was recorded, and no exotherm was observed, confirming that freezing had not taken place. Moreover, even when freezing was purposely initiated and allowed to proceed for 1 minute, no additional damage was evident.

6. *Freezing*

Cells can be preserved for years at a temperature of −196°C, as molecular motion is inhibited in proportion to the reduction in temperature, and virtually all biochemical and physiological processes arrest. To achieve this state, controlled tissue freezing is necessary; the technique is still under intensive investigation. The addition of cryoprotectant agents displaces tissue water and increases the solute concentration, resulting in a depression of freezing point. When freezing occurs, latent heat is released (the exotherm) at the rate of approximately 80 calories (336 J) per gram of water crystallized[57].

Freezing involves numerous changes that are deleterious to tissue survival[52]; some of these are as follows.

(1) *Rate of cooling and/or freezing.* Different types of tissues have different optimum rates of cooling. Exceeding this rate results in insufficient cellular dehydration, the tissue becoming increasingly supercooled, and eventually freezing intra- and extracellularly, sustaining structural damage.

(2) *Site of freezing.* Extracellular crystallization is permitted, but excessive growth of crystals within cells causes irreversible structural damage.

(3) *Solution-effect injury.* Cooling at suboptimal rates results in the so-called solution-effect injury. As the temperature decreases, more and more extracellular water crystallizes as pure ice, with simultaneous solute concentration and cellular dehydration. This dramatic degree of salt concentration and cellular dehydration appears to reduce the viability of the cell.

Freezing of various cell types has been made possible by the addition of cryoprotectant agents, such as glycerol or dimethyl sulphoxide, to the 'freezing medium'. Molecules of the cryoprotectant displace water molecules in the cell, reducing both solution-effect injury and intracellular cell shrinkage.

Not only are there problems with freezing the tissue, but new problems are faced when thawing is attempted. The cryoprotectant must be removed from the thawed cells slowly, so that they never swell osmotically to a damaging size. Each step in both freezing and thawing has a narrow range of acceptable values, and must be carried out appropriately if cellular viability is to be maintained. Presently, organs greater than the size of rat hearts have been poorly preserved by freezing, and extensive work is still necessary to finalize the freezing of organs such that they remain viable after the 'freeze–thaw' period. Techniques for the long-term storage of living cells in some simple tissues (spermatozoa, erythrocytes, lymphocytes, tissue culture cells and bone marrow) have already been developed. These have all used techniques of cryopreservation.

Various types of tissue require different cryoprotectants for optimum protection. Both dimethyl sulphoxide[58] and glycerol[59] are toxic to the myocardium, and may themselves cause as much damage as the actual freezing–thawing process.

The application of our present knowledge to the preservation of large organs has, to date, proved unsuccessful[60]. Rat and hamster hearts frozen at $-6°C$ to $-1°C$ for 5–30 minutes recovered after freezing[61]. Pieces of frog atria beat after cooling to $-70°C$[62]. Puppy hearts frozen at $-2°C$ did not recover[63].

Although a method of preservation based on these techniques may offer the prospect of successful long-term storage in the future, at the present time cryobiological techniques of preservation are not clinically applicable.

Perfusion methods

1. *Total body perfusion using a pump oxygenator*

The donor heart can be preserved for short periods of time in the brain-dead subject by pump oxygenator support. In the first clinical transplant operation performed at our institution the donor underwent total body perfusion after death in order to preserve both the heart and kidneys[64]. We used this simple technique on nearly every occasion until 1981, and have used it on occasions since then. The donor is cooled until the midoesophageal temperature has fallen to approximately 16–20°C, at which point the heart and kidneys are excised, and perfusion discontinued. In our early cases, during suture of the donor heart into the recipient, coronary perfusion was maintained by a line from the recipient heart–lung machine; more recently cardioplegic arrest has been induced, after which the intermittent application of cold (4°C) saline to the heart to maintain a low myocardial temperature has been considered sufficient protection.

Total body perfusion allows protection during preparation for heart (and kidney) excision, but entails a large team of staff, may not prove possible at small peripheral hospitals (and therefore necessitates transfer of the donor to a major centre), and does not result in more than moderate hypothermia, unless cardioplegic arrest and topical cooling is also introduced. If transportation of the donor heart is necessary, some other form of myocardial protection must be introduced.

Its major advantage is in achieving and maintaining a state of whole body hypothermia during which multiple organ excision can be carried out. This may be important in a donor who has become haemodynamically unstable and in whom cardiac arrest or severe hypotension seems imminent. We have used it successfully for the removal of heart, liver and kidneys from a single donor on one occasion recently.

If excision of the heart alone is being considered, it would seem that this technique has few advantages and several disadvantages over cardioplegic arrest and simple ice storage.

2. *Autoperfusion (biological oxygenation)*

The use of an autoperfusing heart-lung preparation as a means of short-term preservation of the heart during its insertion into the recipient must be credited to Demikhov[65], who initially published his work in 1948. The essential feature of the Demikhov preparation is that the systemic circulation is represented by the coronary vessels alone. With artificial maintenance of respiration and temperature, the heart could function normally for many hours.

In 1959, Robicsek and his colleagues[66] developed a modification in which the coronary perfusion pressure was kept stable and the blood volume was self-adjusting. A 'buffer' bag was incorporated to stabilize the pressure in the aorta and allow a second exit for blood not passing to the coronary artery circulation. Hearts were subsequently transplanted into recipient animals following 1–12 hours of storage at normothermia. Thirteen of 19 orthotopic grafts were successful, with the longest survival being 13 days[67, 68].

Biochemical and pathological studies of such an autoperfusing system suggest that integrity of the cell membrane is eventually lost in the myocardium, the lung parenchyma, the red cells, and the capillaries, and that at each level dexamethasone exerts a favourable influence. Progressive metabolic deterioration occurs, with significant changes being detectable 6–12 hours after perfusion has been started; these changes are not due to lack of available oxygen in the blood[69].

Personal observations on the Demikhov preparation have revealed a marked reduction in left ventricular contractility after the initial conversion of the normal canine circulation to that of the heart-lung preparation; a steady improvement occurs during the subsequent 2-hour period of autoperfusion, suggesting satisfactory myocardial perfusion[70]. There is considerable evidence that a heart preserved as a heart-lung preparation for a few hours is subsequently capable of supporting an entire circulatory load after orthotopic transplantation[15, 65, 67, 71, 72], but there seems little immediate hope that an autoperfusing system will be able to maintain cardiac viability of practical clinical value for more than 4–6 hours.

3. *Intermediate host perfusion (parabiosis)*

Parabiosis was probably first performed in 1862 by Paul Bert in Claude Bernard's laboratory in Paris[73]. Viability of the organ is maintained by cross-perfusion from a host animal. The technique has also been used experimentally to resuscitate anoxically arrested hearts[74–76].

The intermediate host animal could theoretically be of the same species (allogeneic) or of another species (xenogeneic). In man, a xenogeneic system would seem most practicable.

Dupree and his colleagues[77] have used a system of 'xenobanking' for the storage of primate hearts. Donor stump-tail monkey hearts were anastomosed to vessels in the abdomen of recipient baboons, whose immune response had been suppressed with a lethal dose of whole body radiation 24 hours prior to receiving the donor hearts. From previous studies, the dose of radiation given (800 rad) was known to allow survival of the host animal for 9–11 days, with nearly complete immunosuppression for 7 days. During this period, electrocardiograms from the donor monkey hearts in the immunosuppressed baboons showed negligible changes, and, apart from minimal oedema in the interstitial spaces, histological section remained essentially normal. Donor hearts were apparently in good condition, therefore, after storage periods longer than those reported using any other method, though the resulting function of the heart was not measured.

Although it is difficult to see a homologous intermediate host storage system being used in man, xenogeneic storage, using an immunosuppressed animal, might prove to be a potential answer to short-term storage of human organs. As with other aspects of this experimental field, such a procedure may not be aesthetically acceptable to many members of the lay and medical communities.

4. *Extracorporeal normothermic perfusion*

The first successful attempt to maintain living organs outside the body for more than a few hours must be attributed to the development by Lindbergh in 1935 of a self-contained, all-glass, pulsatile perfusion apparatus, in which experiments could be carried out under sterile conditions[78]. Carrel and Lindbergh, in 1938, described this apparatus in more detail and reported on the results of over 1000 experiments[79]. Histological examination of guinea-pig hearts revealed that the general morphological architecture was preserved after perfusion for more than 24 hours.

Even today, however, the technical problems remain formidable. A steady increase in the coronary vascular resistance is suggestive of increasing myocardial damage, and can occur as a result of inadequate filtration of the perfusate, the absence of siliconized surfaces on the perfusion apparatus, significant perfusion pressure changes during the period of perfusion, oxygen tensions which are too high or too low, and growth of micro-organisms in the perfusion solution[80].

Lindbergh's original perfusion apparatus has been modified, and has maintained monkey hearts in a pulsating state for periods of up to 72 h, though there was a diminution in the contractions which may have been due to an exhaustion of the supply of nutrient in the medium or an accumulation of toxic by-products[81]. Various types of perfusate have been and are continuing to be studied in relation to the storage of hearts and other organs[82]. Theoretically, blood perfusion would be the optimum method of preservation, but this is at present limited by blood destruction which occurs in all *in vitro* perfusion circuits, leading to altered blood components that damage the myocardium.

Left ventricular performance has been measured in isolated hearts perfused with blood oxygenated by isolated lungs and has been compared with function when the blood was oxygenated by a membrane oxygenator[83]. When the membrane oxygenator was substituted for the isolated lungs, there was invariably an abrupt increase in coronary flow and a decrease in ventricular performance; the increase in coronary flow could always be reversed by the reinclusion of the lungs, although the decline in ventricular performance was sometimes irreversible. The function of the lung as a filter of microemboli is almost certainly a major factor in its beneficial effect.

Following the original work of Hardy's group[84], retroperfusion of the coronary system via the coronary sinus during cardiac arrest has been explored by various investigators. An energy substrate such as glucose can be supplied by this route[85], and has been shown to exert a protective effect upon the heart during 30-minute periods of anoxic arrest at normothermia.

The perfusion systems and solutions available at present do not appear to be sufficiently sophisticated to preserve the myocardium successfully at normothermia; the addition of hypothermia has brought about a significant improvement.

5. *Extracorporeal hypothermic perfusion*

Progress here has been substantial, and, in our unit, has advanced to the point of clinical application[86]. One of the first major advances in this field came from Proctor and Parker[87], who managed to preserve the isolated canine heart for 72 hours with hypothermic perfusion (5 °C) using filtered modified Krebs' solution. Subsequent experiments resulted in the orthotopically transplanted heart supporting the circulation of the recipient dog for 8–14 h, with death occurring from exsanguination rather than from myocardial failure[88].

Using a technique based on that of Proctor, Copeland and his colleagues[89] successfully preserved hearts for 24 hours followed by orthotopic transplantation, with three dogs surviving for 4 days or more and dying of rejection. Guerraty *et al.*[90] have achieved successful dog heart preservation for 24 hours when using low pressure, non-pulsatile hypothermic perfusion and a simple perfusate. Fifteen animals were orthotopically transplanted, of which two died of cardiac failure after 1 and 5 days respectively. Tago and his colleagues[91] preserved 19 beating, blood-perfused hearts at 30 °C for 24 h using a rather complex perfusion system, and appeared to obtain adequate cardiac function in ten out of 16 animals following orthotopic transplantation. Successful 24 h preservation of the rat heart, using the commercially available Eurocollins solution, has been reported by Konertz et al.[92], but myocardial function was determined only by in vitro testing rather than by orthotopic transplantation. Orthotopic transplantation in larger animals is required before this solution can be considered for clinical use.

We have recently developed a hypothermic perfusion system which successfully preserves myocardial viability for 48 hours. The compositions of the two perfusion solutions discussed in this text are shown in Table 5.2. This system has developed through several stages and modifications[93]. Initially, a non-portable apparatus was used and several clear fluid perfusion solutions tested[94].

Table 5.2 Constitution of perfusates used in successful 24 and 48 hours' storage of the heart by continuous extracorporeal hypothermic perfusion at the University of Cape Town

	Solution A		Solution B	
	g/l	mmol/l	g/l	mmol/l
NaCl	6.76	115.70	7.98	143.80
NaHCO$_3$	2.10	25.00	—	—
MgSO$_4$. 7H$_2$O	3.48	14.40	3.48	14.40
CaCl$_2$. 2H$_2$O	0.16	1.10	0.16	1.10
KH$_2$PO$_4$	1.12	8.00	0.235	1.73
K$_2$HPO$_4$	—	—	1.105	6.34
Procaine hydrochloride	0.27	1.10	0.27	1.10
Chlorpromazine	0.005	—	0.005	—
Phenoxybenzamine	0.01	—	0.01	—
Glucose	2.00	11.10	2.00	11.10
Sucrose	2.50	7.00	2.50	7.00
Glycerol	12.60	136.00	12.60	136.00
Taurine	0.50	4.00	0.50	4.00
Osmolality	385 mmol		410 mmol	
pH	7.2–7.4		6.9–7.0	

A simpler portable apparatus (portable system I) was then developed (Figure 5.1), in which the perfusate is both oxygenated and circulated throughout the storage period by the airlift pump principle[95]. The heart is perfused at a low pressure as this results in less oedema than if perfused at a high pressure. At a gas flow of approximately 500 ml per minute, perfusate pH is maintained at 7.0–7.8, and perfusate flow at approximately 60–120 ml/min. The perfusion apparatus is placed in a stainless steel container, insulated with polystyrene and perspex, and packed with ice to maintain the desired temperature of 4–10 °C throughout the preservation period. More recently this apparatus has been further modified (portable system II) to include a larger reservoir and larger volume of solution, thus increasing the pumping efficiency of the system[96].

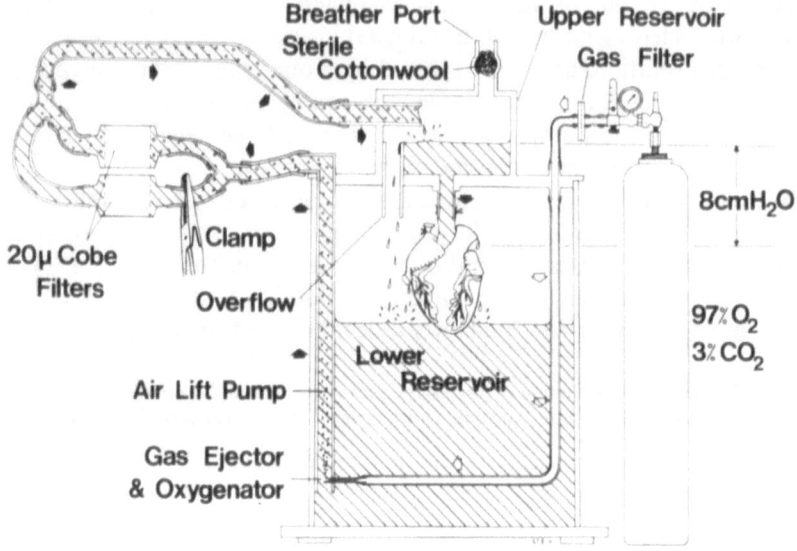

Figure 5.1   Portable hypothermic perfusion apparatus (system I)

Using these three systems good results have been obtained following 24- and 48-hour continuous hypothermic perfusion of the baboon heart (Table 5.3). Following orthotopic allotransplantation, consistent survival of the immunosuppressed recipient baboon until rejection has been obtained[93, 94, 97]. Following autotransplantation[97], baboons have remained alive and well, supported by the preserved heart, for periods of over 2 years before being electively studied and killed.

Using the second system described above, four patients received donor hearts which had undergone periods of ischaemia ranging from 6 hours 55 minutes to 16 hours 50 minutes[86]. In one case the heart was transported by air over a distance of 750 km (470 miles). Heterotopic transplantation was performed in all four patients. In three cases, donor heart function was demonstrated to be good by the progress of the patient, together with cardiac catheterization and angiography. In two of these patients, however, satisfactory donor heart function was delayed for periods of approximately 19 hours, during which time the recipient's own heart, supported by inotropic agents, maintained the circulation. Full recovery of the donor heart occurred, and by the end of the first postoperative day it had taken over full responsibility for the circulation. This delayed recovery has not been seen in any of the baboons in our studies. In the experimental laboratory, however, baboon hearts have been harvested under ideal conditions from healthy animals. A human donor heart has frequently undergone some damage during periods of hypotension, inotropic support and other drug therapy, and we believe that it is these insults, in combination with a prolonged period of hypothermic perfusion, which account for the delay in full recovery.

Table 5.3 Results of orthotopic transplantation and autotransplantation in baboons following heart storage by continuous extracorporeal hypothermic perfusion for periods of 24 and 48 hours at the University of Cape Town

	Solution A			Solution B	
					Portable system II (48 hours)
	Non-portable system (24 hours)	Portable system I (24 hours)	Portable system II (24 hours)	Orthotopic transplants	Autotransplants
Number	6	8*	2	3	4
Mean survival (days)	19.5	26.1	16.0	20.3	(i) 8 days (ruptured suture line)
Causes of death	Rejection	Rejection	Rejection	Rejection	(ii) 1 month (sacrificed)
					(iii) 3 months (sacrificed)
					(iv) 8 months (alive and well)

*In addition, one autotransplanted baboon remained alive and well for over 2 years, at which time it was sacrificed.

Hypothermic perfusion has the advantage over ice storage in that the former provides a continuous supply of oxygen and substrates and a continuous removal of waste products from the organ. Over short periods of time of up to 4 hours the need for perfusion is not critical, but over longer periods perfusion is to be preferred. Its success or failure depends to a very great extent on the chemical components of the perfusate, and, in our experience, it is this which has proved the most time-consuming aspect of the development of a successful perfusion system. Inadequate constituents result in inadequate preservation. Successful low pressure hypothermic perfusion is therefore largely dependent upon the perfusate components and on the perfusate pH, both of which influence the metabolic rate. The degree of oedema which the organ undergoes is influenced both by the pressure at which it is perfused and by the perfusate components.

Although hypothermia allows perfusion to be successful, its addition actually complicates perfusion preservation in homeotherms (mammals) by its inhibition of the sodium-potassium ATPäse[98], and by leading to a change in the saturated membrane lipids, thus altering the normal physiology of the mitochondrial membrane[99]. The mitochondrial membrane ADP–ATP translocator function is also impaired, limiting the supply of high energy phosphates for metabolic needs[100,101]. Though hypothermia reduces cellular energy

consumption, it still remains essential to stimulate sufficient energy production to continue essential cell functions and thus maintain viability. The
damaging effects of continuing cell metabolism, albeit reduced, have been
outlined earlier.

In our own laboratory the regulation of calcium distribution was considered the major factor if successful hypothermic perfusion preservation were
to be achieved. In the hypothermic myocardium, any absence of calcium can
lead to the so-called calcium paradox[101,102], whereas its unregulated presence
in myocardial cells results in enhanced resting myocardial tension (stone
heart), followed by poor or no function at reperfusion[103]. The choice of the
chemical components for our own perfusates was based on the assumption
that calcium distribution must be kept under stringent control.

Five basic factors were considered important.

(1) *Perfusate calcium concentration.* Maintenance of a low perfusate calcium concentration helps to prevent calcium overload in the myocardium. Our own experimental work has shown that perfusing hearts
with a perfusate containing a 2.2 mmol/l calcium concentration results
in poor myocardial protection, whereas perfusing with 1.1 mmol/l calcium appears to be optimal, resulting in excellent protection[104]. If it is
wished to maintain a relatively low calcium concentration in both the
extracellular and intracellular spaces, it seems only logical to have a low
calcium concentration in the perfusate. We believe it is essential, however, to have some calcium in the perfusate to avoid the possibility of
calcium paradox occurring[101]. In the perfused, isolated heart the situation is rather different from that of the cardioplegically arrested heart
during open heart surgery. In the latter case, collateral blood flow provides calcium to the myocardium throughout much of the procedure,
whereas in the isolated perfused heart, unless calcium is provided in the
perfusate, the myocardium will receive no calcium whatsoever. The
consequences are disastrous in that both electrical activity and contractility are impaired, with irreversible ultrastructural changes[101].

(2) *Oxygenation.* Oxygen deprivation reduces the mitochondrial concentration of ATP and citrate, both of which chelate calcium and thus
prevent uncontrolled calcium fluxes followed by calcium leakage into
the cytoplasm, which similarly lacks calcium chelators[21]. Reoxygen-
ation results in a massive energy-dependent calcium uptake into the
mitochondria, resulting in both mitochondrial and myofibrillar
damage[23]. We therefore believe it is essential to continually oxygenate
the perfusate.

(3) *pH.* A high environmental pH, though acceptable in poikilotherms (cold-
blooded animals) at reduced temperatures, appears to be unfavourable
in homeotherms. Reduced temperatures slow down the calcium transport system within the sarcoplasmic reticulum, but the balance between

ATP hydrolysis and calcium uptake remains. A high pH promotes uncoupling, increasing calcium loss from the sarcoplasmic reticulum, whereas a low pH inhibits this loss. A low pH results in coupled calcium transport, although at a reduced rate, with both ATP hydrolysis and calcium uptake remaining in equilibrium, preventing cytoplasmic calcium accumulation. A low pH therefore prevents too high an intracellular calcium[105,106].

(4) *Sodium–calcium exchange.* Sodium competes with calcium for both the high affinity calcium receptor site of the sodium–calcium exchange mechanism and the slow inward channel of the action potential plateau[31,107,108]. If the perfusate sodium concentration is increased, there will be more competition for the sites, resulting in increased efflux of calcium by the sodium–calcium exchange mechanism and decreased calcium inflow via the slow inward channels, thus increasing the calcium concentration in the extracellular space and reducing it intracellularly. A high sodium concentration in the perfusate helps to prevent the intracellular calcium concentration from becoming too high.

(5) *Oedema formation.* The accumulation of oedema in a stored heart has generally been considered a sign of deterioration and indicative of subsequent inadequate function. Our own work would suggest that oedema formation itself is not necessarily damaging, as long as the oedema is gradual in onset and reversible after reperfusion[94]. In fact, gradual oedema formation may play a beneficial role in diluting intracellular calcium. By stimulating a gradual but reversible degree of oedema formation, the cellular and extracellular calcium concentrations are presumably diluted, especially in the extracellular space where oedema formation predominates. Gradual oedema formation can be brought about by including small osmotically active molecules in the perfusate (Table 5.2). This oedema formation may also benefit by diluting other metabolic waste products, such as lactate.

The recent improvement in our preservation system, allowing storage for up to 48 hours, has been brought about mainly by using phosphate as the major buffer in the perfusate rather than bicarbonate. Phosphate buffering maintains a lower perfusion pH (6.95), increases the osmotic effect of the perfusate, and thus reduces the rate of oedema formation. The exact concentration of potassium phosphate in the perfusate appears crucial, as small changes clearly affect subsequent myocardial viability. The concentration in use at present (Table 5.2) appears to be optimal. The benefits brought about by this change of buffer are presumably not only due to the lower pH and reduced rate of oedema formation, but also to the increased availability of phosphate *per se* for use by the cell in the formation of high energy phosphates.

Although experimental 48 h preservation is sufficiently successful for the present demands of transplantation and would allow long distance

transportation, the routine clinical use of extracorporeal hypothermic perfusion still appears to be limited by the state of the myocardium at the onset of
the preservation period. The importance of the agonal period and of the effect
of brain death on the myocardium still require further investigation. Until
these aspects of myocardial preservation are resolved, the use of storage
systems will remain predominantly at the laboratory level. Forty-eight hours
of perfusion preservation are sufficient for our present clinical needs; our
research efforts will in future be directed towards the problem of preventing or
reversing myocardial injury in brain-dead donors.

THE ASSESSMENT OF MYOCARDIAL VIABILITY

Ideally, the transplanted heart must be capable of full function immediately
after its insertion into the recipient. A test of functional viability of the organ
would therefore be a great advantage if storage systems are to become a
clinical reality. A simple, reliable, *in vitro* test of organ viability would
similarly save a great deal in time and animals in the assessment of any new
preservation technique. The ultimate measure of viability of the preserved
heart is its capacity to fully support the circulation after orthotopic transplantation. Ethically this cannot be a test of function in the clinical situation and
the viability should be known at all times throughout the storage period and
also at the time of transplantation.

Any such test of organ viability should be simple, rapid and reproducible.
The search for such a test has explored two main routes.

The first of these is a simple, single measurement or observation that
confirms that the tissues under study are not irreversibly damaged. This may
take the form of, for example, a visual assay of a myocardial enzyme system,
a histochemical change, or the monitoring of a fundamental metabolic event
such as anaerobic glycolysis or lactic acid production.

The second is a functional evaluation of the isolated heart. At present, this
involves multiple haemodynamic and biochemical observations of myocardial
function while the heart is perfused. Such methods are frequently elaborate
and time-consuming, but it is possible that, with further experience, a single
measurement will be found which will indicate the functional state of the
myocardium.

The single, simple observation can be classified as a 'tissue viability test',
whereas the haemodynamic and biochemical studies carried out on the isolated, perfused heart can be considered methods of 'functional evaluation' of
the organ. Whatever the method used, it is crucial that the results obtained
correlate closely with the function of the whole organ after storage and
orthotopic transplantation.

Tissue viability tests

At the present time there is no satisfactory viability test with regard to the myocardium[5]. Tissue reaction to tetrazolium bromide has been investigated, but has not been found reliable[109, 110]. Measurement of the surface pH of the myocardium[111], and inorganic phosphate estimations[112], have also been investigated without success. The estimation of adenine nucleotide levels[113], and the haematoxylin-basic fuchsin-picric acid stain[110] have given more encouraging results. Tissue slice studies of both kidney[56] and heart[114] have proved valuable as a method of determining the viability of injured organs, but are not ideal in the clinical situation.

Functional evaluation of the heart

Most of the investigations relating to myocardial function included in this group have been intended as illustrations of the efficiency of a method of preservation and not as a rapid assessment of a potential donor organ. However, such a test may yet evolve from the techniques of functional evaluation currently being developed.

Several complex systems have been devised[5, 112, 115]. We have developed one such *in vitro* functional testing apparatus (Figure 5.2) which has proved invaluable in the assessment of the success or otherwise of storage procedures on the heart, but which is clearly not suitable as a routine viability test[116]. The state of left ventricular contractility, as indicated by max (dp/dt) and its derivative max (dp/dt)/P, has been emphasized as a major parameter in assessing the performance of the isolated heart in a number of studies[70, 115, 117, 118]. It is easy and quick to measure, reproducible, and gives an absolute figure as a result. Changes in myocardial contractility between the control state, the anoxic or ischaemic state, and the resuscitated state, during experiments involving resuscitation of the heart, can be readily compared. Similarly, improvement or deterioration during a period of preservation can be assessed without difficulty.

Other workers have emphasized alternative individual parameters. In the hypothermic perfusion system developed by Proctor, changes in coronary resistance were found to be a reliable indicator of the subsequent functional capability of the myocardium[87]. The pattern of change of resistance and the final resistance value were both important; in general, the lower the final resistance, the greater the viability of the heart. We have similarly found changes in coronary resistance to be suggestive of changes in viability, but our own work would suggest that this parameter is not always reliable.

A successful outcome to the search for a simple, yet reliable, viability test would not only allow the rapid evaluation of a cadaver donor organ, but would also greatly facilitate the search for reliable methods of resuscitation and preservation; the necessity of demonstrating the efficiency of such a technique by orthotopic transplantation of the organ would be removed. To date, however, no single test has satisfied all of the criteria necessary.

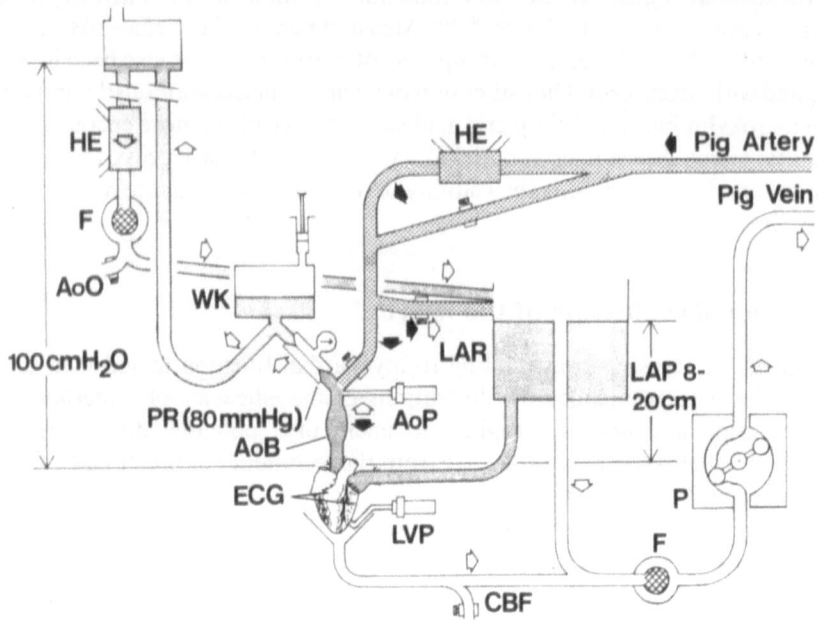

Figure 5.2 System for functional testing of the isolated heart. HE = heat exchanger; F = filter; AoO = aortic output (for monitoring cardiac output); WK = windkessel; PR = non-linear resistance device; AoB = aortic balloon; AoP = aortic pressure monitoring transducer (mmHg); ECG = electrocardiogram needle electrodes; LAR = left atrial reservoir; LAP = left atrial pressure (cmH$_2$O); P = roller pump; LVP = left ventricular pressure monitoring transducer (mmHg); CBF = coronary venous return

References

1. Grover, F. L., Fewel, J. G., Schank, K. P., Ghidoni, J. J., Arom, K. V. and Trinkle, J. K. (1980). Effects of various periods of cold potassium cardioplegic arrest upon myocardial contractility and metabolism. *J. Surg. Res.*, **28**, 328

2. Roe, B. B., Hutchinson, J. C., Fishman, N. H., Ullyot, D. J. and Smith, D. L. (1977). Myocardial protection with cold, ischaemic, potassium induced cardioplegia. *J. Thorac. Cardiovasc. Surg.*, **73**, 366

3. Thomas, F. T., Szentpetery, S. S., Mammana, R. E., Wolfgang, T. C. and Lower, R. R. (1978). Long distance transportation of human hearts for transplantation. *Ann. Thorac. Surg.*, **26**, 344

4. Gillette, P. C., Pinsky, W. W., Lewis, R. M., Bornet, E. P., Wood, J. M., Entman, M. L. and Schwartz, A. (1979). Myocardial depression after elective ischaemic arrest. *J. Thorac. Cardiovasc. Surg.*, **77**, 608

5. Cooper, D. K. C. (1976). The donor heart: the present position with regard to resuscitation, storage and assessment of viability. *J. Surg. Res.*, **21**, 363

6. Lehninger, A. L. (1975). Catabolism and generation of the phosphate bond energy. In *Biochemistry: The Molecular Basis of Cell Structure and Function*. 2nd Edn., p. 361. (New York: Worth)
7. Pegg, D. E. (1981). The biology of cell survival *in vitro*. In Karow, A. M. and Pegg, D. E. (eds.) *Organ Preservation for Transplantation*. 2nd Edn., p. 31. (New York and Basel: Dekker)
8. Leading article. (1973). (Reporting the proceedings of the first international symposium on organ preservation, Cambridge.) *Lancet*, **2**, 715
9. Kirsh, M. M., Behrendt, D. M. and Jochim, K. E. (1979). Effects of methylprednisolone in cardioplegic solution during coronary bypass grafting. *J. Thorac. Cardiovasc. Surg.*, **77**, 896
10. Fox, A. C., Hoffstein, S. and Weissmann, G. (1976). Lysosomal mechanisms in production of tissue damage during myocardial ischaemia and the effects of treatment with steroids. *Am. Heart J.*, **91**, 394
11. Cooper, D. K. C. (1976). Resuscitation of the cadaver donor heart in the dog. III. The influence of the agonal period on the success of resuscitation. *Guy's Hosp. Rep.*, **123**, 363
12. Bogardus, G. M. and Schlosser, R. J. (1956). The influence of temperature upon ischaemic renal damage. *Surgery*, **39**, 970
13. Gott, V. L., Bartlett, M., Johnson, J. A., Long, D. M. and Lillehei, C. W. (1960). High energy phosphate levels in the human heart during potassium citrate arrest and selective hypothermic arrest. *Surg. Forum*, **10**, 544
14. Greenberg, J. J., Edmunds, L. H. and Brown, R. B. (1960). Myocardial metabolism and post-arrest function in the cold and chemically arrested heart. *Surgery*, **48**, 31
15. Webb, W. R. and Howard, H. S. (1957). Cardiopulmonary transplantation. *Surg. Forum*, **8**, 313
16. Stinson, E. B., Dong, E., Angell, W. W. and Shumway, N. E. (1970). Myocardial hypothermia for cardiac transplantation. *Laval Med.*, **41**, 195
17. Lower, R. R., Stofer, R. C., Hurley, E. J., Dong, E. Jr., Cohn, R. B. and Shumway, N. E. (1962). Successful homotransplantation of the canine heart after anoxic preservation for seven hours. *Am. J. Surg.*, **104**, 302
18. Bigelow, W. G., Mustard, W. T. and Evans, J. G. (1954). Some physiological concepts of hypothermia and their application to cardiac surgery. *J. Thorac. Surg.*, **28**, 480
19. Gevers, W. (1977). Generation of protons by metabolic processes in heart cells. *J. Mol. Cell Cardiol.*, **9**, 867
20. Hand, S. C. and Somero, G. N. (1982). Urea and methylamine effects on rabbit muscle phosphofructokinase. *J. Biol. Chem.*, **257**, 734
21. Parr, D. R., Wimshurst, J. M. and Harris, E. J. (1975). Calcium-induced damage of rat heart mitochondria. *Cardiovasc. Res.*, **9**, 366
22. Ganote, C. E., Worstell, J. and Kaltenbach, J. P. (1976). Oxygen-induced enzyme release irreversible myocardial injury: effects of cyanide in perfused rat hearts. *Am. J. Pathol.*, **84**, 327
23. Jennings, R. B. and Ganote, C. E. (1976). Mitochondrial structure and function in acute myocardial ischaemic injury. *Circ. Res.*, **38** (Suppl. 1), 80
24. Melrose, R. G., Dreyer, B., Bentall, H. H. and Baker, J. B. E. (1955). Elective cardiac arrest. *Lancet*, **2**, 21
25. Heggtveit, H. A. (1969). Contributions of electron microscopy to the study of myocardial ischaemia. *Bull. WHO*, **41**, 865
26. Nakae, S., Webb, W. R., Salyer, K. E., Unal, M. O., Cook, W. A., Dodds, R. P. and Williams, C. T. (1967). Extended survival of the normothermic anoxic heart with metabolic inhibitors. *Ann. Thorac. Surg.*, **3**, 37
27. Guth, P. S., Sellinger, O. Z., Amaro, J. and Elaner, L. (1963). Additional permeability effects of chlorpromazine: leaking of lysosomal phosphatase. *Fed. Proc.*, **22**, 626
28. Dawkins, M. J. R., Judah, J. D. and Rees, K. R. (1959). The mechanism of action of chlorpromazine. Reduced disphosphopyridine nucleotide (cytochrome c reductase and coupled phosphorylation). *Biochem. J.*, **73**, 16

29. Judah, J. D. (1960). Effect of antihistamines on mitochondrial swelling and liver injury. *Nature (Lond.).* **185**, 390

30. Lokkegaard, H., Bilde, P. and Dahlager, J. I. (1979). Experimental and clinical studies of extended renal preservation by simple hypothermia. In Pegg, D. E. and Jacobson, I. A. (eds.) *Organ Preservation II.* p. 102. (Edinburgh, London and New York: Churchill Livingstone)

31. Noble, M. I. M. (1979). The calcium cardiac cycle. In Noble, M. I. M. (ed.) *The Cardiac Cycle.* p.28. (Oxford: Blackwell Scientific)

32. Rangel, D. M., Bruckner, W. L., Byfield, J. E., Dinbar, A., Yakeishi, Y., Stevens, G. H. and Fonkalsrud, E. W. (1969). Enzymatic evaluation of hepatic preservation using cell-stabilizing drugs. *Surg. Gynecol. Obstet.,* **129**, 963

33. Fonkalsrud, E. W., Bruchner, W. L., Byfield, J. E., Adomain, G. E., Dinbar, A. and Rangel, D. M. (1970). Enzymatic and ultra-structural evaluation of hepatic preservation in primates. *Arch. Surg.,* **100**, 284

34. Smith, A. D. (1973). Mechanisms involved in the release of noradrenaline from sympathetic nerves. *Br. Med. Bull.,* **29**, 123

35. Buckberg, G. D. (1979). A proposed 'solution' to the cardioplegic controversy. *J. Thorac. Cardiovasc. Surg.,* **77**, 803

36. Freier, D. T. (1979). The role of preservation in renal transplantation. A comparison of methods. *Dial. Transplant.,* **8**, 794

37. Hearse, D. J., Stewart, D. A. and Braimbridge, M. V. (1976). Cellular protection during myocardial ischemia. *Circulation,* **54**, 193

38. Kamiyama, T. M., Webb, W. R. and Baker, R. R. (1970). Preservation of the anoxic heart with a metabolic inhibitor and hypothermia. *Arch. Surg.,* **100**, 596

39. Hearse, D. J., Stewart, D. A. and Chain, E. B. (1974). Recovery from cardiac bypass and elective cardiac arrest. The metabolic consequences of various cardioplegic procedures in the isolated rat heart. *Circ. Res.,* **35**, 448

40. Kunz, W. and Siess, M. (1961). Energiegewinnung am Herzmuskel durch ein Wasserstoffübertragendes Pyrimidinderivat. *Arch. Exp. Pathol. Pharmakol.,* **241**, 529

41. Calman, K. C., Quin, R. O. and Bell, P. R. F. (1973). Metabolic aspects of organ storage and the prediction of organ viability. In Pegg, D. E. (ed.) *Organ Preservation.* p. 225. (Edinburgh and London: Churchill Livingstone)

42. Reitz, B. A., Brody, W. R., Hickey, P. R. and Michaelis, L. L. (1974). Protection of the heart for 24 hours with intracellular (high K^+) solution and hypothermia. *Surg. Forum,* **25**, 149

43. Calman, K. C. and Bell, P. R. (1972). Experimental organ preservation. *Br. J. Surg.,* **59**, 758

44. Jensen, M., Heber, U. and Oettmeier, W. (1981). Chloroplast membrane damage during freezing: the lipid phase. *Cryobiology,* **18**, 322

45. Manax, W. and Lillehei, R. C. (1964). Successful 24-hour *in vitro* preservation of canine kidneys by the combined use of hyperbaric oxygenation and hypothermia. *Surgery,* **56**, 275

46. Wolfe, W. G. and De Vries, W. (1975). Oxygen toxicity. *Ann. Rev. Med.,* **26**, 203

47. Bloch, J. R., Manax, W. G., Eyal, Z. and Lillehei, R. C. (1964). Heart preservation *in vitro* with hyperbaric oxygenation and hypothermia. *J. Thorac. Cardiovasc. Surg.,* **48**, 969

48. Manax, W. G., Eyal, Z. and Lillehei, R. C. (1967). Observations on the homotransplanted canine heart following *in vitro* storage by hypothermia and hyperbaric oxygen. *Vasc. Surg.,* **1**, 30

49. Shumway, N. E., Lower, R. R. and Stofer, R. C. (1966). Transplantation of the heart. In Welch, C. E. (ed.) *Advances in Surgery.* p. 265. (Chicago: Year Book Medical)

50. Lacombe, M., Cachera, J. P., Bui-Mong-Hung, V. M., Laurent, D. and Dubost, C. H. (1967). Orthotopic homotransplantation of preserved hearts in dogs. *J. Cardiovasc. Surg.,* **8**, 298

51. Bui-Mong-Hung, V. M., Leandri, J. and Laurent, D. (1968). Influence of decompression procedure on heart viability after long-term storage using hyperbaric oxygen and hypothermia. *Nature (Lond.),* **219**, 1175

52. Mazur, P. (1981). Fundamental cryobiology and the preservation of organs by freezing. In Karow, A. M. Jr. and Pegg, D. E. (eds.) *Organ Preservation for Transplantation*. 2nd Edn., p. 143. (New York and Basel: Dekker)

53. Farrant, J. (1965). Mechanism of cell damage during freezing and thawing and its prevention. *Nature (Lond.)*, **205**, 1284

54. Rasmussen, D. H. and McCaulay, M. N. (1975). Supercooling and nucleation of ice in single cells. *Cryobiology*, **12**, 328

55. Zavos, P. M. and Graham, E. F. (1981). Preservation of turkey spermatozoa by the use of emulsions and supercooling methods. *Cryobiology*, **18**, 497

56. Wicomb, W. N., Halasz, N. A. and Collins, E. M. (1984). Damaging effect of subzero temperature ($-4°C$) on rabbit renal function. *Cryobiology*, **21**, 6

57. Karow, A. M. (1981). Biophysical and chemical considerations in cryopreservation. In Karow, A. M. Jr. and Pegg, D. E. (eds.) *Organ Preservation for Transplantation*. 2nd Edn., p. 113. (New York and Basel: Dekker)

58. Feuvray, D. and De Leiris, J. (1973). Effects of short-term DMSO perfusions on ultrastructure of the isolated rat heart. *J. Cell. Mol. Cardiol.*, **5**, 63

59. Karow, A. M. and Webb, W. R. (1965). Toxicity of various solute moderators used in hypothermia. *Cryobiology*, **1**, 270

60. Pegg, D. E. (1973). Theory and experiments towards subzero organ preservation. In Pegg, D. E. (ed.) *Organ Preservation*. p. 108. (Edinburgh and London: Churchill Livingstone)

61. Smith, A. U. (1957). Problems in the resuscitation of mammals from body temperatures below 0°C. *Proc. R. Soc. Ser. B*, **147**, 533

62. Luyet, B. (1971). A review of research on the preservation of hearts in the frozen state. *Cryobiology*, **8**, 190

63. Barsamian, E. H., Jacobs, S. W., Collins, S. J. and Owen, O. E. (1959). The transplantation of dehydrated and supercooled hearts. *Surg. Forum*, **10**, 100

64. Barnard, M. S., Van Heerden, J., Hope, A., O'Donovan, T. G. and Barnard, C. N. (1969). Total body perfusion for cardiac transplantation. *S. Afr. Med. J.*, **43**, 64

65. Demikhov, V. P. (1962). *Experimental Transplantation of Vital Organs*. Authorized translation from the Russian by Haigh, B. (New York: Consultants Bureau)

66. Robicsek, F., Stam, R. E., Rees, T. T., Taylor, F. H. and Sanger, P. W. (1959). Transplantation of the heart. 2. Haemodynamic observations on the isolated heart. *Heineman Laboratories Collected Works on Cardiopulmonary Disease*, **1–2**, 96

67. Robicsek, F., Lesage, A., Sanger, P. W., Daugherty, H. K., Galluci, V. and Bagby, E. (1967). Transplantation of 'live' hearts. *Am. J. Cardiol.*, **20**, 803

68. Robicsek, F., Lesage, A., Sanger, P. W., Daugherty, H. K., Moore, M. and Bagby, E. (1968). The maintenance of function of the donor heart in the extracorporeal stage and during transplantation. *Ann. Thorac. Surg.*, **6**, 331

69. Yamada, T., Bosher, L. R. Jr. and Richardson, G. M. (1965). Observations on the autoperfusing heart-lung preparation. *Trans. Am. Soc. Artif. Intern. Org.*, **11**, 192

70. Cooper, D. K. C. (1975). Haemodynamic studies during short-term preservation of the autoperfusing heart-lung preparation. *Cardiovasc. Res.*, **9**, 753

71. Longmore, D. B., Cooper, D. K. C., Hall, R. W., Sekabunga, J. and Welch, W. (1969). Transplantation of the heart and both lungs. II. Experimental cardiopulmonary transplantation. *Thorax*, **24**, 391

72. Whiffen, J. D., Boake, W. C. and Gott, V. L. (1967). Normothermic orthotopic canine heart homotransplantation. *J. Surg. Res.*, **7**, 421

73. Finerty, J. C. (1952). Parabiosis in physiological studies. *Physiol. Rev.*, **32**, 277

74. Angell, W. W. and Shumway, N. E. (1966). Resuscitative storage of the cadaver heart transplant. *Surg. Forum*, **17**, 224

75. Angell, W. W., Dong, E. Jr. and Shumway, N. E. (1968). Four-day storage of the canine cadaver heart. *Rev. Surg.*, **26**, 369

76. Angell, W. W., Rikkers, L., Dong, E. Jr. and Shumway, N. E. (1968). Canine cadaver heart procurement, resuscitation and storage. In Norman, J. C. (ed.) *Organ Perfusion and Preservation*. p. 363. (New York: Appleton-Century-Croft)

77. Dupree, E. L., Mills, M., Clark, R. and Sel, K. W. (1969). Xenogeneic storage of primate hearts. *Transplant. Proc.*, 1, 840

78. Lindbergh, C. A. (1935). An apparatus for the culture of whole organs. *J. Exp. Med.*, 62, 409

79. Carrel, A. and Lindbergh, C. A. (1938). *The Culture of Organs*. (New York: Hoeber)

80. Hobbs, K. E. F. and Ellis, M. (1973). The present status of subzero organ preservation with special reference to the rat heart. In Pegg, D. E. (ed.) *Organ Preservation*. p. 123. (Edinburgh and London: Churchill Livingstone)

81. Perry, V. P., Lindbergh, C. A., Mallinin, T. I. and Mouer, G. H. (1968). Pulsatile perfusion of whole mammalian organs. In Norman, J. C. (ed.) *Organ Perfusion and Preservation*. p. 203. (New York: Appleton-Century-Crofts)

82. Belzer, F. O., Ashby, B. S., May, R. E. and Dunphy, J. E. (1968). Isolated perfusion of whole organs. In Norman, J. C. (ed.) *Organ Perfusion and Preservation*. p. 1. (New York: Appleton-Century-Crofts)

83. Monroe, R. G., Lafarge, C. G., Gamble, W. J., Honda, S. and Kevy, S. V. (1968). Ventricular performance and coronary flow of isolated hearts when perfused through isolated lungs and membrane oxygenators. In Norman, J. C. (ed.) *Organ Perfusion and Preservation*. p. 779. (New York: Appleton-Century-Crofts)

84. Hardy, J. D., Kurrus, F. D., Chavez, C. M. and Webb, W. R. (1964). Heart transplantation in infant calves. Evaluation of coronary perfusion to preserve organ during transfer. *Ann. NY Acad. Sci.*, 120, 786

85. Lolley, D. M., Hewitt, R. L. and Draparas, T. (1974). Retroperfusion of the heart with a solution of glucose, insulin and potassium during anoxic arrest. *J. Thorac. Cardiovasc. Surg.*, 67, 364

86. Wicomb, W. N., Cooper, D. K. C., Novitzky, D. and Barnard, C. N. (1984). Cardiac transplantation following storage of the donor heart by a portable hypothermic perfusion system. *Ann. Thorac. Surg.*, 37, 243

87. Proctor, E. and Parker, R. (1968). Preservation of isolated heart for 72 hours. *Br. Med. J.*, 4, 296

88. Proctor, E. and Jones, G. R. N. (1973). *In vitro* assessment of preserved dog hearts with some reference to preserved dog kidneys. In Pegg, D. E. (ed.) *Organ Preservation*. p. 216. (Edinburgh and London: Churchill Livingstone)

89. Copeland, J. G., Jones, M., Spragg, R. and Stinson, E. B. (1973). *In vitro* preservation of canine heart for 24 to 48 hours followed by successful orthotopic transplantation. *Ann. Surg.*, 178, 687

90. Guerraty, A., Alivizatos, P., Warner, M., Hess, M., Allen, L. and Lower, R. R. (1981). Successful orthotopic canine heart transplantation after 24 hours *in vitro* preservation. *J. Thorac. Cardiovasc. Surg.*, 82, 531

91. Tago, M., Subramanian, R. and Kaye, M. P. (1983). Light and electron microscope evaluation of canine hearts orthotopically transplanted after 24 hours of extra-corporeal preservation. *J. Thorac. Cardiovasc. Surg.*, 86, 912

92. Konertz, W., Zaworka, P., Johannson, W. and Bernhard, A. (1983). Use of Eurocollins solution for 24 hours heart preservation. (Presented at the International Society for Heart Transplantation, Third Annual Scientific Session, New Orleans), *Heart Transplant.* (Suppl.) 24

93. Cooper, D. K. C., Wicomb, W. N., Boyd, S. T., Lanza, R. P., Novitzky, D., Hassoulas, J. and Barnard, C. N. (1983). Orthotopic and heterotopic heart transplantation: aspects of the Cape Town experience. *Transplant. Proc.*, 15, 1232

94. Wicomb, W. N., Cooper, D. K. C., Hassoulas, J., Rose, A. G. and Barnard, C. N. (1982). Orthotopic transplantation of the baboon heart after 20 to 24 hours preservation by continuous hypothermic perfusion with an oxygenated hyperosmolor solution. *J. Thorac. Cardiovasc. Surg.*, **83**, 133

95. Wicomb, W. N., Cooper, D. K. C. and Barnard, C. N. (1982). Twenty-four-hour preservation of the pig heart by a portable hypothermic perfusion system. *Transplantation*, **34**, 246

96. Wicomb, W. N., Novitzky, D. and Cooper, D. K. C. (1984). Forty-eight-hour preservation of the baboon heart by a portable hypothermic perfusion system. (Submitted for publication)

97. Cooper, D. K. C., Wicomb, W. N. and Barnard, C. N. (1983). Orthotopic allotransplantation and autotransplantation of the baboon heart by a portable hypothermic perfusion system. *Cryobiology*, **20**, 385

98. Martin, D. C., Scott, D. F., Downes, G. and Belzer, F. O. (1972). Primary cause of unsuccessful liver and heart preservation: cold sensitivity of the ATPase system. *Ann. Surg.*, **175**, 111

99. Lyons, J. M. and Raison, J. K. ('1970). A temperature-induced transition in mitochondrial oxidation: contrasts between cold- and warm-blooded animals. *Comp. Biochem. Physiol.*, **37**, 405

100. Kemp, A., Groot, G. S. P. and Reitsma, H. J. (1969). Oxidative phosphorylation as a function of temperature. *Biochim. Biophys. Acta*, **180**, 28

101. Zimmerman, A. N. E., Daems, W., Huismann, W. C., Snijder, J., Wisse, E. and Durrer, D. (1967). Morphological changes of heart muscle caused by successive perfusing with Ca^{++}-free and Ca^{++}-containing solutions (Calcium paradox). *Cardiovasc. Res.*, **1**, 201

102. Jynge, P., Hearse, D. J. and Braimbridge, M. V. (1977). Myocardial protection during ischaemic cardiac arrest. *J. Thorac. Cardiovasc. Surg.*, **73**, 848

103. Katz, A. M. and Tada, M. (1972). The 'stone heart': a challenge to the biochemist. *Am. J. Cardiol.*, **29**, 578

104. Wicomb, W. N. (1983). The development of a system of 24-hour preservation of the heart for transplantation. *PhD Thesis*, University of Cape Town. Chapter 8, p. 123

105. Tate, C. A., Chu, A., McMillin-Wood, J. and Barry Van Winkle, W. (1981). Evidence for a Ca^{++}-sensitive factor which alters the alkaline pH sensitivity of SR Ca^{++} transport. *J. Biol. Chem.*, **256**, 2934

106. Duggan, P. F. (1977). Ca^{++} uptake and associated adenosine triphosphatase activity in fragmented sarcoplasmic reticulum. *J. Biol. Chem.*, **252**, 1620

107. Baker, P. F., Blaustein, M. P., Hodgkin, A. L. and Steinhardt, R. A. (1969). The influence of calcium on sodium efflux in squid axons. *J. Physiol.*, **200**, 431

108. Reuter, H. (1974). Exchange of calcium ions in the mammalian myocardium: mechanisms and physiological significance. *Circ. Res.*, **34**, 599

109. Maginn, R. R. and Hadjimichalis, E. (1968). Pretransplant cardiac viability assays. In Norman, J. C. (ed.) *Organ Perfusion and Preservation*. p. 505. (New York: Appleton-Century-Crofts)

110. Cooper, D. K. C. (1974). Studies on resuscitation and short-term preservation of the canine heart. *PhD Thesis*, University of London

111. Couch, N. P. and Middleton, M. K. (1968). Effect of storage temperature on the electrometric surface hydrogen ion activity of ischemic liver and heart. *Surgery*, **64**, 1099

112. Pitzele, S., Sze, S. and Dobell, A. R. C. (1971). Functional evaluation of the heart after storage under hypothermic coronary perfusion. *Surgery*, **70**, 569

113. Calman, K. C. (1974). The prediction of organ viability. *Cryobiology*, **11**, 7

114. Ganote, C. E., Jennings, R. B., Hill, M. L. and Grochowski, E. (1976). Experimental myocardial ischemic injury. II. Effect of *in vitro* ischemia on dog heart slice function *in vitro*. *J. Mol. Cell Cardiol.*, **8**, 189

115. Levitsky, S., Williams, W. H., Detmer, D. E., McIntosh, C. L. and Morrow, A. G. (1970). A functional evaluation of the preserved heart. *J. Thorac. Cardiovasc. Surg.*, **60**, 625

116. Wicomb, W. N., Boyd, S. T., Cooper, D. K. C., Rose, A. G. and Barnard, C. N. (1981). *Ex vivo* functional evaluation of pig hearts subjected to 24 hours preservation by hypothermic perfusion. *S. Afr. Med. J.*, **60**, 245

117. Cooper, D. K. C. (1975). A simple method of resuscitation and short-term preservation of the canine cadaver heart. *J. Thorac. Cardiovasc. Surg.*, **70**, 896

118. Holdefer, W. F. and Edwards, W. S. (1968). Ventricular performance characteristics in a metabolically supported isolated heart preparation: a model for evaluating cardiac storage methods. *Surg. Forum*, **19**, 225

6
Immunological Aspects

INTRODUCTION

Since numerous detailed accounts of transplantation immunology appear elsewhere in the literature[1-3], this chapter will concentrate only on those immunological aspects of cardiac transplantation that are of practical clinical importance today. Five important topics will be discussed: (1) the necessity for donor–recipient ABO blood group compatibility, (2) the role of human leukocyte antigen (HLA) matching, (3) the lymphocytotoxic cross-match test and the problem of preformed antibodies, (4) the value of pretransplant blood transfusions in recipients of cardiac allografts, and (5) the mechanism of allograft destruction.

1. RED BLOOD CELL GROUPS

ABO groups

ABO blood group compatibility between donor and recipient is an essential prerequisite in patients undergoing cardiac transplantation; incompatibility nearly always leads to rapid destruction of the allograft[4,5], although there have been very occasional reports of successful A to O, or B to A kidney grafts[6]. Rejection is thought to be due to antibodies directed against incompatible A or B red cell antigens present on the vascular endothelium of the allograft[7], and may be immediate[6].

A number of transplant centres have shown that group O recipients survive longer after renal transplantation than non-O recipients[8,9]. In our series of cardiac transplant patients, group O recipients survived on average over 6 months longer than non-O recipients (a mean of 25.2 vs. 18.9 months)[10]. Furthermore, both group O and A recipients survived longer on average than patients with blood groups B or AB (group O, 25.2 months; group A, 22.3 months; groups B and AB, 6.7 months). None of these differences, however, reached statistical significance. Patients with blood groups O and A (i.e. non-B antigen patients) who survived 2 months or more, however, survived statistically longer than those with the B antigen (blood groups B and AB) (33.6 vs. 6.7 months, $p < 0.005$ by the Student t-test) (Figure 6.1)[10]. The reason for this five-fold difference in survival between the two groups is unknown, but does not appear to be related to ethnic differences. Presumably, those with blood group B antigen might elicit a greater immune response. To date, however, no other cardiac transplantation centre has confirmed this observation.

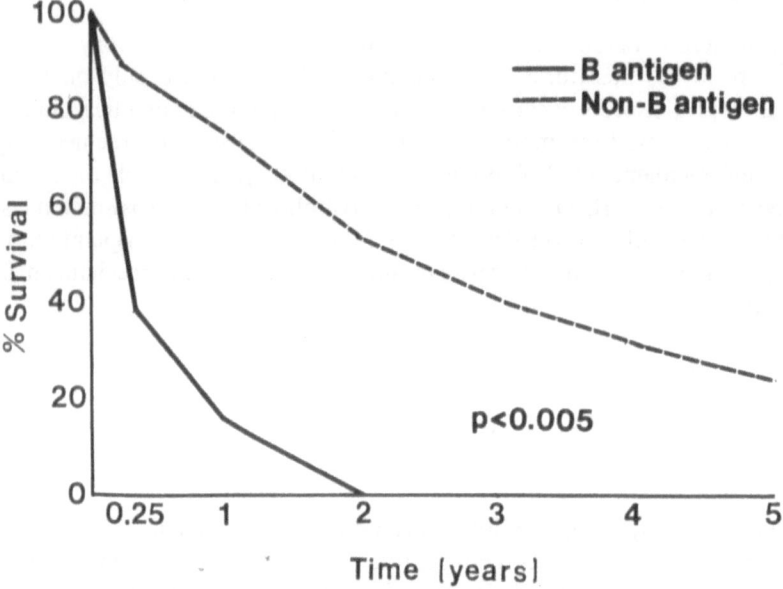

Figure 6.1   Relationship of cardiac allograft survival with the presence of B blood group antigen in recipients surviving 2 months or longer at Groote Schuur Hospital

Rhesus group

Rhesus (Rh) antigens are weak immunogens with regard to organ transplantation and are not considered important[11]. A few studies have found improved renal allograft survival in Rh-positive recipients when compared with Rh-negative recipients[12]. No significant differences in survival between Rh-positive and negative heart transplant recipients have been observed at our own institution.

2. THE HUMAN LEUKOCYTE ANTIGEN (HLA) SYSTEM

The immune response to an allograft is determined primarily by the major histocompatibility complex, known in man as the HLA system. The genes coding for the HLA antigens are located on the short arm of chromosome 6. Knowledge of this system is still evolving, but to date four closely linked HLA loci have been described, designated HLA-A, HLA-B, HLA-C and HLA-D/DR[13].

HLA-A, B and C antigens

HLA-A, B and C antigens have been shown to be expressed on the surface of nucleated cells in the body. To determine a person's HLA-A, B and C pheno-type, the individual's T-lymphocytes are set up in a complement-dependent lymphocytotoxic test against a large number of known antisera. The lympho-cytes are lysed if a cell surface HLA antigen is recognized by specific anti-bodies. For example, if the antiserum known to contain antibodies against HLA-A1 lyse the lymphocytes, then those lymphocytes are coded as HLA-A1.

At the HLA-A locus there are 20 known alleles (different genes that may occupy the same position or locus on a specific chromosome), at the HLA-B 40 alleles, and at the HLA-C eight; each allele produces a corresponding antigen (Table 6.1)[14]. Each individual has two chromosomes 6, one inherited from each parent, and therefore has two of the 20 HLA-A antigens (for example, A1 and A2), two of the 40 HLA-B antigens, and two of the eight HLA-C antigens. If the recipient and donor are not HLA-antigen identical, the immune response of the recipient following organ transplantation is directed primarily against those incompatible antigens on the surface of the donor organ that are not shared by the two individuals.

The role of HLA-A, B and C matching between recipient and donor on allograft survival remains controversial, but recent analyses from large regional and national centres in Europe and North America have found a consistent correlation between HLA-A and B matching and improved renal graft survival[2,3,15]. The survival rate of recipients of well-matched renal allo-grafts is approximately 10–20% higher than that of recipients of poorly matched allografts. The only major analysis of the effect of HLA-C matching on renal allograft survival did not show any significant difference in trans-plant outcome between well-matched and poorly matched donor–recipient groups[16].

There is at present little information on the relationship between HLA-A, B and C matching and survival after transplantation of organs such as the heart, liver and pancreas. Of the 64 donor–recipient pairs in our own series of heart transplant patients to date, only 30 have shared one or two antigens, and one has shared four. The remainder have been complete mismatches. We have not found any significant correlation between HLA-A, B or C compatibility and overall survival, though there was improved survival of the better matched pairs at 1 year (Figure 6.2).

Although the Stanford cardiac transplant group has also found no signifi-cant correlation between HLA matching and survival, they have observed that patients with HLA-A2 or A3 incompatibilities have a significantly higher incidence of graft arteriosclerosis (chronic rejection) than patients with other A locus incompatibilities[17]. In a review of our own patients, however, we did not find this association[18].

Table 6.1 Complete listing of recognized HLA specificities (1980)*

HLA-A	HLA-B	HLA-C	HLA-D	HLA-DR
HLA-A1	HLA-B5	HLA-Cw1	HLA-Dw1	HLA-DR1
HLA-A2	HLA-B7	HLA-Cw2	HLA-Dw2	HLA-DR2
HLA-A3	HLA-B8	HLA-Cw3	HLA-Dw3	HLA-DR3
HLA-A9	HLA-B12	HLA-Cw4	HLA-Dw4	HLA-DR4
HLA-A10	HLA-B13	HLA-Cw5	HLA-Dw5	HLA-DR5
HLA-A11	HLA-B14	HLA-Cw6	HLA-Dw6	HLA-DRw6
HLA-Aw19	HLA-B15	HLA-Cw7	HLA-Dw7	HLA-DR7
HLA-Aw23(9)	HLA-Bw16	HLA-Cw8	HLA-Dw8	HLA-DRw8
HLA-Aw24(9)	HLA-B17		HLA-Dw9	HLA-DRw9
HLA-A25(10)	HLA-B18		HLA-Dw10	HLA-DRw10
HLA-A26(10)	HLA-Bw21		HLA-Dw11	
HLA-A28	HLA-Bw22		HLA-Dw12	
HLA-A29	HLA-B27			
HLA-Aw30	HLA-Bw35			
HLA-Aw31	HLA-B37			
HLA-Aw32	HLA-Bw38(w16)			
HLA-Aw33	HLA-Bw39(w16)			
HLA-Aw34	HLA-B40			
HLA-Aw36	HLA-Bw41			
HLA-Aw43	HLA-Bw42			
	HLA-Bw44(12)			
	HLA-Bw45(12)			
	HLA-Bw46			
	HLA-Bw47			
	HLA-Bw48			
	HLA-Bw49(w21)			
	HLA-Bw50(w21)			
	HLA-Bw51(5)			
	HLA-Bw52(5)			
	HLA-Bw53			
	HLA-Bw54(w22)			
	HLA-Bw55(w22)			
	HLA-Bw56(w22)			
	HLA-Bw57(17)			
	HLA-Bw58(17)			
	HLA-Bw59			
	HLA-Bw60(40)			
	HLA-Bw61(40)			
	HLA-Bw62(15)			
	HLA-Bw63(15)			

*From Terasaki, P. I. (ed.) (1980) *Histocompatibility Testing 1980*. p. 20 (Los Angeles: UCLA Tissue Typing Laboratory)

Although no centre has yet shown convincing evidence of any improved cardiac allograft survival in patients with good HLA antigen matching, our policy with regards to recipient–donor HLA matching has been to offer the heart to the patient with the greatest number of matched antigens with the donor. If the critical physical state of one patient necessitates urgent transplantation, then this patient is given priority regardless of the results of recipient–donor HLA matching.

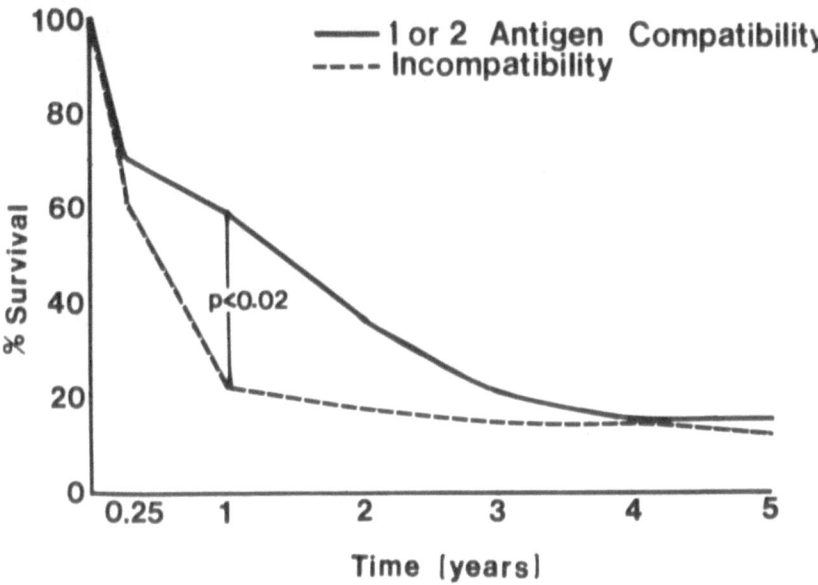

Figure 6.2   Relationship of cardiac allograft survival and donor–recipient HLA-A and B antigen matching at Groote Schuur Hospital

HLA-D and DR 'antigens'

Although the HLA-D determinants or 'antigens' have not yet been formally shown to be antigens (in the sense of being able to give rise to circulating antibodies), the term HLA-D 'antigen' for simplicity is used instead of the more strictly correct HLA-D 'determinant'[19].

A number of B-lymphocyte antigens have been detected which correspond closely to the HLA-D antigen. These B-lymphocyte antigens have therefore been named HLA-DR (HLA-D related) antigens. These HLA-DR antigens are determined by a serological test, as are HLA-A, B and C antigens, though B-lymphocytes rather than T-lymphocytes are used as the target cells.

HLA-D antigens are defined by using special cell culture techniques—the mixed lymphocyte culture (MLC). The MLC can be considered as the *in vitro* homologue of the *in vivo* immune response to an allograft[20]. Up to 6 days, however, are required to complete the MLC test, which is therefore of no practical importance with regard to cardiac transplantation. Though the HLA-D antigens of the recipient can be identified, the test takes too long to type the donor before cardiac transplantation. The status of recipient–donor

D antigen matching can therefore only be known retrospectively and cannot be considered for donor–recipient pair selection in cardiac transplantation. There is some evidence, however, that matching for HLA-D antigens greatly improves the outcome of kidney allografts from living related donors[21,22].

It has been suggested that HLA-DR incompatibility between donor and recipient may well be the major stimulus for the generation of the immune response against a transplanted kidney[23]. Although there are insufficient data to draw any definite conclusions, a number of studies report evidence favouring an important role for HLA-DR antigens in renal transplantation[24-30]. One study demonstrated that matching for HLA-DR antigens extended survival by 18 months in unrelated donor–recipient combinations[29]. Allografts from donors sharing two HLA-DR antigens with the recipient appear to fare significantly better than those with only one or no shared antigens[30]. At the present time there are insufficient data on the relationship between HLA-DR matching and cardiac allograft survival to arrive at any meaningful conclusions.

3. THE LYMPHOCYTOTOXIC CROSS-MATCH TEST AND THE PROBLEM OF PREFORMED ANTIBODIES

As soon as a potential recipient is selected for transplantation, his serum should be set up against a panel of 20 or more T-lymphocytes representing the major antigenic stimuli. The serum should also be tested against a similar panel of B-lymphocytes. HLA-A, B and C antibodies are identified by reactivity (cytotoxic effect in the presence of complement) with donor T-lymphocytes, whereas reactivity with donor B-lymphocytes indicates the presence of HLA-DR antibodies. Preformed antibodies may be present in the recipient following previous organ transplantation, pregnancy or blood transfusions.

Should the recipient's serum be shown to contain preformed lymphocytotoxic antibodies against T cells, difficulty may be met in finding a compatible donor for that particular recipient. If there are no preformed antibodies, selection of a suitable donor should in all likelihood be easy. Nevertheless, we believe a donor-specific lymphocytotoxic cross-match should be performed in every case.

When a possible donor becomes available, a lymphocytotoxic cross-match test must be performed using recipient serum and donor T and B cells. If the recipient serum is shown to contain antibodies that react against and cause lysis of the donor T-lymphocytes[31,32] the recipient is said to be 'presensitized', and there is a very strong chance of hyperacute rejection resulting if transplantation takes place. In one series, 24 out of 30 renal transplant recipients who were presensitized to their donors had immediate and irreversible rejection of the allograft[33].

Although the importance of T cell lymphocytotoxic antibodies in the subsequent destruction of an allograft is accepted, that of B cell lymphocytotoxic antibodies remains uncertain. The role of B cell antibodies in clinical transplantation has received much attention following the first reports of a successful graft outcome in the presence of a positive B cell lymphocytotoxic cross-match[34,35]. Donor-specific B cell lymphocytotoxic antibodies, when present in a potential recipient before transplantation, have been variously reported to: (1) lead to early graft rejection[36,37], (2) bear no relationship to the subsequent transplant outcome[38,39], and (3) correlate with improved graft survival[40]. Furthermore, a distinction has been made according to the temperature at which the test is performed. Antibodies reacting at 37 °C are said to correlate with a poor prognosis, whilst those reacting at 5 °C correlate with an improved prognosis[41]. It has been established, however, that preformed donor-specific B cell lymphocytotoxic antibodies do not lead to the immediate or early allograft failure from hyperacute or accelerated graft rejection which may occur when preformed donor-specific T cell lymphocytotoxic antibodies are present in the recipient serum[41,42], although an isolated case has been reported[43].

The influence of pre-existing, non-donor-specific T cell lymphocytotoxic antibodies (that is, when non-donor-specific T cell lymphocytotoxic antibodies have been demonstrated against a panel of T-lymphocytes) on the subsequent survival of a kidney allograft remains uncertain. From early observations it seemed that patients with broadly reactive antibodies (antibodies with a high frequency of lymphocytotoxicity against a random panel) had impaired graft survival rates[44]. More recently, donor-specific cross-matching has been carried out using both stored recipient sera which have been shown to be previously reactive against a panel of T-lymphocytes, as well as recipient serum obtained immediately before transplantation. The presence of preformed antibodies in stored sera usually did not lead to impaired graft survival, as long as the donor-specific cross-match was negative using all stored and fresh recipient sera[2,45]. Failure to perform the recipient–donor lymphocytotoxic cross-match test using stored sera that have high levels of antibodies may, however, lead to higher rates of hyperacute and accelerated rejection after transplantation[46]. There is, however, some evidence to suggest that antibody formation following rejection of an allograft confers a less favourable prognosis on subsequent graft survival[46].

This evidence is supported by our own observations in one patient following cardiac retransplantation[47]; previously, our understanding of this matter has been based exclusively on data from renal allotransplantation. This patient developed strong multispecific antibodies against T-lymphocytes after rejection at 5 weeks of an HLA non-identical heterotopic cardiac transplant. The heterotopic allograft was excised, and he remained alive supported by his own heart. After some months the antibodies could not be detected, though they recurred following a test transfusion of 500 ml of HLA non-identical blood. When another donor heart became available, the donor-specific T cell lymphocytotoxic cross-match test using both stored and fresh recipient sera was negative. A second heterotopic heart transplant was performed, but the donor heart failed within 5 days, following the onset of a severe irreversible acute rejection episode. At that time, a 32-fold increase in lymphocytotoxic antibodies against donor T cells was demonstrated in the patient's blood.

4. PRETRANSPLANT BLOOD TRANSFUSION

For a number of years blood transfusions were avoided whenever possible in potential transplant recipients in order to minimize the risk of presensitization. It was thought that the development of cytotoxic antibodies to HLA alloantigens would reduce the number of potential donors compatible with that particular recipient[48, 49]. In 1973, however, it was demonstrated in a large renal transplant series that transplant recipients who had never received blood transfusions before transplantation had a significantly lower allograft survival rate than their counterparts who had been transfused[50]. These results have now been confirmed by most renal transplant centres[51–54], though the magnitude of the effect varies markedly from centre to centre.

Although one major centre has reported that favourable renal allograft outcome is directly related to the number of pretransplant transfusions received[55], other groups have not confirmed this, and have instead reported that a single transfusion is as effective as several transfusions and lessens the risk of the potential recipient developing antibodies against HLA antigens[56,57].

One possible explanation for the favourable effect of blood transfusions on allograft survival is that the transfusions differentiate between 'high responders', who would have a high rate of rejection after subsequent organ transplantation, and 'low responders', who would have a low rate. As the high responders develop antibodies following blood transfusion, subsequent transplantation may prove impossible, as no donor can be found against whom the recipient does not have a positive cross-match. Only the low responders are transplanted, with good results[58]. An alternative explanation is that the transfusions induce a state of unresponsiveness similar to immune enhancement[50].

Though well-documented with regard to kidney transplantation, the effect of blood transfusion on patients subsequently undergoing cardiac transplantation is less certain. A beneficial, though not statistically significant, effect was observed and reported by the Stanford group as early as 1973[59]. In a recent review of the patients in our own series, pretransplantation blood transfusions (PTBT) were related to improved survival, though this reached statistical significance only at the 3-year time interval (Figure 6.3)[18]. This lack of *significantly* improved *overall* survival in patients with cardiac transplants may be related to the more widespread use of prophylactic antithymocyte globulin (ATG) in these patients. Improved survival following blood transfusion in recipients of kidney grafts has not been apparent in those patients who have received prophylactic ATG treatment[60].

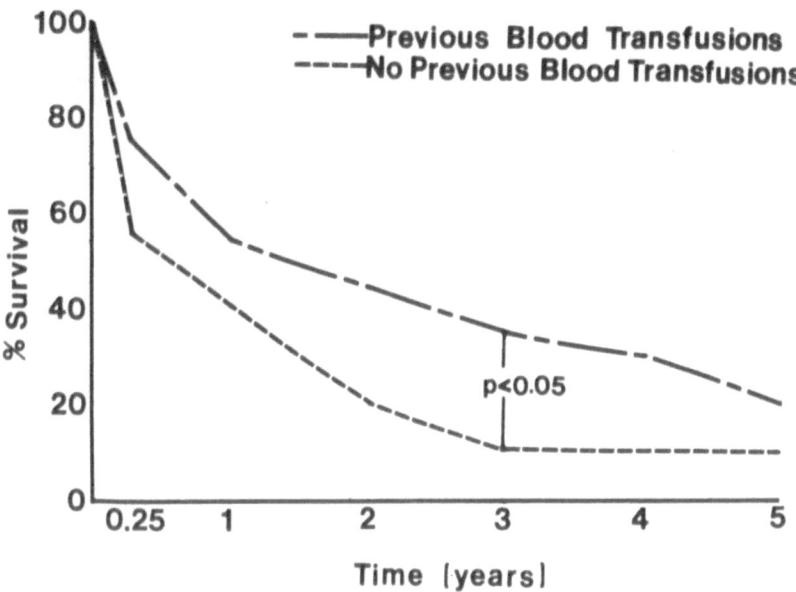

Figure 6.3 Relationship of cardiac allograft survival and pretransplant blood transfusions in recipients at Groote Schuur Hospital

In experimental work in baboons we have found that PTBT, whether given as one or more large transfusions or as small transfusions at frequent intervals, does not result in any significant prolongation of cardiac allograft survival (Table 6.2) (Cooper, unpublished data). These results, however, are at variance with those reported by Van Es *et al.*, who observed a favourable increase in survival of kidney allografts in rhesus monkeys following PTBT[61]. Furthermore, Van Es observed that the length of survival was greater in the monkeys in whom transplantation was performed sooner rather than later after the last transfusion. Unless this is a species or organ-related difference, the lack of correlation between our own results and those of Van Es and his colleagues cannot be adequately explained.

It has already been pointed out that PTBT can sensitize some patients to HLA antigens and thus decrease the chances of finding a negative cross-match donor for those patients. The major limiting factor to the number of transplants performed in most centres, and especially in our own centre, is the availability of donor organs. Any manipulation that might further reduce the number of donors available to any potential recipient should be avoided unless it imparts a clearly beneficial effect which overrides this consideration.

There would, therefore, appear to be no indication at the present time to electively transfuse patients awaiting cardiac transplantation.

Table 6.2 Survival of heterotopic cardiac allografts in baboons receiving pretransplant non-specific and peroperative donor-specific blood transfusions

Group	Survival	Number of baboons	Mean survival time ($\pm SD$) (days)	Median survival time (days)	Mean survival time Statistical difference* from (a) Group 1	(b) Group 3
1	Control (No IS)	10	11.0 (± 5.6)	9.5	—	$p < 0.025$
2	PTBT (Protocol A) (No IS)	8	13.1 (± 7.6)	12.0	NS	NS
3	Post-transplant IS	7	19.9 (± 10.6)	20.0	$p < 0.025$	—
4	PTBT (Protocol B) + post-transplant IS	6	24.0 (± 9.2)	22.0	$p < 0.0025$	NS
5	DST + post-transplant IS	7	22.3 (± 16.7)	18.0	NS	NS

PTBT = Pretransplant non-specific blood transfusion.
Protocol A: Multiple unit blood transfusions on one or two occasions 2–10 weeks before cardiac transplantation.
Protocol B: Single unit blood transfusions at 3–4-day intervals during the 3 weeks before cardiac transplantation.
DST = Peroperative donor-specific blood transfusion.
IS = Maintenance immunosuppression with azathioprine 2.5 mg/kg per day and methylprednisolone 2 mg/kg per day.
*Student t-test for unpaired data.

There is some evidence that the administration of immunosuppressive drugs at the time of blood transfusion reduces or eliminates sensitization[62, 63]. It may prove possible, however, to reverse this state of sensitization. Observations on two cardiac transplant patients in our institution would suggest that the administration of cyclosporin A (CYA) to a sensitized patient leads to the loss of these circulating antibodies (Figure 6.4)[64].

More recently, pretransplant donor-specific blood transfusion (DST) has been shown to correlate with improved graft survival following kidney transplantation from immunologically disparate living-related donors[65, 66]. Transplantation from living-related donors is clearly impossible in patients requiring heart transplantation, and therefore pretransplant DST from the potential donor is not applicable. Clinically, however, it is possible to administer DST at the time of cardiac transplantation, though in baboons we have not found this to be related to any improved survival (Table 6.2).

5. MECHANISM OF ALLOGRAFT DESTRUCTION

The mechanism by which the recipient attempts to destroy the allograft is complex. There is both a cellular response, which is mobilized within hours, and a humoral response, which takes approximately 2 weeks to become effective in the non-sensitized subject. The cellular response is largely a function of the T-lymphocytes, though other cells (K-lymphocytes, macrophages) are involved. The humoral response—the production of antibodies—is a function of B-lymphocytes.

The two major subpopulations of lymphocytes are T-lymphocytes, whose maturation depends on the thymus, and B-lymphocytes, which in mammals are derived probably from bone marrow cells. The T-lymphocytes are further

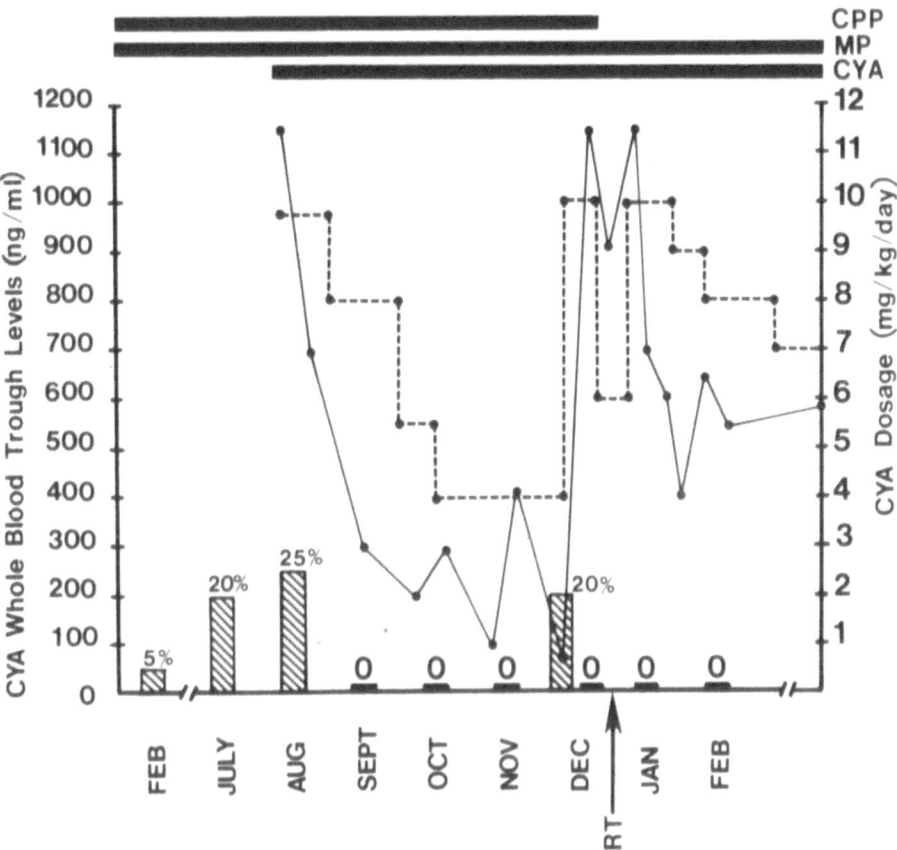

Figure 6.4 Development of lymphocytotoxic antibodies in a patient with a heterotopic heart transplant immunosuppressed with cyclophosphamide (CPP) and methylprednisolone (MP). The antibodies were lost when cyclosporin A (CYA) was added to the regimen, but temporarily returned when the dosage (·----·) of cyclosporin was reduced and the blood trough levels (·——·) of the drug fell below the therapeutic range. Following an increase in cyclosporin dosage, the antibodies again disappeared. An orthotopic cardiac transplant (RT) was then performed, leaving the original heterotopic donor heart *in situ*; the reasons for this choice of operation are discussed elsewhere (Chapter 17). Subsequent immunosuppression has been with cyclosporin and methylprednisolone. No further antibodies have been detected. The cross-hatched columns indicate the percentage of panel cells against which lymphocytotoxic antibodies were present

subdivided into at least three main groups (Figure 6.5): (1) cytotoxic T cells, which cause the cytolysis of allograft cells, (2) helper T cells, which are responsible for enhancing both the humoral and cell-mediated responses, and (3) suppressor T cells, which may inhibit the response (for example, by suppressing antibody formation by B cells).

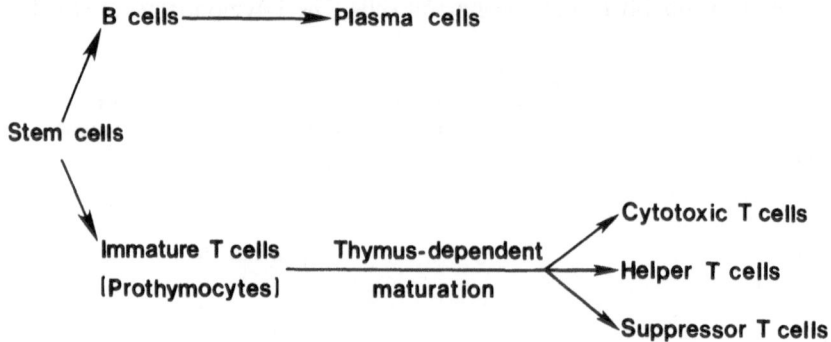

Figure 6.5   Development of basic lymphocyte groups and subgroups

Cytotoxicity in the form of actual cytolysis or of cytostasis (slowing of movement and accumulation of white blood cells in the capillaries) is the final common pathway by which donor cells are killed, and can be induced by (1) T-lymphocytes, (2) killer or 'K' lymphocytes, (3) macrophages, and (4) complement (Figure 6.6). Since macrophages and K cells require antibody for killing, their effect will be delayed until antibody has been produced; T cells, however, can kill incompatible cells directly. Antibodies produced by B cells can also cause cell destruction, but only in the presence of complement.

(1) *T cell cytotoxicity* is thought to be the most important mechanism by which allografts are destroyed[3]. The allogeneic antigens that generate the cytotoxic effects of T cells are not thought to be HLA-A, B or C antigens. Cytotoxic T cells kill donor cells rapidly in an antigen-specific fashion, though without requirement for antibody.

(2) *K cell cytotoxicity*, or antibody-dependent cell-mediated cytotoxicity (ADCC), is another important pathway which can cause destruction of the allograft[67]. The K cell, which may be a subpopulation of the T cell with an Fc receptor (a receptor for the C-terminal fragment of IgG obtained by papain digestion) or a null cell, must attach itself to the exposed Fc fragment of antibody already bound to the target cell in order to produce damage.

(3) The activated *macrophage* can also contribute to graft rejection either non-specifically, by opsonized antibody, or by specific arming factors (lymphokines) produced by T-lymphocytes[68].

(4) Donor organs can be damaged by the action of *complement*-dependent antibody, as occurs in episodes of hyperacute rejection; these donor-specific antibodies trigger the complement cascade to produce cell damage[69].

Each of these types of cytotoxicity may act alone or in concert to destroy an allograft. Current and future improvements in immunosuppression depend on a knowledge of these mechanisms and on our ability to modify them. Optimal combinations of immunosuppressive agents can only be arrived at rationally and effectively by a full understanding of the site and mode of action of each agent.

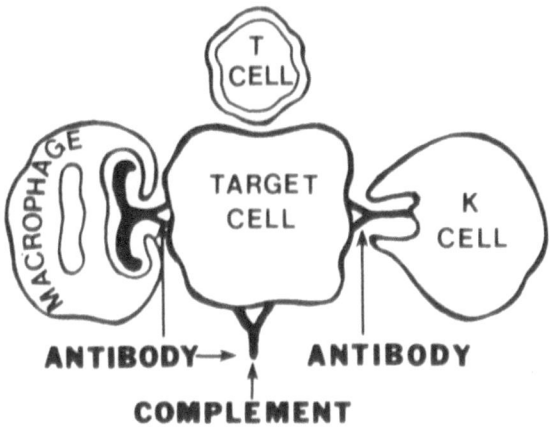

Figure 6.6 The four major ways of donor cell destruction; only T cell cytotoxicity does not require antibody

Antithymocyte globulin (ATG) preparations have been developed with a highly selective effect on circulating T-lymphocytes, which are thought to be the major initiators of acute rejection. While corticosteroid–azathioprine therapy alone has a limited effect on the levels of circulating T-lymphocytes, ATG can lower these levels to less than 1% of normal[3]. This effect is important, since it is relatively unusual for acute rejection to occur in patients with T-lymphocyte levels below 10% of normal (50–150 cells/mm³). ATG has also been shown to decrease K cell cytotoxicity. The combined effect of this agent on both T and K cell reactivity explains its potent antirejection activity relative to steroids and azathioprine. A similar result can be obtained by thoracic duct drainage[70], though this method of immunosuppression has largely been replaced by drug therapy.

Azathioprine also has selective anti-T-cell activity, which may account for the suppression of cell-mediated rejection without alteration of antibody production[71]. Although azathioprine is also active on B cells, this activity is much less intense than on T cells.

Despite much study, the immunosuppressive actions of corticosteroids have not been precisely defined, though they are known to greatly depress K cells, whereas some other immunosuppressive agents such as azathioprine do not[72]. A preferential action of steroids on either B- or T-lymphocytes has not been clearly established[73].

CYA and total lymphoid irradiation (TLI) are both thought to have strong selectivity of action for T-lymphocytes[74-76] and have been used with very promising results. The main target for the action of CYA appears to be the T-helper cell; other T-lymphocyte subpopulations exhibiting suppressor and memory functions are considerably more resistant to its action[77]. There is some evidence that the CYA mechanism of action may be through a blockade or inhibition of the release of interleukins and other lymphokines[78].

CONCLUSIONS

In summary, therefore, before cardiac transplantation is performed, donor–recipient ABO compatibility and a negative donor lymphocyte–recipient sera cross-match must be assured. To date, there is no convincing evidence to show that HLA compatibility improves graft survival, though A2 and A3 incompatibilities may result in early graft arteriosclerosis. Patients with previous high levels of circulating T lymphocytotoxic antibodies may possibly be at risk from accelerated acute rejection, despite a negative donor-specific cross-match at the time of transplantation. Patients with B red cell antigens (blood groups B and AB) and those with no previous history of blood transfusions may be at some disadvantage, although the influence of each of these remains in doubt and is certainly not sufficient to preclude transplantation.

References

1. Hamburger, J. (1982). Transplantation immunology. In Hamburger, J., Crosnier, J., Bach, J. F. and Kreis, H. (eds.) Renal Transplantation: Theory and Practice. 2nd Edn. (Baltimore/London: Williams & Wilkins)
2. Carpenter, C. B. and Stom, T. B. (1980). Transplantation immunology. In Parker, C. W. (ed.) Clinical Immunology. (Philadelphia: Saunders)
3. Thomas, F. and Thomas, J. (1980). Transplantation immunology. In Chatterjee, S. N. (ed.) Renal Transplantation—A Multidisciplinary Approach. (New York: Raven Press)
4. Dausset, J. and Rapaport, F. T. (1966). The role of blood group antigens in human histocompatibility. Ann. NY Acad. Sci., 129, 408
5. Murray, J. E. and Harrison, J. H. (1963). Surgical management of fifty patients with kidney transplants, including eighteen pairs of twins. Am. J. Surg., 105, 205
6. Starzl, T. E., Marchioro, T. L., Holmes, J. H., Hermann, G., Brittain, R. S., Stonington, O. H. and Talmage, D. W. (1964). Renal homografts in patients with major donor–recipient blood group incompatibilities. Surgery, 55, 195
7. Wilbrandt, R., Tung, K. S. H., Deodhar, S. R. and Waddell, W. R. (1969). ABO blood incompatibility in human renal homotransplantation. Am. J. Clin. Pathol., 51, 15

8. Opelz, G. and Terasaki, P. I. (1977). Effect of blood on relation between HLA match and outcome of cadaver kidney transplants. *Lancet*, **1**, 220

9. Joysey, V., Roger, J. H. and Evans, D. B. (1973). Kidney graft survival and matching for HLA and ABO antigens. *Nature (Lond.)*, **246**, 163

10. Lanza, R. P., Cooper, D. K. C. and Barnard, C. N. (1982). Effect of ABO blood group antigens on long-term survival after cardiac transplantation. *N. Engl. J. Med.*, **307**, 1275

11. Van Hooff, J. P., Hendricks, G. F. J. and Van Rood, J. J. (1976). The influence of a number of immunogenic and non-immunogenic factors on the graft prognosis. The relative importance of HLA matching in kidney transplantation. *Academic Thesis*, University of Leiden, p. 69

12. Opelz, G. and Terasaki, P. I. (1979). Cadaver kidney transplants in North America: analysis 1978. *Dial. Transplant.*, **8**, 167

13. Dausset, J. (1981). The major histocompatibility complex in man: past, present and future concepts. *Science*, **213**, 146

14. Nomenclature for factors of the HLA system, 1980 (1980). In Terasaki, P. I. (ed.) *Histocompatibility Testing, 1980*. p. 18. (Los Angeles: UCLA Tissue Typing Laboratory)

15. Opelz, G. (1983). A collaborative transplant study. (Unpublished data)

16. Solheim, B. G., Flatmark, A., Enger, E., Jervell, J. and Thorsby, E. (1977). Influence of HLA-A, B, C and D matching on the outcome of clinical kidney transplantation. *Transplant Proc.*, **9**, 475

17. Pennock, J. L., Oyer, P. E., Reitz, B. A., Bieber, C. P. and Stinson, E. B. (1982). Cardiac transplantation in perspective for the future. *J. Thorac. Cardiovasc. Surg.*, **83**, 168

18. Cooper, D. K. C., Boyd, S. T., Lanza, R. P. and Barnard, C. N. (1983). Factors influencing survival following heart transplantation. *Heart Transplant.*, **3**, 86

19. Svejgaard, A., Hauge, M., Jersild, C., Platz, P., Ryder, L. P., Staub Nielson, L. and Thomsen, M. (1975). *The HLA System: An Introductory Survey*. (New York: Karger)

20. Fournier, C. (1982). Mixed lymphocyte reaction and cell-mediated lympholysis techniques. In Hamburger, J., Crosnier, J., Bach, J. F. and Kreis, H. (eds.) *Renal Transplantation: Theory and Practice*. p. 361. (Baltimore/London: Williams & Wilkins)

21. Cochrum, K. C., Perkins, H. A., Payne, R., Kountz, S. and Belzer, F. O. (1973). The correlation of MLC with graft survival. *Transplant. Proc.*, **5**, 391

22. Walker, J., Opelz, G. and Terasaki, P. I. (1978). Correlation of MLC response with graft survival in cadaver and related donor kidney transplants. *Transplant. Proc.*, **10**, 949

23. Ting, A. (1982). HLA and organ transplantation. In Morris, P. J. (ed.) *Tissue Transplantation*. p. 28. (New York: Churchill Livingstone)

24. Ting, A. (1982). The influence of HLA-DR matching on allograft survival in man. *Heart Transplant.*, **2**, 136

25. Berg, B., Groth, C. G., Lundgren, G. and Moller, E. (1982). The impact of HLA-DR matching on the outcome of cadaveric kidney transplantation. *Transplant. Proc.*, **14**, 178

26. Albrechtsen, D., Bondevik, H., Flatmark, A., Halvorsen, S., Jakobsen, A., Jervell, J., Moen, B. T., Solheim, B., Sodal, G. and Thorsby, E. (1982). HLA matching in first cadaveric renal transplantation in Norway, 1969–1981. *Transplant. Proc.*, **14**, 182

27. Martins da Silva, B., Jeannet, M., Vassali, P., Harder, F. and Largiader, F. (1979). Influence of HLA-DR matching in cadaver kidney transplantation in Swiss-transplant. *Transplant. Proc.*, **11**, 760

28. Festenstein, H., Pachovla-Papasteriadis, C., Sachs, J. A., Jaraque-Mada, D. and Burke, J. M. (1979). Collaborative scheme for tissue typing and matching in renal transplantation: effect of HLA-A, B, D and DR matching and pretransplant blood transfusion on 769 cadaver renal grafts. *Transplant. Proc.*, **11**, 752

29. Persijn, G. C., Gabb, B. W., Van Leeuwen, A., Nagtegaal, A., Hooge-Boom, J. and Van Rood, J. J. (1978). Matching for HLA antigens of A, B and DR loci in renal transplantation by Eurotransplant. *Lancet*, **1**, 1278

30. Goeken, N. E., Thompson, J. S. and Corry, R. J. (1982). A 2-year trial of prospective HLA-DR matching. Effects on renal allograft survival and rate of transplantation. *Transplantation*, **32**, 522

31. Kissmeyer-Nielsen, F., Olsen, S., Peterson, V. P. and Fjeldborg, O. (1966). Hyperacute rejection of kidney allografts, associated with pre-existing humoral antibodies against donor cells. *Lancet*, **2**, 662

32. Weil, R., Clarke, D. R., Iwaki, Y., Porter, K. A., Koep, L. J., Paton, B. C., Terasaki, P. I. and Starzl, T. E. (1981). Hyperacute rejection of a transplanted human heart. *Transplantation*, **32**, 71

33. Patel, R. and Terasaki, P. I. (1969). Significance of the positive crossmatch test in kidney transplantation. *N. Engl. J. Med.*, **280**, 735

34. Ettinger, R. B., Terasaki, P. I. and Opelz, G. (1976). Successful renal allografts across a positive crossmatch for donor B-lymphocyte alloantigens. *Lancet*, **2**, 56

35. Lobo, P. I., Wertervelt, F. B. and Rudolf, L. E. (1977). Kidney transplantability across a positive crossmatch. Crossmatch assays and distribution of B-lymphocytes in donor tissue. *Lancet*, **1**, 925

36. Ayoub, G., Min Sik Park, Terasaki, P. I., Iwaki, Y. and Opelz, G. (1980). B-cell antibodies and crossmatching. *Transplantation*, **29**, 227

37. Buckingham, J. M., Geis, W. P., Giacchino, J. L., Subhash, R., Hano, J. E., Chejfec, G. and Jonasson, O. (1979). B-cell directed antibodies and delayed hyperacute rejection: a case report. *J. Surg. Res.*, **27**, 268

38. Coxe-Gilliland, R. and Cross, D. E. (1979). Warm B-cell antibodies and DRW matching: their influence on transplant outcome at a single center. *Transplant. Proc.*, **11**, 945

39. Morris, P. J. (1978). Histocompatibility antigens in human organ transplantation. *Surg. Clin. N. Am.*, **58**, 233

40. D'Apice, A. J. F. and Taits, B. D. (1979). Improved survival and function of renal transplants with positive B-cell crossmatches. *Transplantation*, **27**, 324

41. Cross, D. E., Coxe-Gilliland, R. and Weaver, P. (1979). DRW antigen matching and B-cell antibody crossmatching: their effect on clinical outcome of renal transplants. *Transplant. Proc.*, **11**, 1908

42. Morris, P. J., Ting, A. and Oliver, D. (1978). Renal transplantation in the presence of positive crossmatch. *Transplant. Proc.*, **10**, 467

43. Dejelo, C. L. and Williams, T. C. (1977). B-cell crossmatch in renal transplantation. *Lancet*, **2**, 241

44. Van Hooff, J. P., Schippers, H. M. A., Van der Steen, G. J. and Van Rood, J. J. (1972). Efficiency of HLA matching in Eurotransplant. *Lancet*, **2**, 1385

45. Cross, D. E., Whittier, F. C., Weaver, P. and Foxworth, J. (1977). A comparison of the antiglobulin versus extended incubation time crossmatching: results in 223 renal transplants. *Transplant. Proc.*, **9**, 1803

46. Salvatierra, O., Perkins, H. A., Amend, W., Feduska, N. J., Dura, R. M., Potter, D. E. and Cochrum, K. C. (1977). The influence of presensitization on graft survival rate. *Surgery*, **81**, 146

47. Lanza, R. P., Campbell, E. M., Cooper, D. K. C., Du Toit, E. and Barnard, C. N. (1983). The problem of presensitized heart transplant recipient. *Heart Transplant.*, **2**, 151

48. Curtoni, E. S., Scudeller, P. I., Mattiuz, G., Savi, M. and Ceppellini, R. (1972). Anti-HLA antibody evaluation in recipients of planned transfusions. *Tissue Antigens*, **2**, 415

49. Terasaki, P. I., Mickey, M. R. and Krasler, M. (1971). Presensitization and kidney transplant failures. *Postgrad. Med.*, **47**, 89

50. Opelz, G., Sengar, D. P. S., Mickey, M. R. and Terasaki, P. I. (1973). Effect of blood transfusions on subsequent kidney transplants. *Transplant. Proc.*, **5**, 253

51. Festenstein, H., Sachs, J. A., Paris, A. M. I., Pegrum, G. D. and Moorhead, J. F. (1976). Influence of HLA matching and blood transfusion on outcome of 502 London transplant group renal-graft recipients. *Lancet*, **1**, 157

52. Fuller, T. C., Demanico, T. L., Cosimi, A. B., Huggins, C. E., King, M. and Russell, P. S. (1977). Effects of various types of RBC transfusions on HLA alloimmunization and renal allograft survival. *Transplant. Proc.*, **9**, 117

53. Svejgaard, A. and Solheim, B. G. (1977). Blood transfusion and kidney transplantation. In *Proceedings of the North Scandinavian Transplantation Meeting. Scand. J. Urol. Nephrol.* (Suppl.), **42**, 79

54. Van Hooff, J.P., Kalff, M. W., Van Pelgeest, A. E., Lansbergen, Q., Hendricks, G. F. J., Castelli, M. and Mackenzie, C. L. S. (1976). Blood transfusion and kidney transplantation. *Transplantation*, **22**, 306

55. Opelz, G. and Terasaki, P. I. (1978). Improvement of kidney-graft survival with increased number of blood transfusions. *N. Engl. J. Med.*, **299**, 799

56. Persijn, G. G., Van Hooff, J. P., Kalff, M. W., Lansbergen, Q. and Van Rood, J. J. (1977). Effects of blood transfusions and HLA matching on renal transplantation in the Netherlands. *Transplant. Proc.*, **9**, 503

57. Williams, K. A., Ting, A., Cullen, P. R. and Morris, P. J. (1979). Transfusions: their influence on human renal graft survival. *Transplant. Proc.*, **11**, 175

58. Van Es, A. A. and Balner, H. (1979). Effects of pretransplant transfusions on kidney allograft survival. *Transplant. Proc.*, **11**, 127

59. Dong, E., Stinson, E. B., Griepp, R. B., Coulson, A. S. and Shumway, N. E. (1973). Cardiac transplantation following failure of previous cardiac surgery. *Surg. Forum*, **24**, 150

60. Cho, S. I., Bradley, J. W., Carpenter, C. B., Cosimi, A. B. and Monaco, A. P. (1983). Antithymocyte globulin pretreatment, blood transfusion and tissue typing in cadaver kidney transplantation. *Am. J. Surg.*, **145**, 464

61. Van Es, A. A., Marquet, R. L., Van Rood, J. J., Kalff, M. W. and Balner, H. (1977). Blood transfusions induce prolonged kidney allograft survival in rhesus monkeys. *Lancet*, **1**, 506

62. Monaco, A. P., Clarke, A. W., Wood, M. L., Sahyoun, A. I., Codish, S. D. and Brown, R. W. (1976). Possible active enhancement of a human cadaver renal allograft with antilymphocyte serum (ALS) and donor bone marrow: case report of an initial attempt. *Surgery*, **79**, 384

63. Anderson, C. B., Sicard, G. A., Rodey, G. E., Anderman, C. K. and Etheredge, E. E. (1983). Renal allograft recipient pretreatment with donor-specific blood and concomitant immuno-suppression. *Transplant. Proc.*, **15**, 939

64. Novitzky, D., Cooper, D. K. C., Du Toit, E., Oudshoorn, M., Langman, E. and Jacobs, P. (1984). Disappearance of preformed lymphocytotoxic antibodies following cyclosporin A administration in two patients with previous heart transplants. (Submitted for publication)

65. Salvatierra, O., Vicenti, E., Amend, W., Potter, D., Iwaki, Y., Opelz, G., Terasaki, P. I., Duca, R., Cochrum, K., Hanes, D., Stoney, R. J. and Feduska, N. J. (1980). Deliberate donor-specific blood transfusion prior to living related renal transplantation. *Ann. Surg.*, **192**, 543

66. Salvatierra, O., Vicenti, E., Amend, W., Potter, D., Garovoy, M., Iwaki, Y., Terasaki, P. I., Duca, R., Hopper, S., Slemmer, T. and Feduska, N. (1983). Four years' experience with donor-specific blood transfusions. *Transplant. Proc.*, **15**, 924

67. Thomas, J., Thomas, F., Kaplan, A. and Lee, H. M. (1976). Antibody-dependent cell-mediated cytotoxicity in chronic renal allograft rejection. *Transplantation*, **22**, 94

68. Hall, B. M., Dorsch, S. and Roser, B. (1978). The cellular basis of allograft rejection *in vivo. J. Exp. Med.*, **148**, 878

69. Descamps, B., Gagnon, R., Van der Gaag, R., Feuillet, M.-N. and Crosnier, J. (1979). Antibody-dependent cell-mediated cytotoxicity (ADCC) and complement-dependent cyto-toxicity (CDC) in 229 sera from human renal allograft recipients. *J. Clin. Lab. Immunol.*, **2**, 303

70. Touraine, J. L., Archimbaud, J. P., Malik, M. C., Dubernard, J. M., Guey, A., Neyra, P., Mongin, D., Baurard, B. and Traeger, J. (1977). Improved results of human renal transplan-tation after thoracic duct drainage and antilymphocyte globulin treatment. In Touraine, J. L. *et al.* (eds.) *Transplantation and Clinical Immunology.* Vol. IX, p. 189. (Amsterdam: Excerpta Medica)

71. Bach, M. A. and Bach, J. F. (1972). Activities of immunosuppressive agents *in vitro*. II. Different timing of azathioprine and methotrexate in inhibition and stimulation of mixed lymphocyte reaction. *Clin. Exp. Immunol.*, **11**, 89

72. Descamps, B., Gagnon, R., Van der Gaag, R., Meyer, O. and Crosnier, J. (1977). Influence of azathioprine–prednisone *in vivo* treatment on lymphocyte-dependent antibody-mediated cytotoxicity (LDAC) in 57 human renal allograft recipients. *Transplant. Proc.*, **9**, 981

73. Bach, J. F. (1975). *The Mode of Action of Immunosuppressive Agents*. p. 379. (New York: American Elsevier)

74. Calne, R. Y. (1979). Immunosuppression for organ grafting. Observations on cyclosporin A. *Immunol. Rev.*, **46**, 113

75. Strober, S., Slavin, S., Gottlieb, M., Zan-Bar, I., King, D. P., Thoppe, R., Fuks, Z., Grumet, F. C. and Kaplan, H. S. (1979). Allograft tolerance after total lymphoid irradiation (TLI). *Immunol. Rev.*, **46**, 87

76. Myburgh, J. A., Smit, J. A., Browde, S. and Hill, R. R. H. (1980). Tranplantation tolerance in primates following total lymphoid irradiation and allogeneic bone marrow injection. *Transplantation*, **29**, 401

77. Borel, J. F. (1982). Immunological properties of cyclosporin A. *Heart Transplant.*, **1**, 237

78. Bunjes, D., Rollinghoff, M., Wagner, H. and Hardt, C. (1981). Cyclosporin A mediates immunosuppression of primary cytotoxic T-cell responses by impairing the release of interleukin 1 and interleukin 2. *Eur. J. Immunol.*, **11**, 657

7
Anaesthesia and Intra-operative Care, including Cardiopulmonary Bypass

INTRODUCTION

Anaesthesia for the first heart transplant[1] was based on the techniques then in general use for anaesthesia for open heart surgery. This approach has been followed in subsequent heart transplants at our institution. The justification for this approach is, we believe, confirmed by the results achieved, with no operative mortality in our series of more than 50 heterotopic transplants. There have been relatively few reports regarding anaesthetic aspects of patients either undergoing heart transplantation[2,3] or subsequent major surgical procedures[4-6].

The operation of heart transplantation remains an emergency procedure. The majority of transplants at our centre have been performed out of ordinary working hours, either at weekends or at night. The donor becomes available only when the criteria of death have been met and consent for donation given. The specific recipient is frequently not selected until HLA antigen matching and lymphocytotoxic cross-matching have been carried out.

THE DONOR

At the time that the donor is taken to the operating theatre, his cardiopulmonary functions will be receiving support as follows: (1) artificial ventilation, (2) intravenous infusions for fluid replacement, acid-base and electrolyte correction, and for the administration of inotropic drugs, and (3) intermittent intramuscular or continuous intravenous vasopressin to maintain an adequate blood pressure and to control the diabetes inspidius that almost always occurs[7].

In the operating theatre, reception of the donor is supervised by an anaesthetist, who will ensure the maintenance of circulatory and respiratory function in spite of brain death. The general principles of intensive care are apposite. Maintenance of renal function is important as, in our unit, kidneys are almost always harvested at the same time as the heart. The donor's trunk is shaved.

Formerly it was our routine to connect the donor to a pump-oxygenator and initiate cardiopulmonary bypass to maintain an adequate circulation and cool the donor organs to low temperatures (16–20°C) before excision. This technique is rarely used today, but is occasionally valuable if donor heart function is unstable and some delay in the readiness of the recipient to accept the donor heart is expected. On these occasions, we cool the donor rapidly to ±20°C. An extra heat exchanger (Sarns) is usually included in the venous line of the extracorporeal circuit to facilitate this rapid cooling, particularly if the donor is of large build.

THE RECIPIENT

The potential recipient is either already resident in the hospital or is admitted urgently once a donor becomes available. In either case, as there is usually a small pool of potential recipients awaiting transplantation, the identity of the specific recipient is not normally known until approximately 1 hour before his transfer to the theatre, when the result of lymphocytotoxic cross-matching becomes known. (The report from Denver of hyperacute rejection on the operating table is a salutary tale in this regard[8].)

The selected recipient is informed, final consent for the procedure taken, and the patient prepared for theatre: (1) intravenous infusions are set up, (2) initial loading doses of immunosuppressive agents (currently cyclosporin A and methylprednisolone) are administered, and (3) the trunk and all four limbs are shaved (the patient has already showered or bathed).

The anaesthetist normally sees the recipient whilst he is in the midst of these procedures. The patient is, not unexpectedly, usually apprehensive at this stage. Introduction of the anaesthetist, examination of the patient from the anaesthetic viewpoint, explanation of the further procedures, establishment of rapport with the patient, and comforting of concerned relatives are carried out as best as may be under these circumstances.

The patient is transferred to the operating theatre suite. The operation on the donor is usually already in progress, and inspection of the donor heart and an assessment of its continuing satisfactory function are carried out before the recipient is anaesthetized. It is occasionally necessary to cancel the transplantation procedure on the recipient due to donor heart failure even at this late stage.

A radial arterial line for monitoring and sampling purposes is established under local anaesthesia. Further intravenous lines are also set up. Care is taken to prevent infection as the patient has already received a loading dose of immunosuppressive therapy. Strict attention to aseptic techniques (as far as possible) is therefore essential. At this stage an intravenous antibiotic is given, currently cephamandole 1 g intravenously.

Induction of anaesthesia

Anaesthesia can then be induced. All recipients clearly have an extremely poor cardiac status[9-11], and therefore drugs that can further depress the already compromised myocardium should be avoided. Attention to maintaining pre-load and afterload to achieve maximal myocardial function is important. At the present time induction is achieved by a narcotic induction technique, followed by the administration of minimal intravenous thiopentone (of the order of 75–100 mg) to achieve hypnosis, and then a lignocaine/succinyl-choline, and perhaps pancuronium, sequence. Oral intubation is performed with blood pressure control by means of intravenous sodium nitroprusside and/or nitroglycerine. Further anaesthesia is inhalational, with judicious increments of intravenous agents, that is, the generally practised anaesthetic techniques that have been found to be satisfactory for routine open-heart surgery.

Dysrhythmias and a fall in cardiac output can occur at this critical stage. In one patient in our series ventricular fibrillation occurred within minutes of inhalational induction. External cardiac massage was performed, and partial pump oxygenator support instituted via the femoral artery and vein. A median sternotomy was then rapidly performed, and superior and inferior vena caval venous catheters inserted via the right atrium. This allowed full cardio-pulmonary bypass support. Orthotopic transplantation was performed with-out incident, and the patient recovered uneventfully. At over 13 years, this patient is at present our longest survivor.

A nasogastric tube and urinary bladder catheter are inserted. (This is in contrast to the practice at Stanford Medical Center, where urinary catheters are not used, but suprapubic catheterization preferred[3].)

The operative procedure

Opening of the pericardium and handling of the heart may be followed by the development of dysrhythmias such as ventricular tachycardia, frequently with a resulting fall in arterial pressure. These can generally be reversed by DC defibrillation; if they prove intractable, the initiation of pump oxygenator support should be provided as soon as possible.

When access to the heart has been established, the patient is fully hep-arinized (checked by activated clotting time) and cardiopulmonary bypass is instituted.

Cardiopulmonary bypass

The extracorporeal circuit, as used at Groote Schuur Hospital (Figure 7.1), consists of Sarns modular roller pumps, Polystan Venotherm VT 5000 oxygenator, William Harvey H-700 F cardiotomy reservoir, and Mayon prepacked tubing.

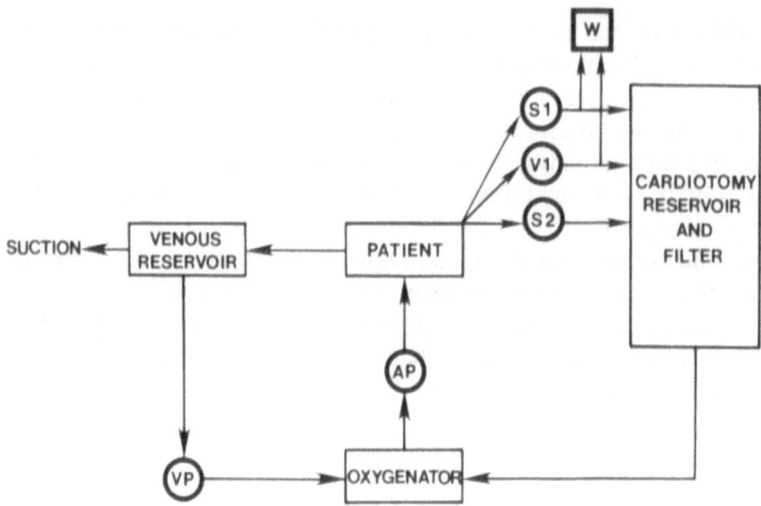

Figure 7.1   Diagram of extracorporeal cardiopulmonary bypass circuit used for routine open heart operations, including orthotopic heart transplantation, at Groote Schuur Hospital, Cape Town. VP = venous pump; AP = arterial pump; S = sucker; V = left ventricular vent; W = waste disposal bag

The machine is primed with 3 litres of a balanced salt solution (Plasmalyte B), to which is added heparin, cephamandole and calcium chloride. Pump flow is calculated on the basis of 2.4 litres per square metre of the body surface area per minute. Because problems can be expected in ensuring adequate venous return when the right atrium is opened, venous suction is sometimes necessary, and so a venous well and pump for venous drainage are included.

For heterotopic heart transplantation we add an extra sucker and an extra vent (Figure 7.2), which can return blood to the cardiotomy reservoir or into a waste bag. (The Harvey cardiotomy reservoir with its four inlets is very suitable when extra suckers are required.) The extra vent will be introduced into the donor left ventricle and gentle suction applied to help prevent myocardial rewarming by recipient collateral blood flow. The additional sucker is used to assist in removing the cold saline which, until revascularization is complete, is poured over the donor heart between each anastomotic procedure (Chapter 8). Our current policy is to cool the patient to 26–28 °C, and to maintain this temperature until the donor heart is revascularized. With the exception of the above modifications the bypass procedure is the same as for any standard open heart operation.

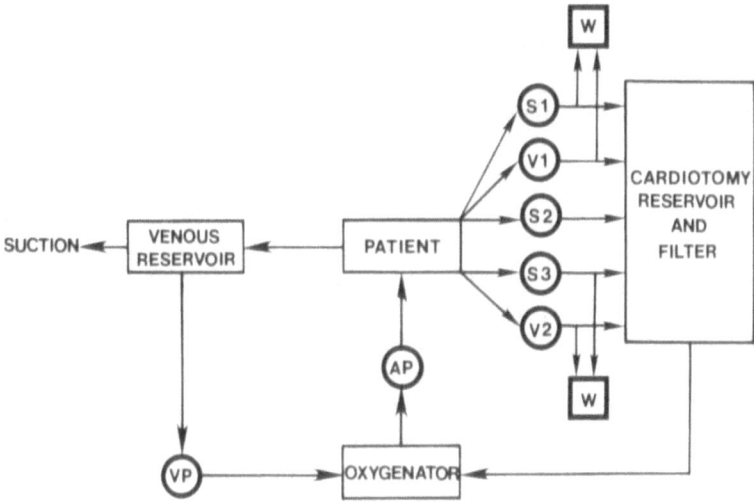

Figure 7.2 Diagram of extracorporeal cardiopulmonary bypass circuit as used for heterotopic heart transplantation at Groote Schuur Hospital, Cape Town. VP = venous pump; AP = arterial pump; S = sucker; V = left ventricular vent; W = waste disposal bag

In the operation of heterotopic heart transplantation it was formerly our policy to allow the recipient heart to beat spontaneously throughout the operation. Body cooling to only 32°C was carried out. In a number of these patients, during cardiopulmonary bypass, ventricular fibrillation of the recipient's heart occurred, sometimes repeatedly, presumably in response to handling and distortion. This condition always responded satisfactorily to DC shock treatment.

On completion of the surgical procedure, a 10–15 J shock is usually sufficient to defibrillate the heart successfully. Rewarming is generally not commenced until the donor heart has been revascularized. This ensures better myocardial protection during the operative procedure, and a rather longer 'recovery phase' for the donor organ during which cardiopulmonary bypass support is maintained. It is usually possible to defibrillate the heart successfully even at temperatures of 28–30°C. After rewarming to 36–37°C has been achieved, cardiopulmonary bypass support is slowly reduced and eventually terminated.

Heterotopic heart transplantation usually requires bypass of 2–2½ hours, lengthened possibly by our cautious approach to supporting the donor heart for up to 1 hour or longer after revascularization, before discontinuing cardiopulmonary bypass. Other units have reported that orthotopic heart transplantation is 'simple by cardiac surgery standards' and involves periods on bypass of approximately 1 hour[4].

Donor hearts have sometimes taken several minutes to begin beating after insertion and revascularization, in spite of appropriate drug therapy, such as the administration of calcium and inotropic agents. On other occasions the heart has contracted satisfactorily for a period, but then has once again either arrested or lapsed into ventricular fibrillation, usually associated with handling and retraction. Drug therapy and/or DC defibrillation have usually been successful in reversing these conditions eventually, but on occasions initial donor heart function has been poor. The experience at Papworth Hospital of spontaneous defibrillation of the donor heart within 2 minutes of releasing the aortic clamp in six out of 12 patients[12] has not been our experience. This observed difference may be related to the condition of the donor heart at the time of excision (Chapter 4), and/or to the adequacy of myocardial protection during the ischaemic period.

Early irreversible failure of the donor heart has, however, occurred in only one patient in our entire series. Following orthotopic transplantation in our initial 1967–73 series, the donor heart in one patient started beating spontaneously in sinus rhythm without apparent difficulty, but would not sustain the circulation in spite of repeated attempts to discontinue pump oxygenator support. This resulted in our only operating theatre death. The cause of donor heart failure could not be determined either in the operating theatre or at postmortem examination.

Following heterotopic transplantation, in some patients the donor heart assumes an immediate predominant role in supplying the systemic circulation (as in the case reported from Stanford[13]). On other occasions, the recipient's original heart has been the major support of the circulation for some hours, during which period the donor heart has recovered good function. At other times there has been a changing relationship between the two hearts in the early post-bypass period, presumably related to iatrogenic procedures which affect the two hearts differently.

Post-bypass period

Electrolyte and acid-base balance is checked, and heparinization reversed. In our experience inotropic and/or chronotropic support (isoprenaline, dopamine, dobutamine, adrenaline) is frequently necessary, at least during the first few hours.

The rate of the denervated donor heart shows no significant response to atropine, digitalis, pancuronium or neostigmine, but does respond to circulating catecholomines[6, 14, 15] (Chapter 10). Following heterotopic heart transplantation, care must be taken to monitor the response of both recipient and donor hearts to the various pharmacological agents administered.

Retreat from the pericardial cavity and chest is in the usual manner. The total period during which the patient remains anaesthetized is not infrequently of the order of 5–9 hours, and is usually longer following heterotopic than following orthotopic transplantation. Not only does the actual surgical procedure take rather longer, but achieving post-bypass haemostasis is also generally more time-consuming after the more complex operation of hetero-topic heart transplantation.

Immediate postoperative care

Reversal of anaesthesia is as for any open heart procedure. The patient remains intubated to allow a few hours' positive pressure ventilation in the intensive care unit (Chapter 9). A chest radiograph is taken before the patient is transferred from the operating table to his bed; this allows a check to exclude a pneumothorax or significant haemothorax, to ensure expansion of the lungs, etc., and to confirm the position of the endotracheal tube and central venous pressure monitoring catheters. In nearly every case, the patient is returned to the intensive care unit in a conscious condition.

References

1. Ozinsky, J. (1967). Cardiac transplantation—the anaesthetist's view: a case report. *S. Afr. Med. J.*, **41**, 1268
2. Garman, J. K. (1981). Anaesthesia for cardiac transplantation. *Cleveland Clin. Q.*, **48**, 142
3. Reitz, B. A., Fowles, R. E. and Ream, A. K. (1982). In Ream, A. K. and Fogdall, R. P. (eds.) *Acute Cardiovascular Management: Anesthesia and Intensive Care.* (Philadelphia: Lippincott)
4. Eisenkraft, J. B., Dimich, I. and Sachdev, V. P. (1981). Anaesthesia for non-cardiac surgery in a patient with a transplanted heart. *Mt. Sinai J. Med.*, **48**, 116
5. Kanter, S. F. and Samuels, S. I. (1977). Anesthesia for major operations on patients who have transplanted hearts—a review of 29 cases. *Anesthesiology*, **46**, 65
6. Samuels, S. I. and Kanter, S. F. (1977). Anaesthesia for major surgery in a patient with a transplanted heart. *Br. J. Anaesth.*, **49**, 265
7. Griepp, R. B., Stinson, E. B., Clark, D. A., Dong, E. and Shumway, N. E. (1971). The cardiac donor. *Surg. Gynecol. Obstet.*, **133**, 792
8. Weil, R., Clarke, D. R., Iwaki, Y., Porter, K. A., Koep, L. J., Paton, B. C., Terasaki, P. I. and Starzl, T. E. (1981). Hyperacute rejection of a transplanted human heart. *Transplantation*, **32**, 71
9. Cooper, D. K. C., Charles, R. G., Beck, W. and Barnard, C. N. (1982). The assessment and selection of patients for heterotopic heart transplantation. *S. Afr. Med. J.*, **61**, 575
10. Hastillo, A., Hess, M. L., Richardson, D. W. and Lower, R. R. (1980). Cardiac transplantation—1980: the Medical College of Virginia Program. *South Med. J.*, **73**, 909
11. Pennock, J. L., Oyer, P. E., Reitz, B. A., Jamieson, S. W., Bieber, C. P., Wallwork, J., Stinson, E. B. and Shumway, N. E. (1982). Cardiac transplantation in perspective for the future: survival, complications, rehabilitation and cost. *J. Thorac. Cardiovasc. Surg.*, **83**, 168
12. English, T. A. H., Cooper, D. K. C. and Cory-Pearce, R. (1980). Recent experience with heart transplantation. *Br. Med. J.*, **281**, 699
13. Melvin, K. R., Pollick, C., Hunt, S. A., McDougall, R., Goris, M. L., Oyer, P. E., Popp, R. L. and Stinson, E. B. (1982). Cardiovascular physiology in a case of heterotopic cardiac trans-plantation. *Am. J. Cardiol.*, **49**, 1301
14. Goodman, D. J., Rossen, R. M., Ingham, R., Rider, A. K. and Harrison, D. C. (1975). Sinus node function in the denervated human heart. Effect of digitalis. *Br. Heart J.*, **37**, 612
15. Leachman, R. D., Cokkinos, D. V. P., Cabrera, R., Leatherman, L. L. and Rochelle, D. G. (1971). Response of the transplanted, denervated human heart to cardiovascular drugs. *Am. J. Cardiol.*, **27**, 272

8
The Surgical Techniques of Orthotopic and Heterotopic Heart Transplantation

INTRODUCTION

There are two standard operations for performing heart transplantation—orthotopic, in which the recipient heart is excised and replaced in the correct anatomical position by the donor heart, and heterotopic (the so-called 'piggy-back' heart transplant), in which the donor heart is placed in the right chest alongside the recipient organ, and anastomosed in such a way to allow blood to pass through either or both hearts. The haemodynamics of this latter operation will be discussed in Chapter 10.

Our own clinical experience was originally with orthotopic transplantation, though in recent years it has been predominantly with the heterotopic technique. We continue to use orthotopic transplantation extensively in our experimental laboratory.

With either transplant technique, we believe that the recipient operation should not be begun until the donor chest has been opened and the donor heart inspected and seen to be suitable for transplantation.

ORTHOTOPIC HEART TRANSPLANTATION

The basic technique of orthotopic heart transplantation was developed in the research laboratory in the late 1950s and early 1960s[1] (Chapter 1). It was the work of Lower and Shumway in 1960[2] which established the operation as a successful procedure in the experimental animal. The operation was first attempted clinically by Hardy and his colleagues in 1964[3] and by Barnard in 1967[4]. In 1968, Barnard[5] subsequently contributed a small but significant modification to the operative technique whereby the incision in the right atrium of the donor heart was extended into the appendage and not into the superior vena cava, thus avoiding the region of the sinoatrial node. The operation has remained essentially unchanged since then, and is the operation of choice in the majority of centres performing heart transplantation today.

Donor heart excision

With the subject supine, a median sternotomy is performed and the pericardium opened longitudinally. The heart is inspected, in possible cases, for external signs of major damage caused by trauma or external cardiac massage. The ascending aorta is partially mobilized to allow subsequent application of a cross-clamp. The superior vena cava (SVC) is mobilized sufficiently to allow ligation cephalad to the sinus node. Two heavy ties are placed around the SVC, but not ligated at this stage. The inferior vena cava (IVC) is mobilized. The donor is fully heparinized. A cannula or needle for infusion of cold cardioplegic agent is inserted into the ascending aorta.

The SVC is doubly ligated (or suture ligated) and divided between the ligatures. (Any indwelling central venous pressure cannula must be withdrawn high into the SVC before this vessel is ligated and divided.) The IVC is clamped at the diaphragm and divided immediately central to the clamp, thus decompressing the right side of the heart. One or more pulmonary veins are opened to decompress the left side of the heart. As no left ventricular vent has been inserted, we believe that adequate decompression of the heart in this way is essential before the aorta is cross-clamped. The ascending aorta is then cross-clamped at the level of the brachiocephalic (innominate) artery, and cardioplegic solution (at 4°C) infused into the root of the aorta. Cold saline (at 4°C) is poured over the heart to cool it rapidly.

During the ischaemic period in which the heart is transferred to the recipient there will be no cardioplegic washout from collateral blood flow (as occurs to a cardioplegically arrested heart during open-heart surgery). It is theoretically, therefore, probably only necessary to give sufficient cardioplegic agent to bring about arrest of the heart. The cardioplegic infusion, however, also contributes towards the rapid cooling of the myocardium, and it is our policy, therefore, to infuse 1 litre.

Once the cardioplegic agent has been administered, the topical cold saline is sucked out of the pericardial cavity, and section of the right pulmonary veins is completed, together with division of the left pulmonary veins. Division of the aorta as high as possible at the origin of the brachiocephalic artery, immediately proximal to the cross-clamp, and of the pulmonary artery at its bifurcation (or of its main right and left branches) completes division of the major vessels.

The apex of the heart is then lifted anteriorly, and the mediastinal tissue posterior to the atria and major vessels is divided by sharp dissection, allowing the heart to be removed from the pericardial cavity.

The approximate time taken from ligation of the SVC to completion of excision of the heart is 5–10 minutes.

Donor heart excision is frequently combined with removal of both kidneys. After the initial preparation of the donor heart, the kidneys are mobilized. Whilst cardioplegic arrest and local cooling of the heart are being induced, the kidneys are removed. Finally, excision of the cold, arrested heart is completed.

Preparation of donor heart

The heart is placed in a bowl of cold (4 °C) saline while it is prepared ready for insertion into the recipient.

The right atrial cavity is opened, beginning posterolaterally at the IVC orifice and continuing the incision into the base of the right atrial appendage, thus avoiding the areas of the coronary sinus and the sinoatrial node[5] (Figure 8.1). The tissue between the orifices of the four pulmonary veins in the posterior aspect of the left atrium is excised, leaving one large opening (Figure 8.2).

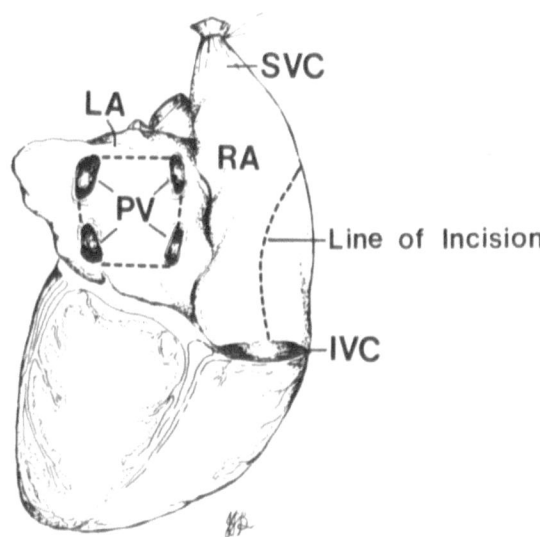

Figure 8.1 Orthotopic transplantation. Excised donor heart (posterior view), showing lines of incision.

Abbreviations used in figures in this chapter are: LA = left atrium; RA = right atrium; SVC = superior vena cava; IVC = inferior vena cava; PV = pulmonary vein; RV = right ventricle; PA = pulmonary artery; AO = aorta; LV = left ventricle; CS = coronary sinus

The heart can then be transferred to the surgical team preparing the recipient.

Once the heart has been placed in the empty pericardial cavity of the recipient, the aorta and pulmonary artery can be trimmed to the ideal length.

The recipient operation

With the patient lying supine, a median sternotomy is performed, the pericardium opened longitudinally, and its edges retracted.

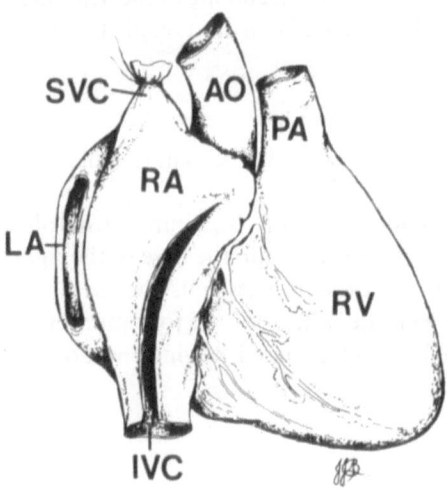

Figure 8.2 Orthotopic transplantation. Donor heart (right antero-lateral view) prepared for implantation

Initiation of cardiopulmonary bypass

After heparinization, cardiopulmonary bypass is initiated via cannulae inserted into the ascending aorta at the level of the brachiocephalic artery, and into the SVC and IVC via the lateral wall of the right atrium (Figure 8.3). A left ventricular vent is inserted into the apex. Snares or clamps are placed around the SVC and IVC to bring about total cardiopulmonary bypass. Total body cooling to at least 32°C, and preferably lower (26–28°C), helps prevent early rewarming of the donor heart as it lies in the pericardial cavity during insertion. The aorta is then cross-clamped immediately proximal to the aortic cannula.

Excision of the recipient heart

The heart is excised by dividing the right and left atrial walls and atrial septum, leaving a cuff of atrial wall to allow easy suture of the donor heart. Both atrial appendages should be excised to prevent thrombus formation occurring in these cavities subsequently. The aorta and main pulmonary artery are divided as close to their respective valves as possible (Figure 8.3). Subsequently these vessels may be trimmed before being sutured to their counterparts of the donor heart.

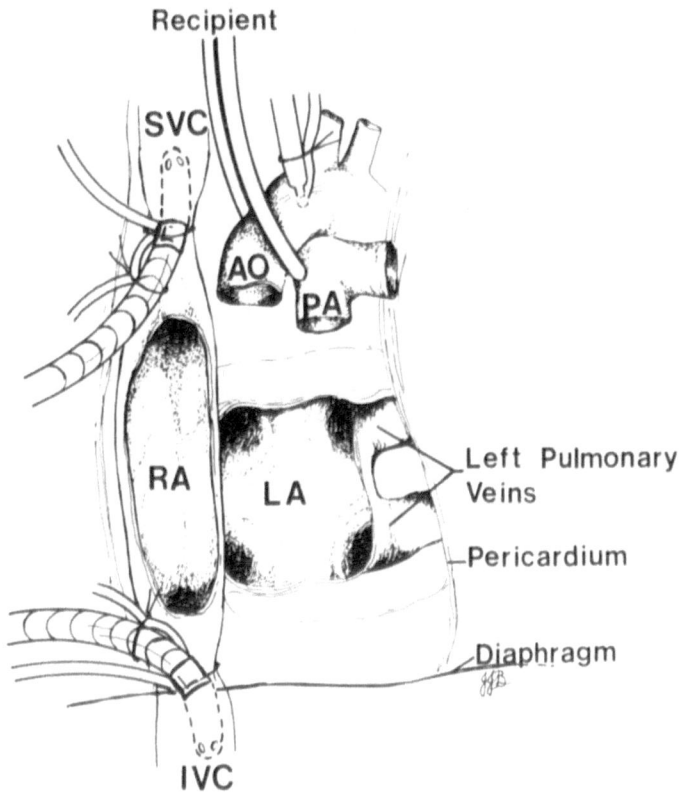

Figure 8.3 Orthotopic transplantation. View of recipient pericardial cavity after excision of the recipient heart

Anastomosis of left atria

The donor heart is then placed (or held by an assistant) over the left side of the divided sternum, parallel to the remnants of the excised recipient heart. Its posterior surface lies anteriorly so that the free walls of both recipient and donor left atria lie adjacent to each other. Using a double-ended 4/0 polypropylene suture, the left atrial walls are anastomosed by a continuous suture, beginning at their midpoints laterally (Figure 8.4). At a convenient stage the donor heart is drawn down into the pericardium and the suture tightened. The suture is continued around the superior and inferior borders of the left atrium on to the atrial septum, and tied in the middle of the septum (Figure 8.5).

It is essential to maintain myocardial temperature as low as possible, preferably below 15 °C, throughout the ischaemic period, though tissue damage from freezing must be avoided. Between the performance of each suture line, therefore, the pericardium should be temporarily filled with cold saline to maintain a low myocardial temperature, or, ideally, a system of continuous myocardial cooling should be utilized. Further cold cardioplegic agent should be infused through the coronary tree at similar intervals, primarily for its cooling effect.

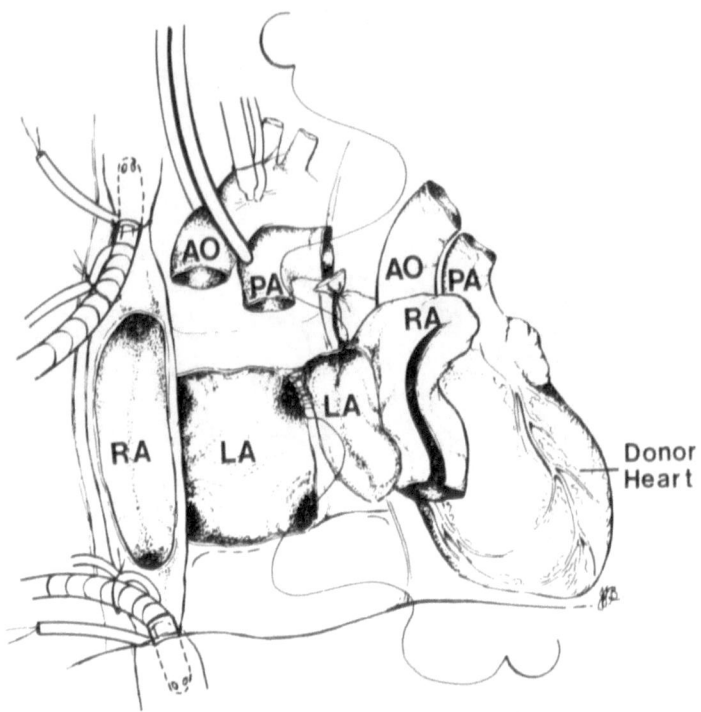

Figure 8.4 Orthotopic transplantation. Donor and recipient hearts, showing the beginning of the anastomosis between the two left atria

Infusion of large doses of cardioplegic agent at this stage, particularly if the agent contains a calcium blocking agent, has, in our experience, led to a delay of several minutes or longer in the return of adequate myocardial contractions after the resumption of myocardial blood flow; we believe, however, that effective myocardial protection is essential, and that the overuse of cardioplegic agent and topical cold saline is preferable to underuse.

Anastomosis of right atria

A suture of 5/0 polypropylene (or of 4/0 polypropylene if the right atrial walls are particularly thick) is then placed at the junction of the superior right atrial free wall with the septum, and continued around the superior, septal and inferior borders of the right atrium, and tied at the midpoint of the right atrial free wall laterally (Figure 8.6). The atrial septum has therefore been sutured twice, once on the left atrial side and once on the right.

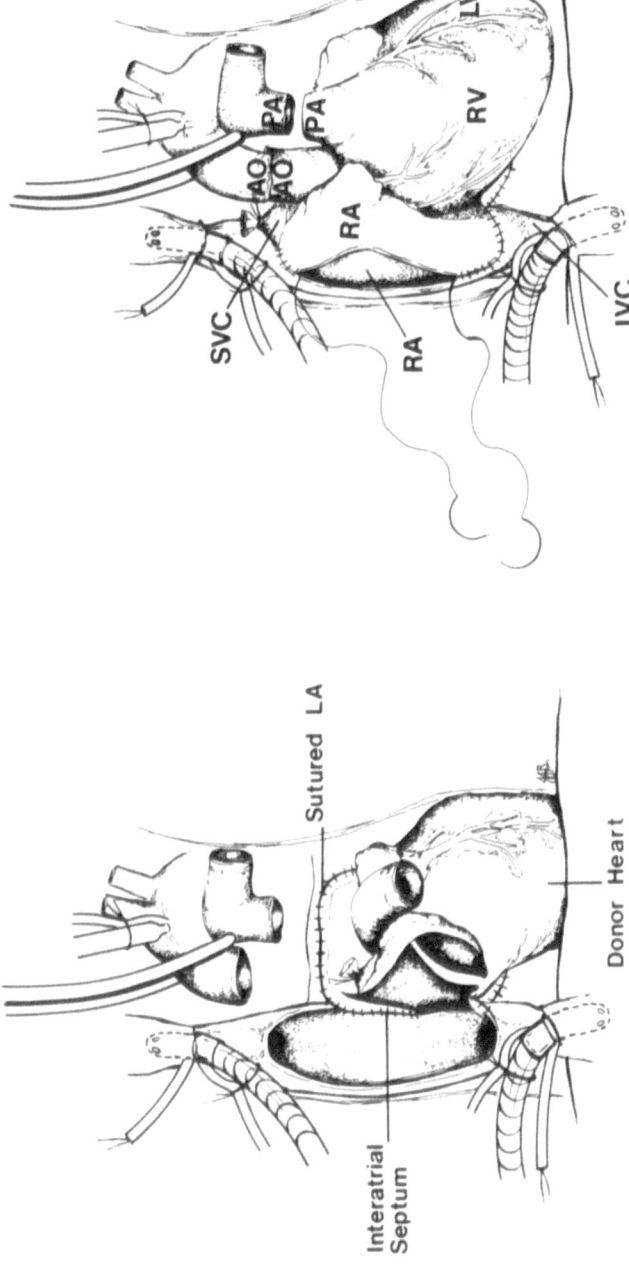

Figure 8.6 Orthotopic transplantation. The septal anastomosis has been completed; the free walls of the two right atria are being anastomosed

Figure 8.5 Orthotopic transplantation. Completed left atrial free wall suture line; the anastomosis between the two septa is being performed

Anastomosis of aortae

The aortae are anastomosed by continuous suture using 4/0 polypropylene (Figure 8.7).

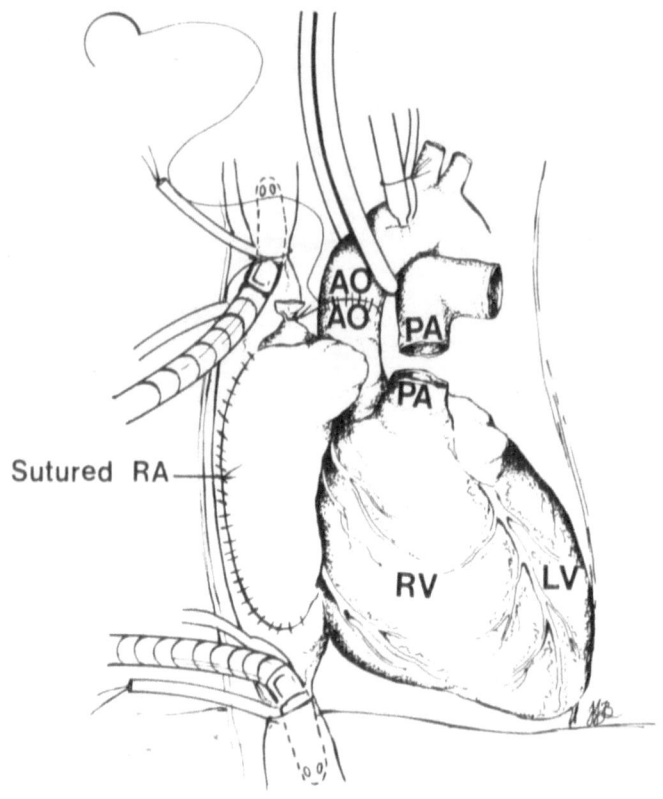

Figure 8.7 Orthotopic transplantation. The right atrial suture line has been completed; beginning of aortic anastomosis

A left ventricular vent is then inserted, either at the apex or, preferably, through the left atrial appendage, thus avoiding any damage to the ventricular myocardium. An air vent is inserted into the root of the aorta, either through the remnant of the recipient aorta or through the donor aorta. Frequently, the original cannula inserted into the donor aorta for infusion of cardioplegic solution can be used for this purpose. The aortic cross-clamp is then released, allowing the coronary arteries of the donor heart to be once again perfused with oxygenated blood. The SVC and IVC snares or clamps are released to allow coronary sinus return to drain through the venous cannulae to the pump oxygenator (Figure 8.8). The apex of the heart should be lifted up, the venous pressure allowed to rise, and the lungs ventilated temporarily in an effort to

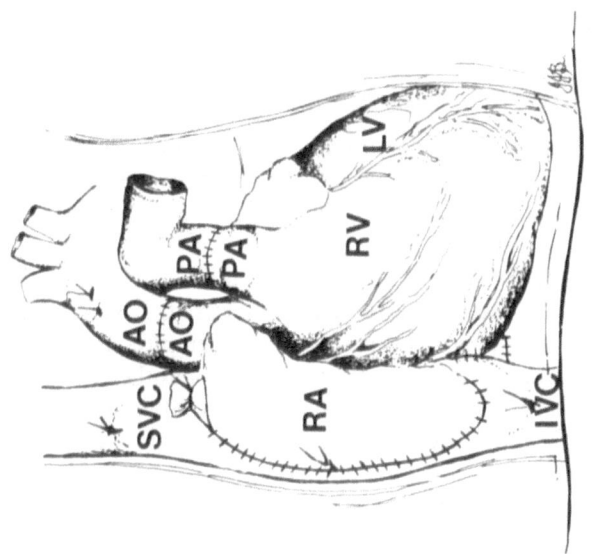

Figure 8.9 Orthotopic transplantation. Completed operation

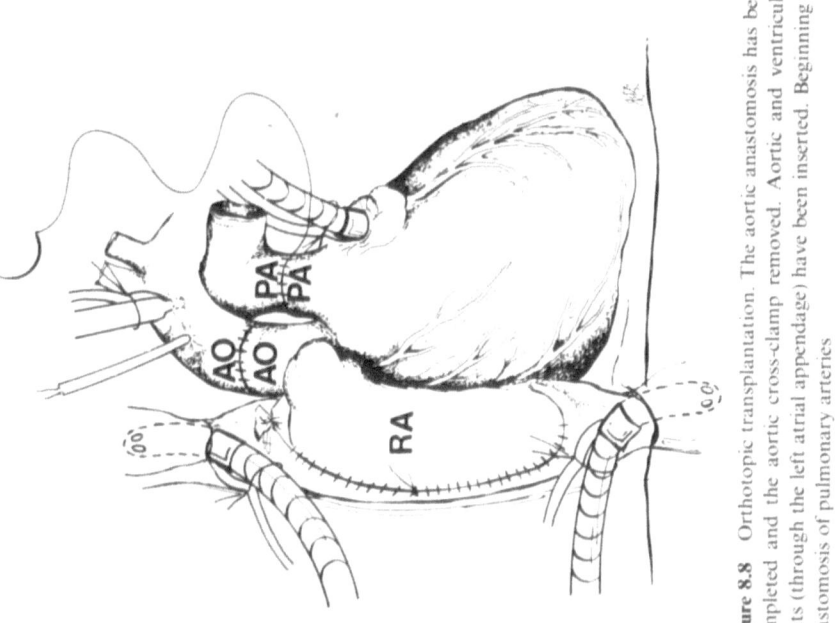

Figure 8.8 Orthotopic transplantation. The aortic anastomosis has been completed and the aortic cross-clamp removed. Aortic and ventricular vents (through the left atrial appendage) have been inserted. Beginning of anastomosis of pulmonary arteries

expel air from the heart through the ventricular vent. The venous pressure is subsequently reduced again to facilitate the performance of the pulmonary artery anastomosis.

Total body rewarming can now begin.

Anastomosis of pulmonary arteries

The two pulmonary arteries are then anastomosed using a continuous suture of 4/0 polypropylene (Figure 8.8). It is usually necessary to place suction catheters in one or both vessels during the procedure to ensure a clear field, free from blood.

By this time vigorous ventricular fibrillation or spontaneous coordinated myocardial contractions have usually occurred. If ventricular fibrillation is present, electrical defibrillation should be attempted. Further vigorous efforts to expel air from the cavities of the heart should then be repeated.

It has been our policy to provide at least 30 minutes' pump oxygenator support of the heart after release of the aortic clamp to allow full recovery of the donor heart from its ischaemic episode, before challenging it with responsibility for support of the circulation. During this period a careful check for bleeding is made on all suture lines, and further sutures inserted if necessary.

Discontinuation of pump oxygenator support

When myocardial function is clearly satisfactory, and adequate rewarming has taken place, the ventricular vent is removed. The SVC cannula is withdrawn into the right atrium, and the IVC cannula removed. Cardiopulmonary bypass is discontinued, and the aortic air vent removed. If cardiac performance is satisfactory, then the aortic and SVC cannulae are removed and protamine sulphate administered (Figure 8.9).

Two drains are inserted, one into the posterior pericardial cavity and the other into the anterior mediastinum after closure of the pericardium. The sternum is reunited with at least six stainless steel wire or other strong sutures, and the tissues anterior to the sternum repaired.

Comment

The two potential major complications of this operation are bleeding, in view of the extensive areas of anastomosis, and systemic air emboli. Great care must be taken to dispel all air from the left atrial and ventricular cavities before the donor heart resumes coordinated contractions after reperfusion.

Every effort must be made to maintain donor myocardial temperature as low as possible (yet avoid freezing injury) during transfer of the heart from donor to recipient, and this should be continued until blood reperfusion is commenced. The limitations of simple hypothermia and other storage methods in maintaining myocardial viability are discussed elsewhere (Chapter 5).

HETEROTOPIC HEART TRANSPLANTATION

Heterotopic heart transplantation has a long history in the experimental laboratory[1] (Chapter 1), but was not attempted clinically until 1974[6]. Based on extensive experimental work by Losman and Barnard[7], a form of heterotopic transplantation was carried out whereby the donor heart acted solely as a left ventricular assist device[6]. This operation involved anastomoses between the donor and recipient left atria and aortae; donor coronary sinus venous return was drained via the donor right atrium and right ventricle into the recipient circulation by anastomosing the donor pulmonary artery to the recipient right atrium. Two such operations were performed. Both patients suffered recurrent attacks of recipient heart dysrhythmias, including ventricular fibrillation, during which time the donor heart satisfactorily supported the circulation alone. As a result of this experience, however, the technique was modified to allow bypass and support of both recipient ventricles[6,8].

Heterotopic heart transplantation has both advantages and disadvantages over orthotopic transplantation (Chapter 20). Few other centres involved in heart transplantation have performed this operation. This may, in part, be due to lack of familiarity with the various technical steps of the procedure, which is a little more complex than orthotopic transplantation.

Donor heart excision

Donor heart excision is very similar to that described previously for orthotopic transplantation, but a greater length of SVC should be retained. The SVC is, therefore, mobilized along the whole of its length and two ligatures passed around it cranial to the azygos vein, which itself is doubly ligated and divided. Otherwise, excision follows the lines as described for orthotopic transplantation.

Preparation of the donor heart

The heart is placed in a bowl containing saline or cardioplegic solution at 4 °C, where it is prepared for implantation into the recipient (Figure 8.10).

The orifices of both right pulmonary veins and of the IVC are closed with continuous, double-layered sutures of 5/0 polypropylene, care being taken to ensure that coronary sinus drainage is not obstructed during closure of the IVC.

The bridge of tissue between the left superior and inferior pulmonary veins is excised to make a single opening into the left atrium; this opening may need to be extended to achieve a diameter of approximately 3.5–4 cm, or the equivalent of a normal mitral valve orifice. The midpoint of the posterior wall of this opening may be marked with a suture to act as a reference during subsequent implantation into the recipient.

A longitudinal 5 cm incision, just to the right of the interatrial septum, is made in the posterior aspect of the SVC and right atrium; at least half the length of this incision must involve the right atrial wall. The ligated azygos vein can be used as a reference marker for the posterior wall of the SVC.

Approximately 10 minutes are required to prepare the heart in this way. The organ is then transferred to the recipient surgical team.

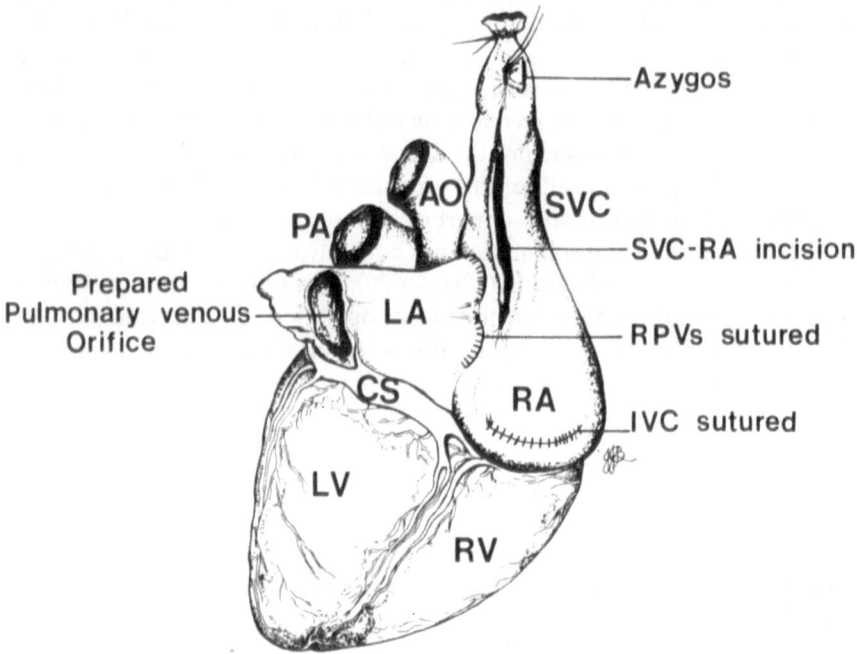

Figure 8.10   Heterotopic transplantation. Donor heart (posterior view) prepared for implantation

The recipient operation

With the patient supine, a midline sternotomy is performed and the peri-cardium opened longitudinally. A right-sided pleuropericardial flap is created (Figure 8.11), first by dividing the mediastinal pleura immediately posterior to the sternum and then by extending this incision medially over the diaphragm to a point 2 cm from the right phrenic nerve; a similar reflection of the pleuropericardium is made superiorly, extending the incision towards the SVC, again taking care to avoid the phrenic nerve. In this way a rectangular flap is created that comprises the parietal pericardium and mediastinal pleura. Haemostasis of the edges of this flap must be carried out carefully as no further opportunity to do this will arise. The flap is allowed to fall back over the hilum of the right lung (Figure 8.12), creating a single large right pleuro-pericardial cavity.

Initiation of cardiopulmonary bypass

The patient is fully heparinized. An aortic cannula is inserted at the level of the origin of the brachiocephalic artery, and venous cannulae into the SVC (through the right atrial appendage) and IVC (through the inferior right atrial wall). Cardiopulmonary bypass is initiated and a left ventricular apical vent introduced. The patient is cooled.

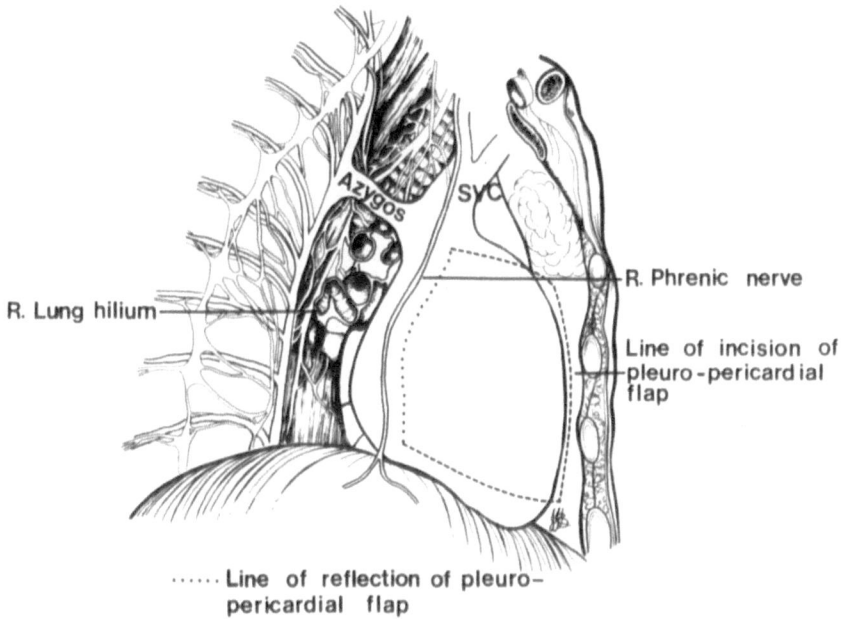

Figure 8.11 Heterotopic transplantation. Recipient: right-sided view of mediastinum; the line of the pleuropericardial incision is indicated

For most open heart procedures our cardiopulmonary bypass system includes two suction catheters and one ventricular suction vent, which return blood to the pump oxygenator; for heterotopic heart transplantation we have available three suction catheters and two vents (Chapter 7).

The recipient heart can be continuously perfused by the pump oxygenator, and therefore allowed to beat throughout the period of insertion of the donor heart. If the recipient heart is to remain beating, however, the temperature of the circulating blood must not be lowered much below 32°C (possibly to 28°C), or ventricular fibrillation is likely to occur, which may result in less satisfactory myocardial protection. Alternatively, the recipient aorta can be cross-clamped and the recipient heart protected by the infusion of cardio-plegic agent and by the topical application of cold saline throughout the operation. Cross-clamping of the recipient aorta may facilitate the technical steps of the operation by preventing recipient coronary sinus blood return to the operating field, and also allows the blood temperature to be reduced to lower levels, thus facilitating the maintenance of a low donor myocardial temperature. Systemic hypothermia of 26–28 °C is maintained, largely to diminish rewarming of the donor heart by its proximity to the recipient organs during its ischaemic period. Our own preference at present is for cardioplegic arrest and hypothermic protection of the recipient heart, as this allows rather better myocardial protection of the donor heart, which we feel has a high priority.

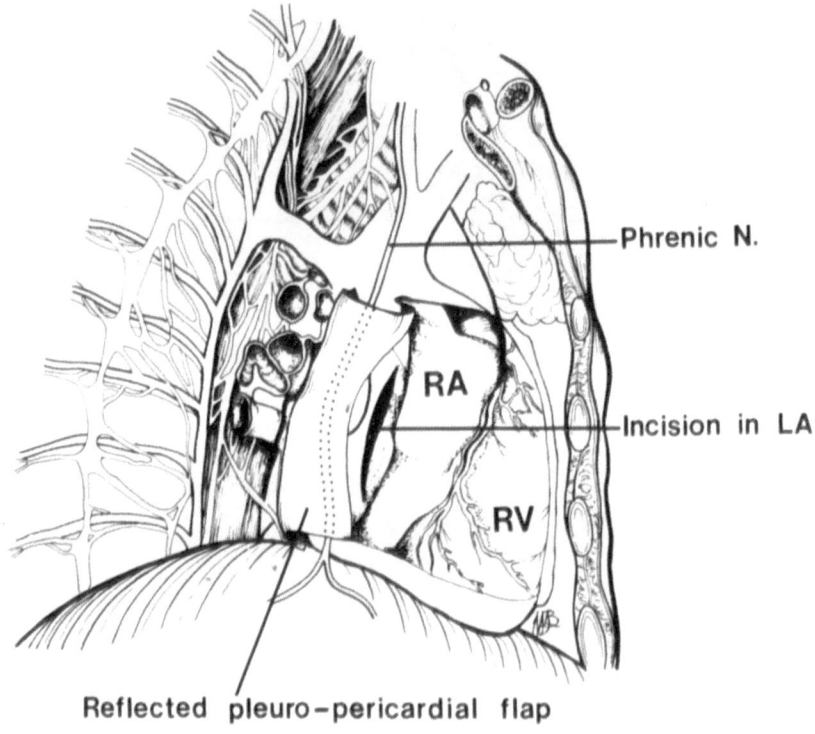

Phrenic N.

RA

Incision in LA

RV

Reflected pleuro–pericardial flap

Figure 8.12 Heterotopic transplantation. Recipient: reflection of pleuropericardial flap to lie anterior to the hilum of the right lung

The operation will therefore be described with the recipient heart arrested throughout (although the aortic cross-clamp is not indicated in the accompanying figures).

A catheter for cardioplegic solution infusion is placed in the root of the recipient aorta, which is then cross-clamped immediately proximal to the pump oxygenator cannula. Cardioplegic solution is rapidly infused into the root of the aorta, and cold saline poured over the heart to fill the pleuropericardial cavity.

Anastomosis of left atria

An incision, as for mitral valve surgery, is made into the recipient left atrium immediately posterior to the interatrial groove, extending from the superior to the inferior extremes of the groove (Figure 8.13).

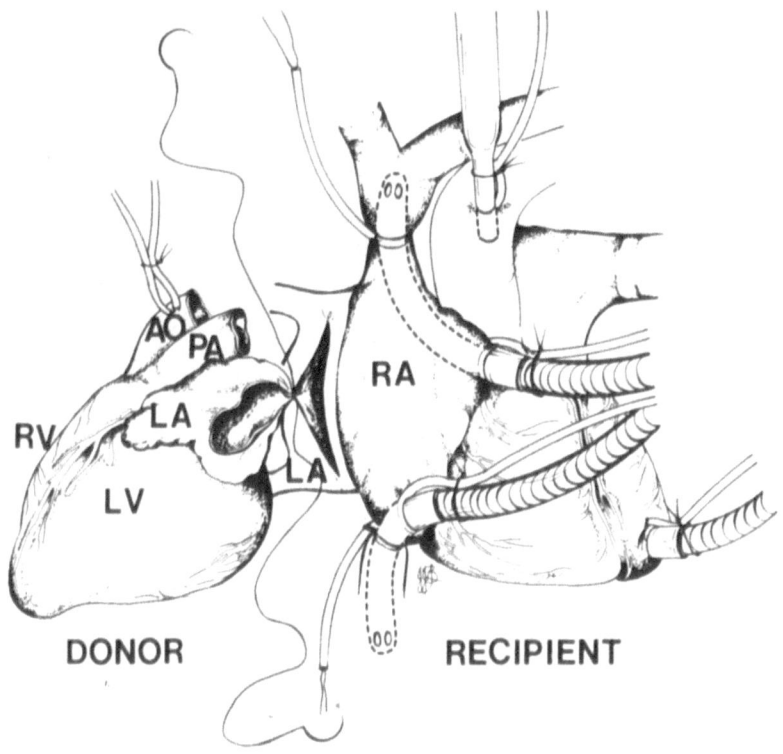

Figure 8.13 Heterotopic transplantation. Donor and recipient hearts, showing the beginning of the posterior suture line of the left atrial anastomosis

The donor heart is then placed in the right thoracic cavity anterior to the collapsed right lung and lying alongside the recipient heart. Using double-ended 4/0 polypropylene, the midpoint of the posterior lip of the incision in the recipient left atrium is sutured to the midpoint of the posterior lip of the opening in the donor left atrium. The two atria are anastomosed by a continuous suture, first along the posterior aspect and then along the anterior aspect. The completed anastomosis will be totally inaccessible at the end of the operation and therefore it is essential that it be haemostatic.

A wide communication between the two left atria has been created, forming a common atrium from which blood can enter either donor or recipient left ventricles.

Until recently it was our policy to introduce an apical vent into the donor left ventricle at this stage. Gentle suction was applied to help prevent myocardial rewarming by recipient blood, which returns to the common atrium by collateral flow. As a recipient left ventricular vent is already *in situ*, which almost certainly drains blood returning to the common atrium, the insertion of a vent into the donor heart at this stage is probably unnecessary. Before reperfusion of the heart by release of the aortic occlusion clamp, however, a vent is inserted into the donor left ventricle via the left atrial appendage and mitral valve, to remove air from this chamber.

Donor myocardial protection

Until the donor heart is revascularized, between each anastomosis, cold saline (4°C) is poured over both hearts to help maintain an adequate state of myocardial hypothermia. Further increments of cold cardioplegic solution should be infused into both recipient and donor ascending aortae at similar time intervals. The cannula inserted into the donor aorta for the initial infusion of cardioplegic agent before excision can be used again for this purpose. Once cardioplegic infusion has begun and all air displaced from the aorta, a cross-clamp is applied to occlude the distal end of this vessel, thus ensuring that the donor coronary arteries are adequately perfused.

Anastomosis of right atria

Clamps or snuggers (snares) are placed around the SVC and IVC, though, if venous drainage by the two indwelling cannulae is good, the application of snares may not be necessary; partial cardiopulmonary bypass may suffice. A 5 cm longitudinal incision is made into the lateral aspect of the recipient SVC and right atrium just anterior to the interatrial groove, beginning 2–3 cm above the vena caval–right atrial junction and continued 2–3 cm into the right atrium (Figure 8.14).

The donor SVC is extended alongside its counterpart. An eyelid retractor is used to retract the anterior lip of the incision in the recipient right atrium. The midpoint of the posterior lip of the incision in the recipient atrium is sutured to the most caudal point of the incision in the donor atrium, using a double-ended 5/0 polypropylene suture (Figure 8.15). The two right atria are then anastomosed by a continuous suture carried in each direction, first posteriorly (Figure 8.16) and then anteriorly. At the completion of this anastomosis the ligated donor azygos vein remnant will lie at the midpoint of the anterior suture line (Figure 8.17), over which a small metal ring is tied down as a fluoroscopic reference for the passage of endomyocardial biopsy forceps into the donor heart during the postoperative period.

The manoeuvre of suturing the midpoint of the posterior lip of the recipient atrial wall to the most inferior aspect of the incision in the donor atrium ensures that this anastomosis will remain wide, allowing free flow of blood from one chamber to the other, and permitting the easy passage of endo-myocardial biopsy forceps.

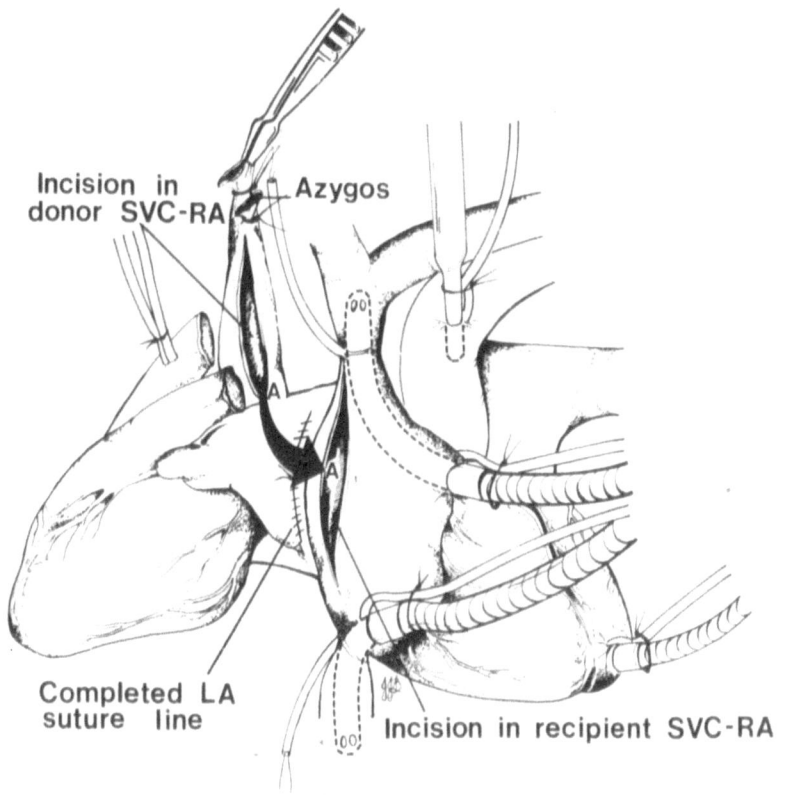

Figure 8.14 Heterotopic transplantation. Completed anterior left atrial suture line. The SVC–RA incision in each heart is shown; note that the inferior point of the incision in the donor SVC–RA (A) will be sutured to the midpoint in the posterior lip of the incision in the recipient SVC–RA (A)

Anastomosis of aortae

The donor aorta is trimmed to the minimum length required to allow anasto-mosis to the recipient aorta and yet avoid distortion or kinking of the left or right atrial anastomoses. An unnecessarily long donor aorta will allow the donor heart to drop back into the right pleural cavity, compressing the right lung. A short donor aorta will lift the donor heart anteriorly and superiorly, and allow for maximal expansion of the right lung posterior to the trans-planted organ. Temporary inflation of the lungs at this stage will help in estimating optimal length.

A longitudinal incision, equal in length to the diameter of the donor aorta, is made into the recipient aorta at a convenient point; it should be sited to the right of the midline. End-to-side anastomosis of donor to recipient aorta is made using a continuous suture of 4/0 polypropylene (Figure 8.17).

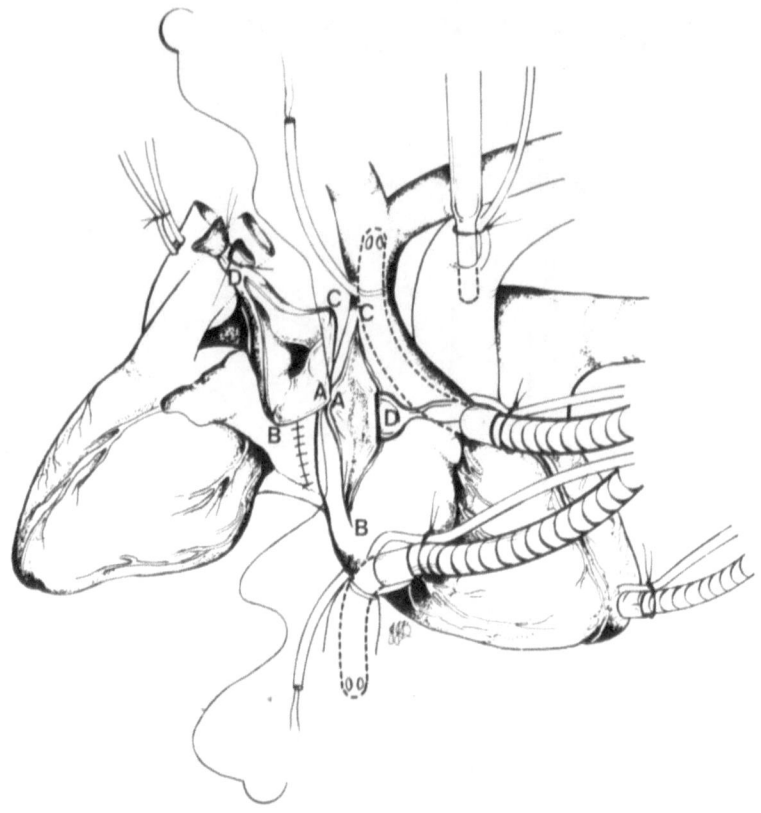

Figure 8.15 Heterotopic transplantation. The first suture in the anastomosis between the donor and recipient SVC–RA has been inserted (A:A)

The cardioplegic catheters in both aortae are converted to use as air vents, and the caval cannulae unsnugged. The cross-clamp is removed from the recipient aorta, and from this point both donor and recipient myocardiums are continuously perfused with blood from the pump oxygenator. To avoid continuous spillage of blood into the surgical field, a sucker is introduced into the donor pulmonary artery. The patient can now be rewarmed to 37°C.

Anastomosis of pulmonary arteries

In our experience, the donor pulmonary artery (PA) will not adequately reach to the recipient PA without undue tension or distortion of the other anastomoses; a conduit is therefore inserted. Originally, a length of donor descending aorta was excised and utilized for this purpose, but more recently we have used a pre-clotted woven Dacron graft. The size of graft chosen will depend largely on the diameter of the donor PA; this is usually of the order of 22 mm. (With a similarly sized polytetrafluorethylene ('Gor-tex') graft, difficulty has been found in positioning it to configurate with the surrounding anatomy without kinking.)

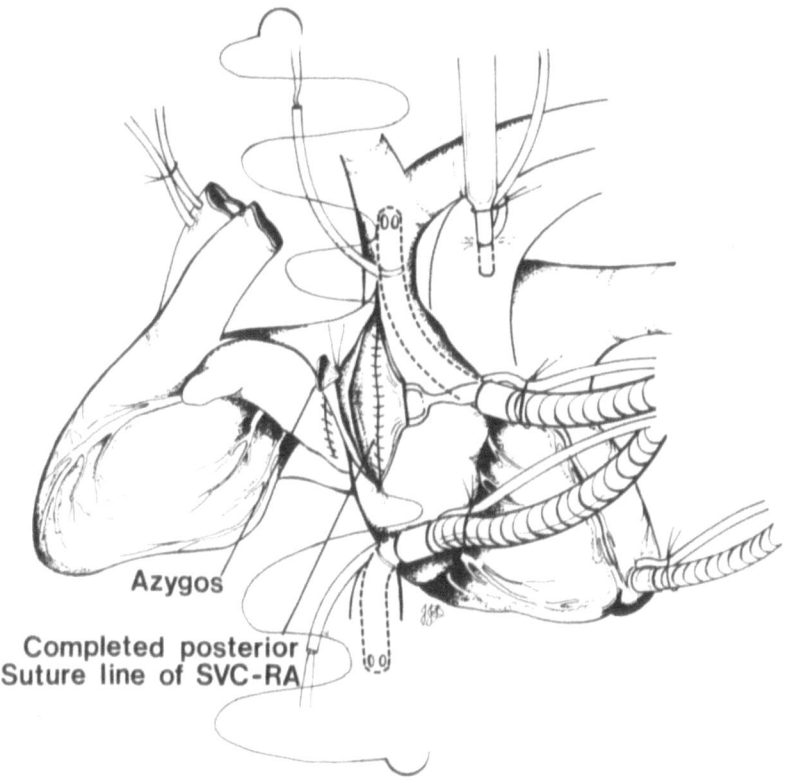

Azygos

Completed posterior
Suture line of SVC-RA

Figure 8.16 Heterotopic transplantation. Completed posterior right atrial suture line

A longitudinal incision of suitable length is made in the recipient main PA. The Dacron graft is anastomosed end-to-side to the recipient PA using continuous 4/0 polypropylene, the first stitch being placed at the distal end of the incision (Figure 8.18). The graft is tailored to the correct length to bridge the gap between the two pulmonary arteries. The end-to-end anastomosis to the donor PA is again performed using continuous 4/0 polypropylene (Figure 8.19). To ensure a bloodless field during this procedure, it is sometimes necessary to insert a flexible sucker along the lumen of the Dacron graft into the recipient PA; both recipient and donor PA suckers are removed before completion of the final anastomosis.

As rewarming occurs the donor heart will either begin spontaneous sinus rhythm or lapse into vigorous ventricular fibrillation, requiring electrical defibrillation. After evacuation of air from *both* donor and recipient left ventricles the donor left ventricular vent is removed. Further attempts to expel air from the recipient left ventricle are made before removal of the second vent.

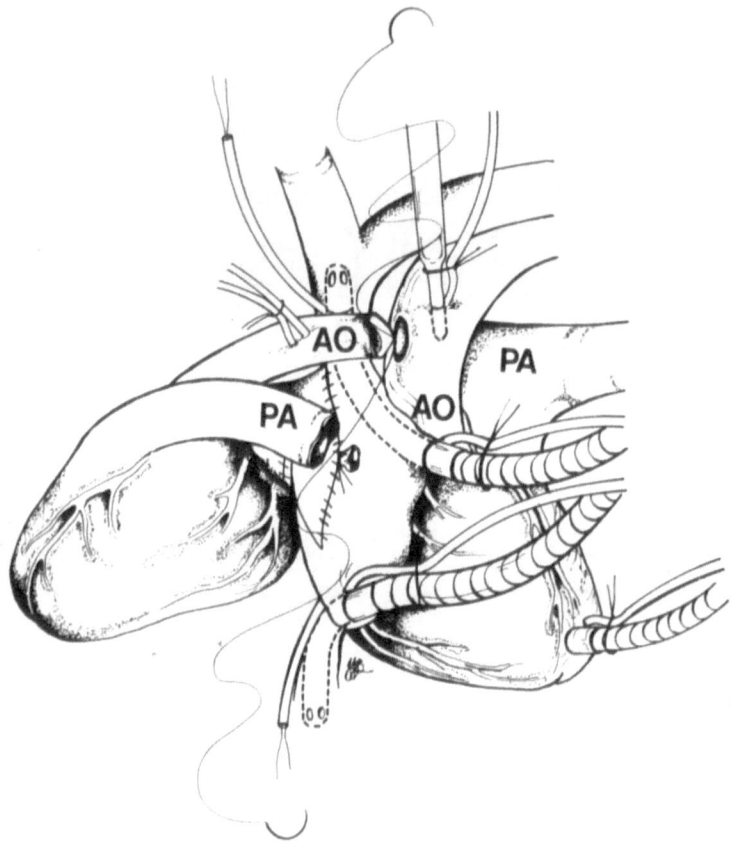

Figure 8.17 Heterotopic transplantation. The SVC–RA anterior suture line has been completed; beginning of aortic anastomosis. When the recipient heart is continuously perfused throughout the operation, a side-biting clamp is applied to the aorta for the performance of this anastomosis

Discontinuation of pump oxygenator support

As with orthotopic transplantation it has been our policy to allow at least 30 minutes for donor heart recovery, especially if the ischaemic time has been long. During this period a careful inspection is made of the accessible suture lines to confirm haemostasis; the PA and aortic anastomoses can usually be inspected satisfactorily, but it is frequently difficult to inspect the anterior right atrial suture line, and impossible to see the deeper suture lines. The venous cannula in the SVC is withdrawn into the right atrium, the IVC cannula removed, and, if the haemodynamic status of each heart is stable, cardiopulmonary bypass is discontinued and the patient decannulated (Figure 8.20). The heparin is neutralized with protamine sulphate. Three drains are inserted, one into the pericardial cavity posterior to the recipient heart, a second anterior to this heart, and a third to ensure adequate drainage of the right pleural cavity.

Before closure of the chest the anaesthetist is requested to ventilate both lungs fully to ensure expansion of the right lung, particularly of the lower lobe, which has been compressed by the donor heart throughout the procedure. The sternum is united with at least six wire or other strong sutures.

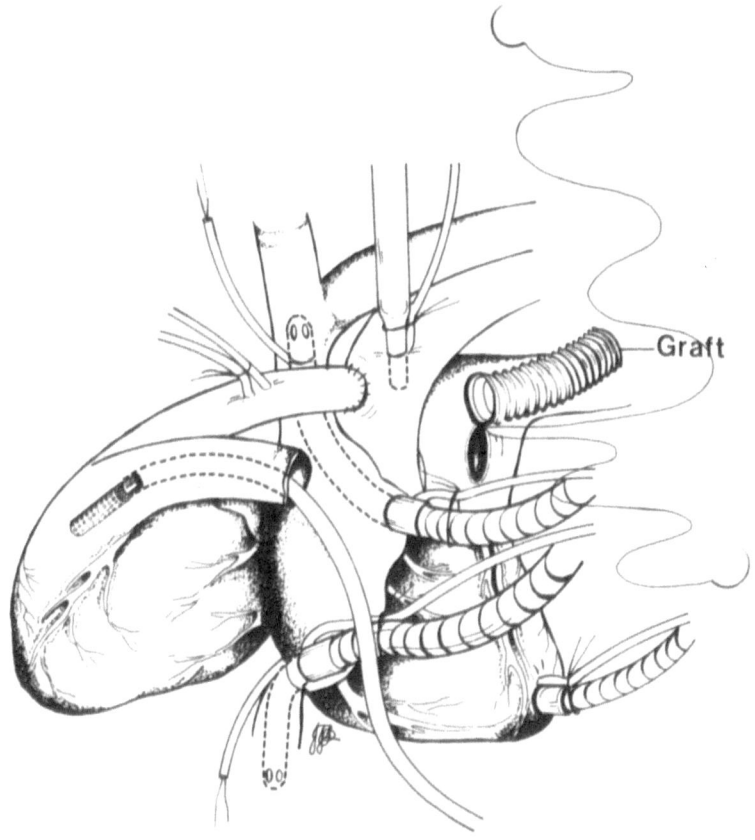

Figure 8.18 Heterotopic transplantation. The aortic anastomosis has been completed; recipient pulmonary artery (PA) incision and beginning of anastomosis of Dacron graft

In our experience the recipient operation in its entirety requires approximately 4–5 hours for completion.

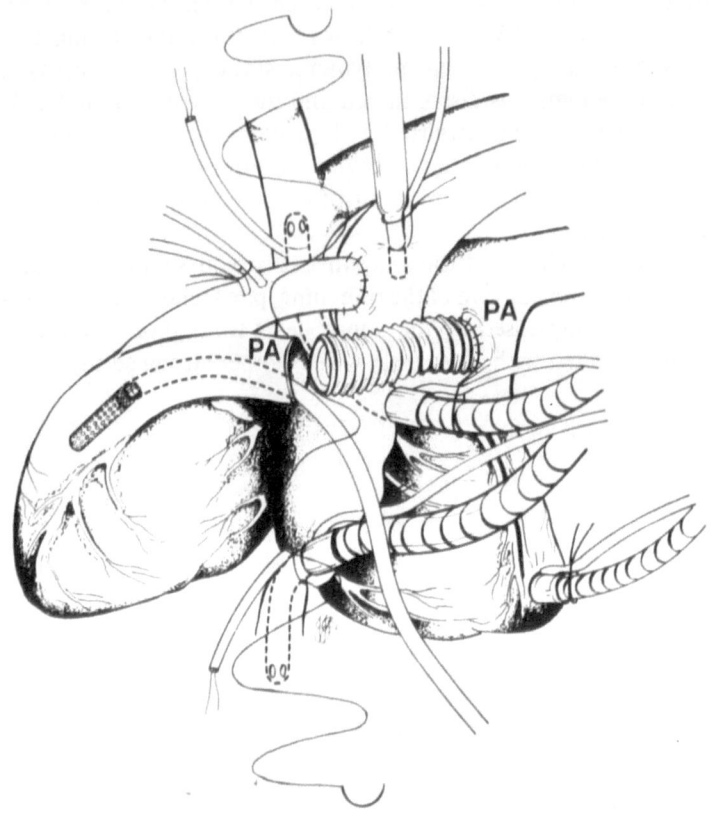

Figure 8.19   Heterotopic transplantation. Completed distal (recipient) PA-graft anastomosis; beginning of proximal (donor) PA-graft anastomosis. A suction catheter has been inserted through the pulmonary valve into the donor right ventricle

COMMENT

This operation has been combined on occasion with other procedures to the recipient heart, such as resection of a left ventricular aneurysm, coronary artery bypass graft, or mitral annuloplasty. Although this technique involves the inclusion of a vascular prosthesis into a patient who will subsequently be heavily immunosuppressed, we have seen no infectious complications related to the presence of this graft.

Neither the left nor the right atrial anastomosis must be restrictive. If the right atrial anastomosis is confined to the superior venae cavae, then inadequate flow into the donor right atrium may result. Any subsequent contraction at the suture line may lead to difficulty in manipulating biopsy forceps into the donor right ventricle; in such cases left ventricular biopsies must be obtained by the arterial route. The incision in each heart must be extended well down into the atrial wall.

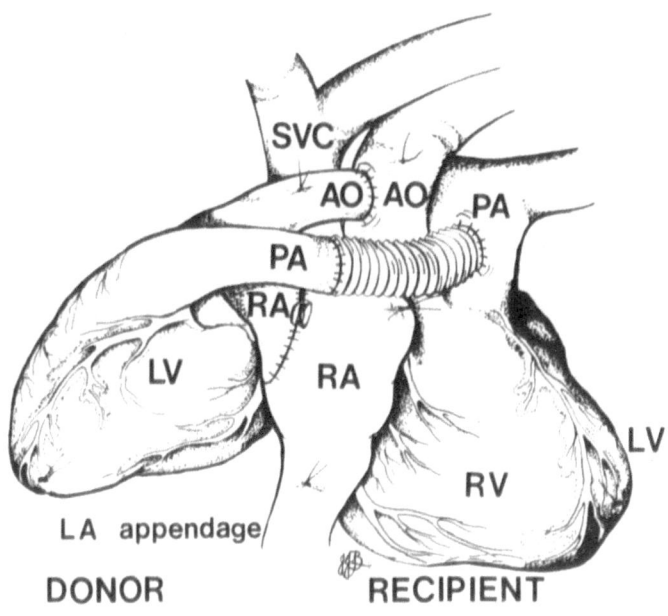

Figure 8.20   Heterotopic transplantation. Completed operation

Heterotopic heart transplantation by the technique described above connects the donor heart in parallel with the recipient heart. Preferential flow to donor or recipient ventricle will be directly related to the respective ventricular compliance. Ejection of blood is asynchronous, depending on the different heart rates, but does not substantially interfere with the performance of either heart[9].

Some collapse of the right lower lobe is always present at the end of the operation, but with adequate physiotherapy this lobe expands over the course of the next few days; this has not increased the incidence of postoperative pulmonary infection in this lobe. The presence of the heterotopic allograft in the right chest (Figures 8.21 and 8.22) leads to a slight reduction in right lung volume, but in no case has this been associated with symptoms of impaired ventilatory capacity. We have transplanted large adult hearts into two 14-year-old boys without problems in this respect.

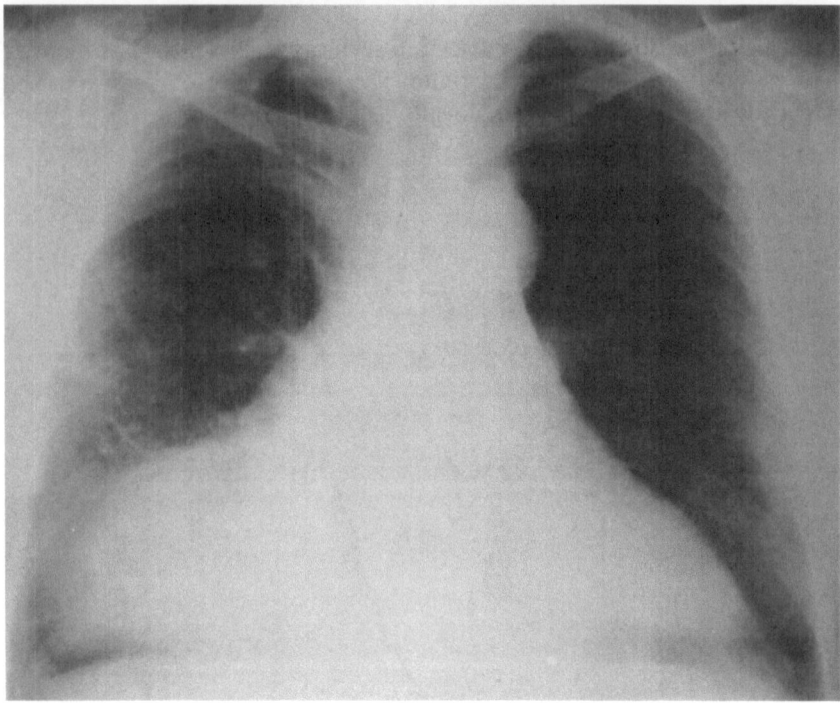

Figure 8.21   Postero-anterior chest radiograph of patient with heterotopic heart transplant; the donor heart lies in the right chest

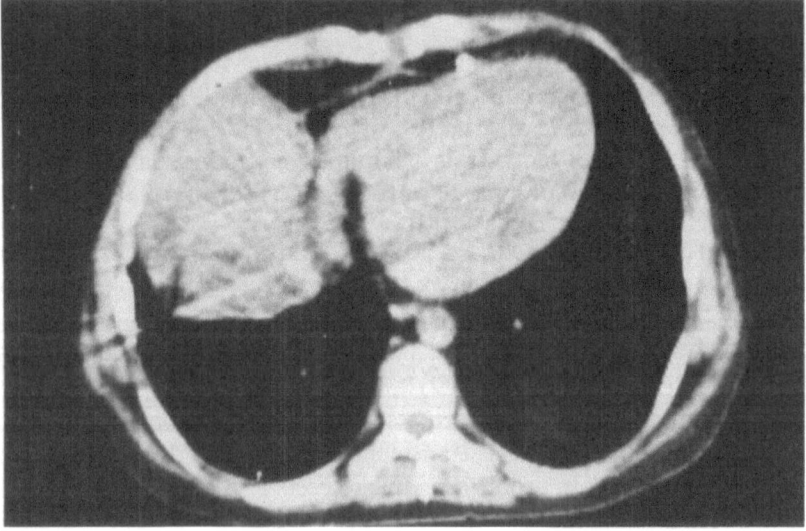

Figure 8.22   Computerized axial tomographic scan of the chest (viewed from below) showing the donor heart in the right chest anteriorly

References

1. Cooper, D. K. C. (1968). Experimental development of cardiac transplantation. *Br. Med. J.*, **4**, 174
2. Lower, R. R. and Shumway, N. E. (1960). Studies on orthotopic transplantation of the canine heart. *Surg. Forum*, **11**, 18
3. Hardy, J. D., Chavez, C. M., Kurrus, F. E., Webb, W. R., Neely, W. A., Eraslan, S., Turner, M. D., Fabian, L. W. and Labecki, J. D. (1964). Heart transplantation in man: developmental studies and report of a case. *J. Am. Med. Assoc.*, **188**, 113
4. Barnard, C. N. (1967). A human cardiac transplant: an interim report of a successful operation performed at Groote Schuur Hospital, Cape Town. *S. Afr. Med. J.*, **41**, 1271
5. Barnard, C. N. (1968). What we have learnt about heart transplants. *J. Thorac. Cardiovasc. Surg.*, **56**, 457
6. Barnard, C. N. and Losman, J. G. (1975). Left ventricular bypass. *S. Afr. Med. J.*, **49**, 303
7. Losman, J. G. and Barnard, C. N. (1977). Haemodynamic evaluation of left ventricular bypass with a homologous cardiac graft. *J. Thorac. Cardiovasc. Surg.*, **71**, 695
8. Novitzky, D., Cooper, D. K. C. and Barnard, C. N. (1983). The surgical technique of heterotopic heart transplantation. *Ann. Thorac. Surg.*, **36**, 476
9. Beck, W. and Gersh, B. J. (1976). Left ventricular bypass using a heterotopic cardiac allograft: hemodynamic studies. *Am. J. Cardiol.*, **37**, 1007

9
Immediate Postoperative Care and Maintenance Immunosuppressive Therapy

IMMEDIATE POSTOPERATIVE CARE

The immediate postoperative care of a patient who has undergone heart transplantation, whether it be orthotopic or heterotopic, is identical to that of any patient who has undergone open heart surgery. Special precautions need to be taken, however, to minimize the risk of infection. Maintenance immunosuppressive therapy is begun immediately before the operation and is continued afterwards.

Patient monitoring

The patient will return from the operating theatre intubated and ventilated with a volume-cycled ventilator capable of providing intermittent mandatory ventilation and positive end-expiratory pressure. *In situ* arterial and central venous (CVP) cannulae allow monitoring of pressures, and other intravenous lines allow replacement of blood and fluid as well as administration of vasoactive drugs if necessary. A urinary catheter, rectal temperature probe, and electrocardiogram (ECG) electrodes are also in position. If heterotopic heart transplantation was performed, the ECG electrodes are positioned to allow clear monitoring of complexes from both hearts. *In situ* drainage catheters will drain both the posterior pericardial cavity and anterior mediastinum in the case of an orthotopic transplant, as well as the right pleural cavity in the case of a heterotopic transplant.

It has not been our policy to monitor either left atrial or pulmonary artery 'wedge' pressures in our patients; neither left atrial cannulae nor Swan Ganz catheters have been employed. The complex anatomy of heterotopic heart transplants renders measurement of cardiac output difficult. Following orthotopic transplantation, if donor heart function is clearly satisfactory, we do not feel that measurements of left heart pressures or cardiac output are necessary. Such observations may be essential, however, if donor heart function is poor, requiring intravenous inotropic drug therapy.

The nursing staff will monitor arterial and central venous pressures, rectal temperature, respiratory and ventilator parameters, the heart rate(s), and peripheral pulse rate. They will also keep careful records of blood loss from the drains, urinary output, and blood, plasma and fluid input.

Most centres involved in heart transplantation consider it an advantage to extubate the patient as soon as possible to minimize the risk of chest infection. It is argued that the presence of an indwelling endotracheal tube, which prevents the normal cough reflex, and the intermittent introduction of tracheal suction catheters are factors that predispose to infection. Extubation should be carried out as soon as the patient is awake enough to cooperate with the nursing and physiotherapy personnel and can cough when requested, as long as his or her haemodynamic state is satisfactory. We have not seen any early postoperative chest infection, however, in patients in whom, for one reason or another, there has been a delay in extubation until 24 or even 48 hours have elapsed. There would appear to be a greatly increased risk of chest infection should the patient require ventilation beyond this time.

Chest drains are removed when there is no risk of further bleeding and, in the heterotopic heart transplant patient, in the absence of a right pneumothorax or significant pleural effusion. Removal can generally be carried out within 48 hours, but has on occasion been delayed. We have experienced no complications from leaving the drains in longer, if indicated.

Initially chest radiographs are taken at least every 12 hours until the chest drains have been removed and the patient is being mobilized, and then at daily intervals to augment the clinical examination of the chest. The radiographs are taken primarily to confirm bilateral lung re-expansion and absence of pleural effusion, particularly after heterotopic transplantation, and the absence of areas of consolidation that suggest infection. Frequent chest radiographs are obtained throughout the hospital stay of the patient to exclude early changes suggestive of infection.

Precautions to prevent infection

Meticulous attention to sterility is required by the nursing staff for all procedures affecting the patient. All personnel attending the patient should wash their hands before touching the patient or his bed. Sterile gloves should be worn whenever preparing an injection, especially if it is to be administered intravenously, or changing infusion bottles.

Several specimens are taken each day for laboratory study to monitor possible early infection. Tracheal aspirate, blood, urine, and swabs from the throat and from around the various drains and cannulae are sent daily for the first few days for culture to exclude significant bacterial growth. Urine and throat gargle viral culture media are sent for virological studies. Blood cytomegalovirus titres are estimated weekly.

All arterial and intravenous cannulae are removed as soon as possible to reduce the risk of introducing infection into the blood either through or alongside the cannulae. With careful attention, a CVP line can be left *in situ* for several weeks, if required, in patients who require such a line for any purpose, such as the daily intravenous administration of antithymocyte globulin. The alternative is to set up a new intravenous line each day to give this agent. It has been our policy to withdraw the indwelling CVP cannula approximately 1 cm per day, clean the surrounding skin with iodine or other effective antiseptic, and apply a new sterile dressing on each occasion. Withdrawing the cannula daily may help to prevent the accumulation of bacteria at the cutaneous entry side. With meticulous care to this matter, an intravenous infusion may be maintained infection-free for several weeks.

The patient should be nursed in a clean-air environment. The number of hospital personnel entering the room should be kept to a minimum. All personnel should ideally change into 'operating room' garments before entering the patient's room, or at least cover their outer clothing with a clean surgical gown, and wear masks and caps. We believe that these procedures reduce the risk of introducing infection into the room from the outside.

Physiotherapy

To ensure early re-expansion of the lungs and to keep the airways clear of secretions, physiotherapy is commenced within 2 h of operation and continued every 4 h for 2 days, and then as often as necessary until the patient is fully mobilized, at which time it may be reduced or discontinued altogether. In the intubated patient this takes the form of vigorous vibration of the thoracic cage, postural drainage, and hyperinflation of the lungs by manual Ambu bagging to expand the lungs and loosen secretions, followed by tracheobronchial suction. A mucolytic agent may be injected into the airways of patients with viscid secretions. In the extubated patient, nebulization of the airways by a Bird ventilator, together with positive end-expiratory pressure, followed by assisted expectoration, should be carried out every 4 h to prevent atelectasis and to keep the airways free of excessive secretions.

Within 2 h of operation passive muscular exercises are introduced, particularly to the legs to prevent deep vein thrombosis and to strengthen the musculature. Active exercises are introduced as soon as the patient can cooperate. As soon as possible, usually within 48 h, the patient should be assisted to sit and stand out of bed at intervals of a few hours, and encouraged to become fully mobile over the next few days.

These patients have frequently been relatively inactive or even bedridden for some weeks or months before transplantation due to their underlying myocardial failure. Their muscles may have become weak and wasted. Furthermore, the steroid drugs, which are given to prevent rejection, particularly if given in large doses, contribute in most patients to a further wasting of the musculature that is so extreme in some to warrant the description of 'steroid myopathy'. Frequent and regular attention is required from the physiotherapist if this muscle wasting is to be kept to a minimum and eventually reversed. Each patient is prescribed a programme of exercises which he is expected to perform every 2 h throughout the waking hours. This exercise programme concentrates on strengthening the arms and legs. Static dynamic bicycle riding is generally begun under the physiotherapist's supervision within the first 3 or 4 days, as long as the patient's general condition does not contraindicate this more vigorous form of exercise. Initially the bicycle workload is set low and the period of time the patient spends on it strictly restricted to 2 minutes, but both factors are steadily increased as the patient's recovery continues. Bicycle riding is carried out four times each day and the period of exercise increased up to 15 minutes per session.

During a severe acute rejection episode, when the myocardium is oedematous and undergoing cellular infiltration and myofibre injury, we believe it is only sensible to restrict the exercise of the patient in an effort to minimize permanent myocardial damage. Vigorous exercise such as bicycle riding should be omitted, though gentle exercise and walking should continue.

Prevention of psychological isolation

Though the patient is physically isolated in his or her intensive care unit room for several days or weeks, or even months in some cases, this psychological isolation should be minimized by providing adequate visual and auditory communication systems with the outside. Visiting relatives and friends should be encouraged to use this communication system, but only one or two close relatives should be allowed to enter the isolation room; these relatives must take the same precautionary measures as the hospital staff. It is equally important to prevent boredom by providing such facilities as television and/or video, which the patient may make use of if he feels inclined. The occupational therapist may play an important role at this stage.

DRUG THERAPY OTHER THAN IMMUNOSUPPRESSION

Antibiotic therapy

In our unit, all patients undergoing open heart surgery receive cephamandole 1 g intravenously at the time of induction of anaesthesia, which is repeated when cardiopulmonary bypass is initiated, and continued after operation every 6 h for 2 days or until the patient has been extubated. This has also been our policy in patients undergoing heart transplantation. Prolonged prophy-lactic antibiotic therapy is to be avoided in the immunosuppressed patient, as there is a greater risk of this leading to fungal overgrowth, an important cause of infection in such patients, and to the growth of bacteria resistant to that particular antibiotic. Further antibiotics should only be given when signs of clinical infection are present and when the causative organism(s) has been identified, if this proves possible. Further guidelines on infection and anti-biotic policy are given in Chapter 13.

Vasoactive drug therapy

If inotropic support is indicated we prefer dobutamine hydrochloride, though isoprenaline hydrochloride is administered if an increase in donor heart rate is considered desirable. Relative sinus bradycardia with a rate falling to 30–40 beats/minute has been seen in some patients during the first week or two. In all cases this has spontaneously and steadily increased to at least 50 beats/min within a few days. Persistently low heart rates suggest that a degree of heart block may have been induced at operation; more detailed ECG studies should be carried out to clarify this point. If an atrioventricular conduction defect is confirmed, pacing of the heart should be considered. An epicardial system is preferable to reduce the risk of septicaemia and thrombosis.

We have also observed the need for temporary inotropic support in the occasional patient with pulmonary infection, particularly in mycobacterial infections such as tuberculosis, presumably as a result of an increase in pulmonary vascular resistance.

Intravenous vasodilator therapy with, for example, sodium nitroprusside, may be indicated in the early postoperative period to reduce afterload, as in any patient who has undergone open heart surgery. The administration of the immunosuppressive agent, cyclosporin A, is associated with hypertension in a significant number of patients. This may require control with vasodilators administered orally, such as prazosin, or calcium antagonists, such as nifedipine.

Pain relief

Large doses of morphine and other central nervous system or respiratory depressant drugs should be avoided before extubation; intravenous doses of 2.5 mg of morphine given when necessary rarely cause significant respiratory depression. After extubation adequate pain relief or, preferably, pain avoid-ance is essential if the patient is to be encouraged to cough adequately to prevent secretion accumulation in his airways.

Dysrhythmias

Most patients undergoing heart transplantation have received digoxin before operation. After transplantation digoxin is normally unnecessary, but may be indicated for rhythm disturbances of the donor heart, which are relatively uncommon in hearts that have not suffered damage from prolonged ischaemia during implantation, or of the recipient heart in patients with heterotopic heart transplants. These latter dysrhythmias can often be ignored, unless they lead to haemodynamic embarrassment of the donor heart, which rarely occurs. It should be remembered that the denervated donor heart is less sensitive to the effects of digoxin than is an innervated heart. Other therapeutic agents that have an effect in correcting dysrhythmias may be indicated, though again the response of the denervated donor heart may differ from that of an innervated heart. Calcium antagonists, such as verapamil hydrochloride, and β-blocking agents have a greater effect on the denervated heart than on an innervated heart. After heterotopic transplantation, the effect of such drugs on each heart should be monitored and the dosage carefully balanced to prevent unwanted effects in either heart.

Fluid retention

A diuretic is frequently necessary during the first few postoperative days, particularly in patients who were in severe cardiac failure before operation. We generally use intravenous frusemide until the patient is clearly free of peripheral oedema, and then continue with oral frusemide or other diuretics if such therapy is indicated for a longer period of time; the fluid-retention effect of corticosteroids may make this necessary in some patients. Cyclosporin A (CYA) therapy, particularly if given intravenously, may be associated with an acute oliguria, which may respond to frusemide therapy, though, in addition, reduction in the CYA dosage or omission of this drug is required for a period of time. It may be difficult to distinguish oliguria from CYA toxicity from acute tubular necrosis from other courses. This topic is discussed further in Chapter 18.

Prevention of steroid-induced peptic ulceration

Corticosteroids are associated with numerous complications, several of which may be life-threatening (Chapter 18). Cimetidine is begun immediately after operation to help prevent gastric erosion or stress ulcer. The drug is initially administered intravenously (200 mg 6-hourly) while the patient is still intubated, and subsequently given orally (200 mg at 6-hourly intervals during the day and 400 mg at night). As an additional safeguard it has been our policy to give an antacid, such as aluminium hydroxide or magnesium trisilicate, during the first month or two after transplantation when steroid dosage may remain high.

Anticoagulation

Full anticoagulation is unnecessary in patients with orthotopic heart transplants unless there are other specific indications. It is our policy, however, to give an anti-platelet agent indefinitely.

Patients with heterotopic heart transplants, however, are at risk from thrombus formation in the ventricles of the recipient heart which are likely to be functioning very inadequately, with resulting systemic or pulmonary embolism (Chapter 20). In the presence of an adequately functioning donor heart, the recipient's own heart may not generate enough left ventricular pressure to open the aortic valve consistently. Not infrequently, thrombus formation has already occurred prior to transplantation in these myopathic ventricles and further clots may develop following transplantation. If the aortic valve of the recipient heart is observed never to open, which is, in fact, rare, especially in the early postoperative months, the risk of systemic embolism might be considered to be non-existent, but this assumption would be incorrect. In most of these hearts the mitral valve is incompetent as a result of the left ventricular dilatation that usually occurs from longstanding cardiac failure, whether this be from cardiomyopathy or ischaemic heart disease. Thrombus may subsequently collect in the recipient left ventricle and spread through the incompetent mitral valve into the common left atrium, from where it may be ejected by the donor left ventricle as an embolus.

It is essential therefore to fully anticoagulate patients in whom the recipient heart remains *in situ*. Warfarin sodium administration is begun once the chest drains have been removed and is continued for the lifetime of the patient. An antiplatelet agent such as sulphinpyrazone (200 mg 8-hourly) or dipyridamole (100 mg 6-hourly) is also administered. Disprin or other salicylates have been avoided in view of the risk of gastric erosion, which is already increased in patients receiving corticosteroids.

Prevention of chronic rejection

It is generally considered that a diet low in lipids may reduce the rate of progression of chronic rejection (accelerated graft arteriosclerosis) (Chapters 16 and 17). This diet should be initiated as soon as practicable in the postoperative period.

Hypercholesterolaemia

In patients with underlying ischaemic heart disease who are known to be hypercholesterolaemic, therapy with a cholesterol-reducing agent, such as cholestyramine, may reduce the rate of progress of atheroma in peripheral vessels; in patients at risk this therapy is begun in the early postoperative period. Whether such therapy slows the development of graft arteriosclerosis remains in doubt.

Antituberculous therapy

Long-term antituberculous therapy is essential in patients who have con-tracted this disease in the past. In patients with features on chest radiographs of previous tuberculosis infection it has become our policy to administer isoniazid for the first 6 months as prophylaxis against recurrence.

Vitamins

We have also administered vitamins B, which may be depleted in patients with preoperative liver failure, and C, to promote healing, to our patients during their hospital stay.

MAINTENANCE IMMUNOSUPPRESSIVE THERAPY

Before 1983, when cyclosporin A became available to us, we used what is commonly referred to as 'conventional' immunosuppressive therapy (a com-bination of azathioprine and methylprednisolone with or without antithymo-cyte globulin). Cyclosporin therapy, which was introduced into clinical renal transplant practice by Calne in 1978[1], has been regarded as 'experimental' during the past few years. Our own limited experience with CYA supports the good experience of the cardiac transplant group at Stanford University[2] and the many renal and liver transplant centres which have had access to this drug[3]. It would therefore seem no longer sensible to refer to azathioprine and methylprednisolone therapy as 'conventional', as it would appear that CYA will increasingly become the basic immunosuppressive agent of choice.

The various pharmacological immunosuppressive agents available to those involved in transplantation have been discussed by a number of authors, notably by Salaman[4], and detailed accounts of their structure and mode of action can be found elsewhere[5-9].

1. Azathioprine, corticosteroids, and antithymocyte globulin

Azathioprine

Azathioprine is one of a large group of antimetabolite compounds that compete for and block specific receptors, thus affecting DNA and RNA synthesis, and interfering with protein synthesis. Azathioprine was introduced into experimental and clinical practice with regard to renal transplantation by Calne in 1961[10]. Specifically, it is a purine antagonist that is similar in structure to 6-mercaptopurine. Since these agents are only effective against prolifer-ating cells, they are most effective when given *after* antigen exposure[11]. All immune responses requiring cell proliferation may be inhibited by the drug, including antibody production and graft rejection. It is rather ineffective when used as the sole immunosuppressant following human renal transplantation[12,13]. It has not been used alone after cardiac transplantation.

Azathioprine's main toxic effect is on the bone marrow, which results in leukopenia, thrombocytopenia and, occasionally, anaemia, though leukopenia has rarely proved a problem following cardiac transplantation. Following withdrawal or reduction of the drug, recovery of the bone marrow is usually rapid in patients with cardiac allografts. Very occasionally azathioprine causes liver dysfunction, though we have not experienced this to any significant degree in the patients under our care; substitution of azathioprine with cyclophosphamide is recommended in such cases.

It has been our policy to begin azathioprine immediately before operation with a loading dose of approximately 3–4 mg/kg intravenously. After transplantation it is given initially intravenously and subsequently orally at the maximal tolerated level as judged by the absence of bone marrow and hepatic toxicity. The intravenous and oral doses are identical. In our experience the average dose for adults ranges between 1.5 and 4.5 mg/kg/per day; the total white blood count should be maintained in the range of 3000–5000 cells/mm³.

Corticosteroids

Steroids were introduced into clinical renal transplant practice in 1963[14], though the evidence that they protect tissue allografts is surprisingly sparse[6]. It is the glucocorticoids, rather than the mineralocorticoids, which possess immunosuppressive activity. Prednisone or prednisolone have been most commonly used in transplantation. They inhibit a variety of intracellular enzymes that depress protein, RNA, and DNA synthesis. There is extensive death of small lymphocytes in the blood, thymus, lymph nodes and spleen, though the mechanism for this effect is not well understood. Much of the immunosuppressive action of steroids is, however, attributed to their anti-inflammatory properties. Cell-mediated immunity is depressed in most species.

The timing of steroid administration is probably not critical. It is often assumed that high-dose therapy must be started immediately rejection has been diagnosed if the graft is to be saved, and yet this may not be true. In the rat heart allograft model a single bolus of methylprednisolone is more effective in prolonging graft survival when given late than when given early in the rejection process[15].

There are many different regimens for administering steroids to transplant patients. Our own regimen has been to begin with relatively large intravenous doses for the first 6 days, following with a moderately high oral dose, which is steadily reduced over the first 3 months. A regimen of 600 mg of methylprednisolone sodium succinate on the day of operation (in three divided doses of 200 mg each—preoperative, peroperative and postoperative) is reduced by 100 mg/day until discontinued, by which time oral methylprednisolone of 64 mg/day has been introduced. Depending on the patient's progress, the oral dose is steadily reduced towards a goal of 32 mg/day at 3 months, and to 20 mg/day at 1 year, though these goals are frequently not achieved.

A low-dose maintenance steroid regimen has been found to be just as effective as a high-dose regimen in both patients[16-18] and animals[19] with kidney grafts. There is also evidence from experimental work at our own centre that survival of heart grafts in baboons is the same whether the baboons receive a low-dose or a high-dose regimen (Table 9.1); the low-dose regimen appeared to be associated with less infectious complications[20].

Table 9.1 Survival of heterotopic cardiac allografts in baboons receiving various immuno-suppressive regimens or immunoregulatory procedures

Group	Treatment	Number of baboons	Mean survival time ($\pm SD$) (days)	Median survival time (days)	Mean survival time *Difference from:	
					Group 1	Group 2
1	Control	10	11.0 (± 5.6)	9.5	—	$p < 0.025$
2	AZA 2.5 mg/kg per day MP 2 mg/kg per day	7	19.1 (± 10.6)	20.0	$p < 0.025$	—
3	AZA 2.5 mg/kg per day MP 0.5 mg/kg per day	8	18.3 (± 7.6)	17.5	$p < 0.025$	NS
4	AZA 2.5 mg/kg per day MP 0.5 mg/kg per day 1 g i.v. bolus methylprednisolone (days 5, 6 and weekly)	6	15.2 (± 6.9)	15.0	NS	NS
5	AZA 5 mg/kg per day MP 2 mg/kg per day	8	25.6 (± 24.9)	16.0	$p < 0.05$	NS
6	AZA 2.5 mg/kg per day MP 2 mg/kg per day Cyclophosphamide 1 mg/kg per day	5	15.0 (± 5.1)	15.0	NS	NS
7	AZA 2.5 mg/kg per day MP 2 mg/kg per day Propranolol 1–2 mg/kg per day	6	17.8 (± 13.8)	17.0	NS	NS
8	Pre-transplant splenectomy AZA 2.5 mg/kg per day MP 2 mg/kg per day	6	10.7 (± 2.5)	10.5	NS	$p < 0.05$
9	Niridazole 50 mg/kg per day	7	13.9 (± 5.1)	11.5	NS	NS
10	Niridazole 25 mg/kg on alternate days, reducing to 8 mg/kg every 3 days AZA 2.5 mg/kg per day MP 2 mg/kg per day	7	26.3 (± 11.5)	30.0	$p < 0.01$	NS
11	AZA 2.5 mg/kg per day MP 2 mg/kg per day Niridazole metabolite 10–25 mg/kg per day	3	22.0 (± 9.2)	24.0	$p < 0.025$	NS

*Student's t-test for unpaired data; AZA = azathioprine; MP = methylprednisolone.

This experimental work prompted us to use a low-dose regimen in five consecutive patients undergoing heterotopic heart transplantation or retransplantation. Recipients received our standard intravenous methylprednisolone of 600 mg on the day of operation, reducing by 100 mg doses daily, at which time they were given a maintenance oral dose of 32 mg/day instead of the usual 64 mg/day. Although four of the five patients survived the initial 6-month period, all four suffered at least one episode of severe, and in three cases early, acute rejection. The one death was from viral pneumonia on the 35th day in a patient who had suffered no significant acute rejection. Two patients received very large total doses of steroids, as they both required long courses of intravenous methylprednisolone in the treatment of multiple episodes of severe acute rejection. The total dosage they received exceeded that of many of our previous patients who received a higher maintenance dose of methyl-prednisolone. In one, after his fourth severe acute rejection episode, main-tenance methylprednisolone dosage was increased to 64 mg/day and he suffered no further acute rejection. There are so many variables in the treatment of any one patient undergoing heart transplantation that it is difficult to arrive at any meaningful conclusions from this small experience, particularly with so few patients. Nevertheless, our short experience with the low-dose regimen was not encouraging.

Early in the Groote Schuur Hospital experience, it was our policy to give booster doses of steroids (1 g methylprednisolone i.v.) at weekly intervals during the first 2–3 months following transplantation, based on the hypothesis that such booster doses might prevent acute rejection episodes from occur-ring, or at least abort rejection at an early stage[21]. In recent years we returned to this policy. Though we have no confirmatory statistical evidence, it has been our impression that patients who received a weekly 1 g dose of i.v. methylprednisolone suffered fewer acute rejection episodes than those who did not. Salaman has reported a beneficial effect from similar booster doses of steroids in rats with kidney grafts, if given when rejection is anticipated[19]. In baboons with heart grafts, however, we have been unable to show that this therapy increases survival (Table 9.1)[22].

Antithymocyte globulin

Antithymocyte globulin (ATG) has been shown to prolong renal allograft survival[23–25], and was first introduced into a cardiac transplant programme by the Stanford group in 1973[26]. Although we originally used equine anti-lymphocyte globulin (EALG), in recent years we have used rabbit antithymo-cyte globulin (RATG); each has been given on a daily basis by intravenous infusion for the first 4–6 weeks following transplantation.

The immunosuppressive effect of antilymphocyte globulin (ALG) was first demonstrated in the rat skin graft model[27]. The properties of ALG depend to a large extent on its method of preparation. It can be prepared against a wide variety of antigens, including those on thoracic duct or blood lymphocytes and thymocytes. ALG is prepared by immunizing, most commonly, rabbits or horses with human lymphocytes or thymocytes. A clear description of the steps involved in its preparation is given by Touraine *et al.*[28]. The dosage varies widely, depending on the preparation used.

In recent years, RATG (ATG Fresenius) has been the globulin of choice at our institution. This is administered immediately before operation in a dose estimated to reduce the circulating T-lymphocytes to the therapeutic range of 50–150 cells/mm^3. The usual dose has been approximately 2.5–5.0 mg IgG/kg per day; we have always given this drug intravenously. After operation the T-lymphocytes are counted daily using the sheep red cell rosetting test, and the dosage of antithymocyte globulin estimated accordingly. We have found it relatively easy to determine the dose necessary to maintain the T-lymphocytes at the desired level. In our unit, this particular RATG has been given in doses of up to 1000 mg/day (approximately 12 mg IgG/kg per day), though the daily dosage has varied widely from patient to patient. The drug is diluted in 100–200 ml normal saline and is given as a single daily infusion over a period of 1–2 hours. When severe acute rejection is occurring and the T-lymphocytes multiplying rapidly, it may be preferable to administer it in divided doses to distribute its therapeutic effect more evenly across a 24 h period.

Allergic reactions to RATG have been unusual in our experience, though two patients experienced anaphylactic reactions. It has been our policy to give an antihistamine such as promethazine hydrochloride (12.5 mg) intravenously immediately before the infusion of the RATG. The Stanford group has preferred the intramuscular administration of this agent, but repeated injections cause local inflammation and pain[26]. Although the use of ATG remains controversial we have found it to be an effective adjunct to azathioprine and corticosteroids.

The several potential complications of each of these three 'conventional' immunosuppressive agents—azathioprine, corticosteroids and ATG are discussed in Chapter 18.

Adjunctive therapy

Heparin. Until 1981 it was our policy to heparinize the patient for the first 2 weeks after transplantation (beginning after removal of the chest drainage tubes) and during episodes of acute rejection. (Warfarin sodium therapy was begun towards the end of this initial 2-week period for continued anticoagulation of patients with heterotopic allografts.) Heparinization was thought to be beneficial by helping to prevent immunologically-induced intravascular thrombosis. This policy was discontinued in the light of reports that showed no beneficial effect in patients with kidney grafts[29].

Other. With azathioprine and a steroid such as methylprednisolone as the standard immunosuppressive therapy, much experimental and clinical work has been carried out towards improving its efficacy by adding a further drug or by replacing azathioprine with an alternative immunosuppressive agent. Salaman has comprehensively reviewed this subject[4].

Conclusion

In our experimental laboratory we have investigated several agents known to have immunosuppressive effects either *in vitro* or *in vivo*. We have been fortunate in being able to carry out this work in primates using the Chacma baboon heterotopic heart transplant model[20, 22, 30]. Using a modification of the Mann technique[31] for heterotopic heart transplantation in the neck, we have studied the effect of several agents, or procedures such as splenectomy, on allograft survival. The results are outlined in Table 9.1. No agent or procedure that we have investigated to date has been found to increase allograft survival significantly. Our experimental results with regard to the effect of pretransplantation blood transfusion on cardiac allograft survival have already been summarized (Chapter 6).

Until cyclosporin became available to us, therefore, we had no personal evidence, nor could we find any good evidence in the literature, to change our immunosuppressive regimen from a combination of azathioprine, methylprednisolone and antithymocyte globulin.

2. Cyclosporin A

Cyclosporin was initially isolated from the fermentation broth of a soil fungus, *Trichoderma polysporum Rifai*[32]. The cyclosporins have a narrow spectrum of antibiotic activity[33], reducing the growth rate of a few yeasts and fungi. Full reviews of the immunosuppressive properties of this drug have been published elsewhere[3, 34–36]. Cyclosporin appears to act by blocking the T helper cell function and has little or no effect on B cells. It does not depress the bone marrow as do antimetabolites.

Although some renal transplant groups administer CYA alone[37], only adding a steroid if acute rejection occurs, most groups favour a combination of CYA and low-dose steroids[38]. Most heart transplant centres, including our own, also use a combination of CYA and steroids[39–41].

Ideally, CYA should be begun 6 hours before operation, at least one dose of 18 mg/kg being administered orally. After the operation we administer a total of 12 mg/day given in two divided doses until blood levels are obtained. The dose is then adjusted to maintain therapeutic levels in the blood (see below). The drug comes in liquid form and is commonly given in a chocolate drinking solution that the pharmaceutical company (Sandoz Ltd, Basle, Switzerland) provides. If the patient is unable to take oral drugs, then CYA can be given intravenously, but in much reduced dosage of approximately 5 mg/kg/day, divided into two doses. The intravenous dose is diluted in normal saline (100 mg/CYA in 100 ml saline) and administered over a 2–3 hour period to reduce its renal toxic effect. Both the oral and intravenous forms can induce oliguria from toxicity on the proximal renal tubules. In our experience the intravenous administration of CYA appears to be more readily followed by acute anuria and therefore we have preferred to avoid this form of administration whenever possible. It is usually possible to give the drug orally to patients recovering from cardiac transplantation even on the first postoperative day. Intramuscular administration is not recommended, since the drug is very poorly absorbed.

Whether CYA is given orally or intravenously it is essential to measure the blood levels frequently (preferably daily, but at least three times each week) during the first 4 weeks until the dosage has been adjusted to achieve the correct therapeutic blood level. Blood levels are then estimated at least weekly for one further month and on a monthly basis thereafter. Blood should be drawn immediately before administration of the drug to give a 'trough' level, and 2 or 4 hours afterwards to give a 'peak' level. Cyclosporin levels are measured by a radioimmunoassay technique[42]. Dosage should be adjusted to maintain the trough level between 300 and 500 ng/ml. The peak level is of less importance, but very high peak levels (above 1000 ng/ml) should be avoided if possible. The higher peak and lower trough levels that occur when cyclosporin is given intravenously may require a reduction in the dosage and an increase in the frequency of administration.

It has become our policy to estimate the blood levels on the first postoperative day and reduce the dosage accordingly. In our limited experience we have found that there is a high risk of inducing significantly impaired renal function if the dosage is not adjusted rapidly to maintain blood trough levels within the therapeutic range. Maintenance doses of approximately 6 mg/kg per day are generally achieved within 1–2 months.

We have noted at our institution that rather lower dosages of CYA are required to maintain adequate blood trough levels in the early postoperative period in patients with cardiac transplants than in patients with renal transplants. This may be related to the fact the CYA is excreted through the liver, and that the rate of excretion may therefore be reduced in patients who have had longstanding hepatic congestion secondary to cardiac failure. A number of other drugs affect the blood levels of CYA, in particular, ketoconazole and cimetidine, which increase its concentration, and phenytoin, rifampicin and phenobarbitone, which decrease its concentration.

In view of the toxic effect of CYA on the proximal tubules, careful monitoring of the blood urea, serum creatinine, and creatinine clearance is essential. The blood urea remains slightly elevated during CYA administration, though the serum creatinine may remain within normal levels. The most sensitive test would appear to be the creatinine clearance, which falls when toxicity occurs. We have attempted to adjust the dosage of the drug to maintain a creatinine clearance of more than 60 ml/minute. Cyclosporin dosage is reduced if the clearance should fall below this level. Diuretic therapy may help to maintain the creatinine clearance above this level.

Hepatotoxic effects of CYA have been reported with increasing levels of various liver enzymes[3], though we have not found this to be a significant problem in administering the drug. The potential complications of use of this drug are discussed more fully in Chapter 18.

In combination with CYA, we have administered a relatively low dose of methylprednisolone. On the day of operation the patient receives 125 mg i.v. every 8 hours (on induction of anaesthesia, during the operation, and after the operation). On the first postoperative day the patient receives 125 mg i.v. of methylprednisolone in the morning and evening, and a total of 1 mg/kg per day orally in two divided doses on subsequent days. This is reduced steadily by approximately 1–2 mg/day during the course of the first month if the patient's progress with regard to episodes of acute rejection permits. We therefore expect methylprednisolone dosage to be 0.3–0.4 mg/kg per day by 1 month, and less than 0.2 mg/day by 1 year.

Using this regimen, our initial experience with CYA has been good. Though we have experienced problems with the renal toxic effects, our patients have suffered very few major rejection episodes. Mild acute rejection episodes have been relatively common, but severe episodes certainly less frequent than when immunosuppression has been with azathioprine, corticosteroids and RATG. The immunosuppressive efficacy of CYA allows steroid dosage to be reduced at 1 month to levels not reached with conventional immunosuppression for at least 3–6 months, and commonly not until the end of the first year. This is a major advance that reduces the debilitating effects and complications associated with high-dose steroid therapy. It will be interesting to see whether corticosteroid therapy might be discontinued completely in some, if not all, patients receiving CYA who remain well for longer than 2 or 3 years after cardiac transplantation. The long-term effects of CYA therapy, however, remain uncertain, and a number of questions relating to its effect on renal function, blood pressure, and the development of graft arteriosclerosis, remain unanswered.

References

1. Calne, R. Y., White, D. J. G., Thiru, S., Evans, D. B., McMaster, P., Dunn, D. C., Craddock, G. N., Pentlow, B. D. and Rolles, K. (1978). Cyclosporin A in patients receiving renal allografts from cadaver donors. *Lancet*, **2**, 1323
2. Oyer, P. E., Stinson, E. B., Jamieson, S. W., Hunt, S. A., Billingham, M., Scott, W., Bieber, C. P., Reitz, B. A. and Shumway, N. E. (1983). Cyclosporin A in cardiac allografting: a preliminary experience. *Transplant. Proc.*, **15**, 1247
3. White, D. J. G. (ed.) (1982). *Cyclosporin A*. (Amsterdam: Elsevier Biomedical)
4. Salaman, J. R. (ed.) (1981). *Immunosuppressive Therapy*. (Lancaster: MTP Press)
5. Schwartz, R. S. (1968). Immunosuppressive drug therapy. In Rapaport, F. T. and Dausset, J. (eds.) *Human Transplantation*. p. 440. (New York: Grune & Stratton)
6. Santos, G. W. (1972). Chemical immunosuppression. In Najarian, J. S. and Simmons, R. L. (eds.) *Transplantation*. p. 206. (Philadelphia: Lea & Febiger)
7. Bach, J. F. (1976). The pharmacological and immunological basis for the use of immunosuppressive drugs. *Drugs*, **11**, 1
8. Hurd, E. R. (1977). Drugs affecting the immune response. In Holborow, E. J. and Reeves, W. G. (eds.) *Immunology in Medicine*. p. 1067. (London: Academic Press)

9. Berenbaum, M. C. (1975). The clinical pharmacology of immunosuppressive agents. In Gell, P. G. H., Coombs, R. R. A. and Lachman, P. J. (eds.) *Clinical Aspects of Immunology*. p. 689. (Oxford: Blackwell Scientific)

10. Calne, R. Y. (1961). Inhibition of the rejection of renal homografts in dogs by purine analogues. *Transplant. Bull.*, **28**, 65

11. Hersh, E. M., Cargone, P. P. and Freireich, E. J. (1966). Recovery of immune responsiveness after drug suppression in man. *J. Lab. Clin. Med.*, **67**, 566

12. Gleason, R. E. and Murray, J. E. (1967). Report from Kidney Transplant Registry: analysis of variables in the function of human kidney transplants. *Transplantation*, **5**, 360

13. Kries, H., Lacombe, M., Noel, L. H., Descamps, J. M., Chailley, J. and Crosnier, J. (1978). Kidney graft rejection: has the need for steroids to be re-evaluated? *Lancet*, **2**, 1169

14. Goodwin, W. E., Kaufman, J. J., Mims, M. M., Turner, R. D., Glassock, R., Goldman, R. and Maxwell, M. M. (1963). Human renal transplantation. I. Clinical experiences with six cases of renal homotransplantation. *J. Urol.*, **89**, 13

15. Salaman, J. R. and Couhig, E. (1980). Timing of anti-rejection therapy. *Transplantation*, **29**, 468

16. McGeown, M. G., Kennedy, J. A., Loughridge, W. G. G., Douglas, J. F., Alexander, J. A., Clarke, S. D., McEvoy, J., Hewitt, J. C. and Nelson, S. D. (1977). One hundred kidney transplants at the Belfast City Hospital. *Lancet*, **2**, 648

17. Chan, L., French, M., Beare, J., Oliver, D. O. and Morris, P. J. (1980). Prospective trial of low-dose versus high-dose prednisolone in renal transplant patients. *Transplant Proc.*, **12**, 323

18. McGeown, M. G., Douglas, J. S., Brown, W. A., Donaldson, R. A., Kennedy, J. A., Loughridge, W. G. G., Mehta, S., Nelson, S. D., Doherty, C. C., Johnstone, R., Todd, G. and Hill, C. (1980). Advantages of low-dose steroid from the day following renal transplantation. *Transplantation*, **29**, 287

19. Salaman, J. R. (1983). Influence of steroid dosage in the survival of cardiac allografts in the rat. *Transplantation*, **35**, 510

20. Cooper, D. K. C., Rose, A. G. and Barnard, C. N. (1982). Low-dose versus high-dose steroid therapy in the prevention of acute rejection in baboon heterotopic cardiac allografts. *Transplantation*, **34**, 107

21. Barnard, C. N. (1969). A new approach to the treatment of rejection: experience with the third human-to-human heart transplantation performed in Cape Town. *Prog. Cardiovasc. Dis.*, **12**, 201

22. Cooper, D. K. C., Novitzky, D., Lanza, R. P., Rose, A. G., Wicomb, W. N. and Barnard, C. N. (1984). Immunosuppression in the baboon cardiac allograft model: effects of splenectomy, bolus methylprednisolone, propranolol, high-dose azathioprine, cyclophosphamide, and a niridazole metabolite. *Transplantation*. (In press)

23. Nagaya, H. and Sieker, H. O. (1965). Allograft survival: effect of antiserums to thymus glands and lymphocytes. *Science*, **150**, 1181

24. Davis, R. C., Cooperband, S. R. and Mannick, J. A. (1969). Preparation and *in vitro* assay of effective and ineffective antilymphocyte sera. *Surgery*, **66**, 58

25. Levey, R. H. and Medawar, P. B. (1966). Trial of rabbit antihuman ALG in cadaver kidney transplantation. *Ann. NY Acad. Sci.*, **129**, 164

26. Baumgartner, W. A., Reitz, B. A., Oyer, P. E., Stinson, E. B. and Shumway, N. E. (1979). Cardiac homotransplantation. *Curr. Probl. Surg.*, **16**, 1

27. Woodruff, M. S. A. and Anderson, N. F. (1963). Effects of lymphocyte depletion by thoracic duct fistula and administration of lymphocyte serum on the survival of skin homografts in rats. *Nature (London)*, **200**, 702

28. Touraine, J. L., Malik, M. C. and Traeger, J. (1981). Antilymphocyte globulin and thoracic duct drainage in renal transplantation. In Salaman, J. R. (ed.) *Immunosuppressive Therapy*. p. 55. (Lancaster: MTP Press)

29. Griffin, P. J. A. and Salaman, J. R. (1981). A controlled trial of heparin in renal transplant rejection. *Transplantation*, **32**, 306

30. Boyd, S. T., Cooper, D. K. C., Baigrie, R., Rose, A. G. and Barnard, C. N. (1981). An investigation of the immunosuppressive effects of niridazole and metronidazole in rat and baboon heterotopic allograft models. *Transplantation*, **31**, 326

31. Mann, F. C., Priestley, J. T., Markowitz, J. and Yater, W. M. (1933). Transplantation of the intact mammalian heart. *Arch. Surg.*, **26**, 219

32. Borel, J. F., Feurer, C., Gubler, H. U. and Stahelin, H. (1976). Biological effects of cyclosporin A: a new antilymphocytic agent. *Agents Actions*, **6**, 468

33. Dreyfuss, M., Harri, E., Hofmann, H., Kobel, H., Pache, W. and Tscherter, H. (1976). Cyclosporin A and C: new metabolites from *Trichoderma polysporum*. *Eur. J. Appl. Microbiol.*, **3**, 125

34. Green, C. J. (1981). Cyclosporin A. In Salaman, J. R. (ed.) *Immunosuppressive Therapy*. p. 75. (Lancaster: MTP Press)

35. Morris, P. J. (1981). Cyclosporin A. *Transplantation*, **32**, 349

36. Borel, J. F. (1982). Immunological properties of cyclosporin A. *Heart Transplant.*, **1**, 237

37. Calne, R. Y., Rolles, K., White, D. J. G., Thiru, S., Evans, D. B., Henderson, R., Hamilton, D. L., Boone, N., McMaster, P., Gibby, O. and Williams, R. (1981). Cyclosporin A in clinical organ grafting. *Transplant. Proc.*, **13**, 349

38. Starzl, T. E., Hakala, T. R., Rosenthal, J. T., Iwatsuki, S. and Shaw, B. W. (1983). The Colorado–Pittsburgh cadaveric renal transplantation study with cyclosporine. *Transplant. Proc.*, **15**, 2459

39. Oyer, P. E., Stinson, E. B., Jamieson, S. W., Hunt, S. A., Perlroth, M., Billingham, M. and Shumway, N. E. (1983). Cyclosporine in cardiac transplantation: a 2½-year follow-up. *Transplant. Proc.*, **15**, 2546

40. Hardesty, R. L., Griffith, B. P., Debski, R. F. and Bahnson, H. T. (1983). Experience with cyclosporine in cardiac transplantation. *Transplant. Proc.*, **15**, 2553

41. Wallwork, J., Cory-Pearce, R. and English, T. A. H. (1983). Cyclosporine for cardiac transplantation: UK trial. *Transplant. Proc.*, **15**, 2559

42. Donatsch, P., Abisch, E., Homberger, M., Traber, R., Trapp, M. and Voges, R. (1981). A radioimmunoassay to measure cyclosporin A in plasma and serum samples. *J. Immunoassay*, **2**, 19

10
Physiology and Pharmacology of the Transplanted Heart

INTRODUCTION

The primary function of the heart is to deliver oxygenated blood to the tissues of the body, in accordance with their metabolic requirements. In order to meet these rapidly changing metabolic demands, the response of the heart and peripheral circulation is integrated by a number of intrinsic and extrinsic control mechanisms[1-3].

The major factors which determine the cardiac output and its distribution are outlined in Figure 10.1[1]. Many of these factors are intricately regulated by the central nervous system (sympathetic and parasympathetic), humoral mechanisms (circulating catecholamines) and intrinsic metabolic and electrolyte alterations. These regulatory mechanisms ensure a controlled, integrated response of the heart and peripheral circulation to increased stress.

PHYSIOLOGY OF THE TRANSPLANTED HEART

Cardiac transplantation results in complete denervation of the heart, which is permanent[4-10], thereby depriving the heart of the important neural regulating mechanisms. Nevertheless, the actions of a number of other compensatory mechanisms allow the circulatory system to meet the increased demands placed upon it at times of stress, thus enabling a large proportion of transplant recipients to be rehabilitated successfully and returned to an active life[11,12].

The resting state

Heart rate

Following the abolition of the usually dominant inhibitory vagal influences (by denervation), the resting rate of the transplanted heart is generally higher than normal[4–10, 13–15], and does not reflexly alter in response to the Valsalva manoeuvre[4, 5], carotid sinus massage[5], alterations in body position[4, 5, 16], or drugs such as phenylephrine, atropine or amyl nitrate[4–6].

Cardiac dynamics

Although the cardiac index of the transplanted heart is lower than that of normally innervated control hearts, it remains in the normal range; resting cardiac dynamics are essentially normal[6, 7, 10].

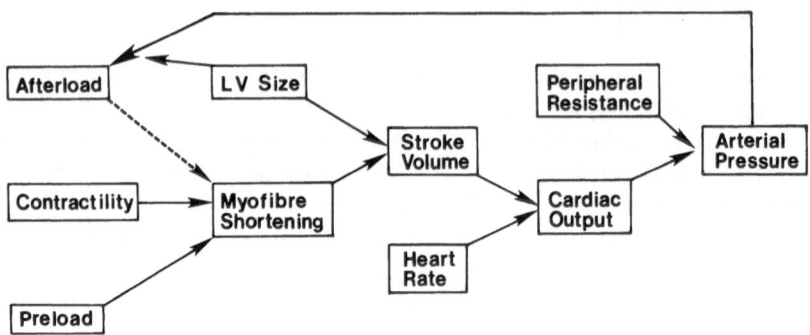

Figure 10.1 Diagram showing the interactions between the various components regulating cardiac activity (after Braunwald[1]). Solid lines represent an increasing effect; the dotted line indicates a depressant effect. The numerous factors which affect these components themselves have not been included. Note, however, that left ventricular (LV) size is a determinant of both the afterload and the stroke volume. The preload, by altering LV size, may therefore influence the afterload

Response to exercise

Isometric exercise

Isometric exercise increases systemic arterial blood pressure in normal healthy subjects[17, 18]. Sustained isometric contractions of more than 15% of the voluntary maximum (irrespective of the size of the muscle involved) result in the accumulation of muscle metabolites which stimulate reflex afferents, causing sympathetic activation and vagal inhibition. Thus, heart rate increases, peripheral vasoconstriction occurs and cardiac output increases slightly.

Following cardiac transplantation, patients performing isometric exercise increase their systolic and diastolic blood pressures in a manner identical to that of control subjects[15, 19, 20]. The cardiac acceleration observed in control subjects does not occur, but cardiac output in both control subjects and transplant recipients rises slightly, though not significantly. The major alteration, accounting for the observed rise in blood pressure, is an increase in the peripheral vascular resistance. Peripheral resistance rises equally in both groups[19, 20].

Dynamic exercise

Dynamic exercise differs from static, isometric exercise in that not only is peripheral perfusion pressure increased, but cardiac output must be increased and appropriately distributed in order to deliver nutrients to, and remove metabolites from, the periphery.

The fact that transplant recipients are able to perform significant amounts of dynamic exercise is well recognized[6, 10, 13, 16]. The transplanted, denervated heart is able to increase its output significantly in response to exercise, but it does appear that maximal work capacity may be less than that achieved by age-matched control subjects[10, 16]. There are some striking differences in the mechanisms whereby normal and transplanted hearts increase their cardiac output in response to an increase in demand.

(1) *Heart rate.* In the normal situation, the heart rate is determined not only by the intrinsic rate of spontaneous depolarization in the sinoatrial node, but also by extrinsic neural (sympathetic and parasympathetic) and humoral (circulating catecholamines) mechanisms. With the onset of exercise (and even occasionally preceding exercise) heart rate rises rapidly, remains elevated for the duration of exercise and subsides promptly after the cessation of exercise. These alterations are mediated predominantly by the neural mechanisms (sympathetic stimulation and parasympathetic inhibition).

The heart rate of the transplanted heart, which is generally higher at rest than that of controls, does rise with dynamic exercise, but the pattern of response is different from that of controls. The heart rate of transplant recipients rises much more gradually after the onset of exercise, never reaches the same peak heart rate, and subsides more slowly after cessation of exercise[4, 5, 8, 9, 14]. This change in heart rate is mediated predominantly by a rise in the levels of circulating catecholamines[8, 21-23]. Changes in heart rate correlate with changes in the levels of circulating noradrenaline[8], and can be inhibited by β-receptor blockers. If the effects of circulating catecholamines are blocked pharmacologically, a small rise of about 10 beats per minute still occurs in response to exercise[21, 22]. This is probably related to the chronotropic effect of right atrial distension produced by increased venous return.

(2) *Cardiac output and work.* In normally innervated hearts, changes in heart rate account for most of the increased cardiac output which occurs, whilst stroke volume remains virtually unchanged. Vasodilatation of the blood vessels supplying the exercising muscles results in a decreased peripheral vascular resistance and an increased venous return. With more strenuous exercise, the increased preload (due to the increased venous return) results in an increase in the stroke volume (the Frank–Starling mechanism), thus further increasing the cardiac output[1-3, 24-26].

The transplanted heart, despite the initial lack of cardioacceleration, is able to increase its output rapidly in response to dynamic exercise[5-10, 13, 14]. In contradistinction to the normally innervated heart, the Frank–Starling mechanism appears to play a major role early in this response, as the left ventricular end-diastolic pressure[5–8, 10, 13] and volume[8] rise early in exercise, and stroke volume and cardiac output increase concomitantly (before any change in heart rate). Peripheral circulatory changes are similar to those which occur in the normal subject.

At higher work loads, the chronotropic and inotropic effects of circulating catecholamines, such as noradrenaline, play a more prominent role[6, 8, 9], increasing the heart rate, circumferential fibre shortening[8], and ejection fraction[9] of the transplanted heart, causing a further increase in the cardiac output[6, 8, 9]. These effects may be enhanced by the known sensitivity of the denervated heart to catecholamines[5, 27, 28].

It is apparent, however, that despite these compensatory mechanisms, the cardiac output of the transplanted heart, both at rest and at peak exercise, may be lower than that of normally innervated control hearts[6, 10, 15]. Similarly, the duration of the period of exercise which can be maintained is less than in control subjects[10, 16]. Even if work load is increased gradually to allow the somewhat delayed compensatory mechanisms of the denervated, transplanted heart to take effect, transplant recipients produce more lactate and are able to utilize less oxygen than controls, suggesting that they are undergoing a greater degree of anaerobic metabolism[16]. Furthermore, transplant recipients performing exercise have a demonstrably increased arteriovenous oxygen difference compared with controls, indicating an increased extraction of oxygen from haemoglobin by the tissues, and suggesting that cardiac output is comparably lower than in controls[6, 8].

It has been suggested that these findings, which imply suboptimal cardiac function, may be the result of subclinical rejection[16], as dogs with auto-transplants are able to perform maximally[29].

(3) *Training effects.* Adequate physical training does not cause a reduction in resting heart rate of the transplanted heart (though it does in control subjects), but the heart rate at submaximal work rates is significantly reduced when compared to pretraining levels. Work capacity is markedly improved. Thus, cardiac innervation is not required to produce increased work capacity following physical training[14].

PHYSIOLOGY FOLLOWING HETEROTOPIC HEART TRANSPLANTATION

When heterotopic heart transplantation is performed, the parallel linkage of the compliant donor transplanted heart with the failing non-compliant recipient heart leads to complex changes. As there is no pressure difference between the anastomosed atria, filling of the transplanted and recipient ventricles is determined by their relative compliance (Figure 10.2). Filling of the more compliant donor ventricle therefore accounts for most of the venous return, and the contribution of this ventricle to the total cardiac output is consequently far greater. Thus, diastolic compliance as well as systolic mechanical function determine preferential flow through the donor ventricle. This situation may be altered by the onset of rejection, which can markedly decrease the compliance of the donor ventricle, and would therefore tend to reverse the pattern of distribution of the venous return.

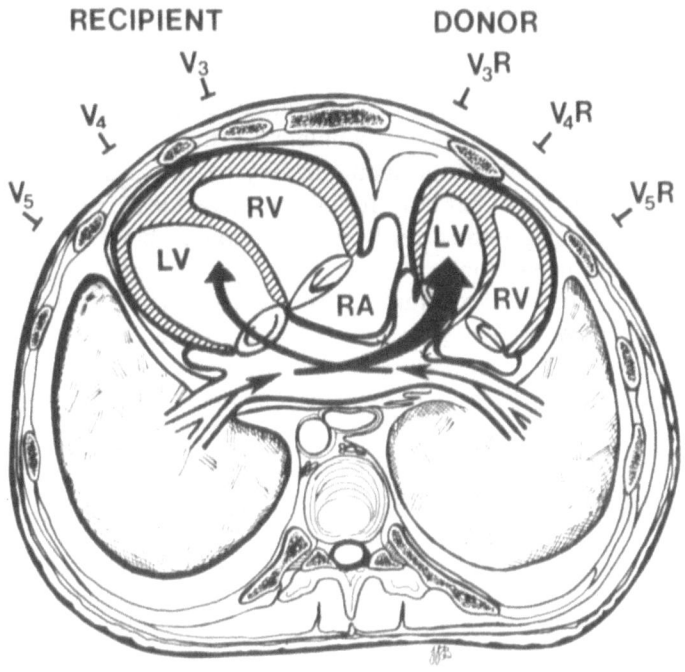

Figure 10.2   Diagram of a transverse section through the thorax of a patient with a heterotopic heart transplant. The donor heart is situated in the right pleural cavity. (The sites of electrocardiographic electrode placement are also indicated.) Blood flow from the common left atrial chamber is governed by the relative compliances of the two left ventricles. Unless rejection of the donor heart is occurring, the compliance of the donor left ventricle will be greater than that of the diseased recipient left ventricle; blood in the common left atrial chamber will therefore drain predominantly to the donor left ventricle

Complex beat-to-beat alterations in preload and afterload occur, and these can also strikingly affect the performance of the recipient heart. If the hearts are allowed to beat spontaneously and happen to contract synchronously[30], or if they are paced synchronously[31], then the contribution of the recipient heart to the stroke volume of the synchronized beat falls dramatically. The recipient ventricle is frequently unable to raise its peak left ventricular pressure above aortic pressure and, therefore, ejection from this ventricle does not occur[30-32]. The bolus of blood in this ventricle may be shunted via an incompetent mitral valve through the common left atrium into the donor ventricle and ejected into the aorta[32].

Conversely, recipient heart function is optimized if the two hearts beat (or are paced) sequentially[30, 31]. At least one patient has had a double atrial-triggered pacemaker implanted in order to assure sequential contraction of the hearts and optimize recipient heart function[33].

Subsequent work, however, has shown that although the ejection fraction and output of the recipient heart is increased during sequential pacing, there is no real advantage to be gained from this procedure as the donor heart is capable of maintaining a normal cardiac output in the absence of any recipient heart function[31, 32]. Furthermore, the total output of the spontaneously beating recipient heart is not significantly different from the total output of the sequentially paced heart, as the spontaneously beating heart seldom beats synchronously with the donor heart for prolonged periods[31]. Sequential atrial pacing is therefore not used routinely when heterotopic heart transplants are performed at our institution[34].

There is evidence to suggest that recipient heart function may deteriorate over a period of time following heterotopic heart transplantation[32, 34]. Whether this is the result of the increased afterload on the recipient heart, or is simply a reflection of progression of the original disease process, is uncertain.

ELECTROPHYSIOLOGY OF THE TRANSPLANTED HEART

Recent evidence suggests that the long-term survivors of heart transplantation have a high incidence of minor electrophysiological abnormalities[35]. The commonest findings are an abnormality of sinus node function (delayed sinus node recovery time) and delayed conduction through the atria, with resultant first-degree atrioventricular (AV) block. The clinical significance of these findings is, however, uncertain[35].

There is also a high incidence of dual AV nodal pathways, but no episodes of sustained re-entrant tachycardia have been reported[35]. Although His-ventricular conduction may occasionally be prolonged, higher degrees of AV block than first-degree block have also not been reported[35], and denervation appears to have little influence on the resting electrophysiologic characteristics of the atrioventricular conduction system[36].

Denervation does not protect the transplanted heart from arrhythmias[37, 38]. In one study, atrial arrhythmias occurred in 72% of patients and ventricular arrhythmias in 57%. Arrhythmias appear to be related to periods of acute rejection[37, 38], and respond to treatment of the rejection, or to antiarrhythmic drugs such as quinidine. The increased sensitivity of the transplanted heart to catecholamines[31], and the lack of suppressant vagal tone, may be significant factors in the pathogenesis of the arrhythmias[37, 38].

PHARMACOLOGY OF THE TRANSPLANTED HEART

Data concerning the pharmacology of the transplanted heart are limited. A number of general principles may, however, be applied.

Firstly, drugs whose effect on the heart is mediated via the autonomic nervous system (sympathetic and parasympathetic) will have no effect on the transplanted heart. Secondly, denervation of the heart may result in an enhanced response to certain drugs (e.g. β-receptor stimulants). Thirdly, drugs which are negatively inotropic or which have an effect on the peripheral vasculature may have a profound effect on cardiac performance, as the transplanted heart relies mainly on the Frank–Starling mechanism and on changes in contractility for its stress response.

A few drugs should be considered in more detail.

Digoxin

In normally innervated hearts, digoxin has a significant effect on AV nodal conduction, prolonging both the effective refractory period and the functional refractory period, irrespective of cycle length[39]. There is a lesser effect on sinus node function, with slight increases in cycle length, sinus node recovery time, and sinoatrial conduction time occurring in response to digoxin[40]. These effects appear to be mediated via the autonomic nervous system, as digoxin has only a minimal effect on the AV node of the denervated, transplanted heart[39], and has virtually no effect on sinus node function[40] (although sinoatrial exit block has been produced in one patient).

The therapeutic implications of these findings are that the effect of digoxin on AV conduction in the transplanted heart is blunted, and the amount of slowing of the ventricular response in atrial fibrillation is less than occurs in innervated hearts.

In normally innervated hearts, digitalis in higher dosage has been shown to augment sympathetic nerve activity[41], and this may predispose to digitalis-induced ventricular arrhythmias. Whether arrhythmias caused by digoxin toxicity are less common in the transplanted heart is, however, unknown.

The effects of digoxin on the force of contraction and on the peripheral circulation (vasoconstriction) remain unchanged.

Calcium antagonists

The calcium antagonists, nifedipene, verapamil and diltiazem, all have direct binding sites on the myocardium, and therefore have an effect on the denervated heart. These drugs should, however, be used with caution as they are all negatively inotropic, and all, to a greater or lesser degree, have effects on the peripheral vasculature. Use of these agents in transplant recipients may therefore produce exaggerated haemodynamic changes.

Inotropic agents

Cardiac denervation results in depletion of myocardial catecholamines. Increased sensitivity to circulating catecholamines ensues, as can be evidenced by the enhanced inotropic and chronotropic response of the transplanted heart to agents such as adrenaline, noradrenaline and isoprenaline[5, 27, 28]. This sensitivity appears to be mediated by a change in the state of the β-receptors. Other inotropic agents (e.g. dopamine and dobutamine), whose actions are mediated via β-receptors, could be expected to have a similarly enhanced effect.

β-Receptor blockers

The catecholamine-depleted, transplanted heart is dependent on circulating catecholamines[28]; the response to circulating catecholamines is critical in the exercise capability and the heart rate response of transplant recipients[22]. β-Blockers, by inhibiting one of the major compensatory mechanisms of the denervated heart, dramatically reduce the exercise tolerance of transplant recipients[22].

Antiarrhythmic agents

Ventricular and supraventricular arrhythmias of the transplanted heart appear to be associated most commonly with acute rejection. Treatment of the rejection is normally sufficient to abolish these arrhythmias[37, 38]. Quinidine gluconate has been used successfully as an antiarrhythmic agent in the transplanted heart, suggesting that innervation is not required for a cardiac response to antiarrhythmic therapy[38]. Most antiarrhythmic agents are, however, negatively inotropic and should be used with due caution.

Reference

1. Braunwald, E. (1974). Regulation of the circulation. *N. Engl. J. Med.*, **290**, 1124, 1420
2. Braunwald, E. and Ross, J. (1979). Control of cardiac performance. In Berne, R. M. (ed.) *Handbook of Physiology*. Section 2. Vol. 1, p. 533. (Bethesda, Md: American Physiological Society)
3. Braunwald, E. (1971). Structure and function of the normal myocardium. *Br. Heart J.*, **33** (Suppl.), 3
4. Beck, W., Barnard, C. N. and Sohrire, V. (1969). Heart rate after cardiac transplantation. *Circulation*, **40**, 437
5. Carleton, R. A., Heller, S. J., Najafi, H. and Clark, J. G. (1969). Haemodynamic performance of a transplanted human heart. *Circulation*, **40**, 447
6. Stinson, E. B., Griepp, R. B., Schroeder, J. S., Dong, E. and Shumway, N. E. (1972). Haemodynamic observations one and two years after cardiac transplantation in man. *Circulation*, **45**, 1183
7. Beck, W., Barnard, C. N. and Schrire, V. (1971). Haemodynamic studies in two long-term survivors of heart transplantation. *J. Thorac. Cardiovasc. Surg.*, **62**, 315

8. Pope, S. E., Stinson, E. B., Daughters, G. T., Schroeder, J. S., Ingels, N. B. and Alderman, E. L. (1980). Exercise response of the denervated heart in long-term cardiac transplant recipients. *Am. J. Cardiol.*, **46**, 213

9. McLaughlin, P. R., Kleiman, J. H., Martin, R. P., Doherty, P. W., Reitz, B., Stinson, E. B., Daughters, G. T., Ingels, N. B. and Alderman, E. L. (1978). The effect of exercise and atrial pacing on left ventricular volume and contractility in patients with innervated and denervated hearts. *Circulation*, **58**, 476

10. Clark, D. A., Schroeder, J. S., Griepp, R. B., Stinson, E. B., Dong, E., Shumway, N. E. and Harrison, D. C. (1973). Cardiac transplantation in man: review of first three years' experience. *Am. J. Med.*, **54**, 563

11. Christophersen, L. K., Griepp, R. B. and Stinson, E. B. (1976). Rehabilitation after cardiac transplantation. *J. Am. Med. Assoc.*, **236**, 2082

12. Hunt, S. A., Rider, A. K., Stinson, E. B., Griepp, R. B., Schroeder, J. S., Harrison, D. C. and Shumway, N. E. (1975). Does cardiac transplantation prolong life and improve its quality? An updated report. *Circulation*, **54** (Suppl. 3), 56

13. Cory-Pearce, R., Wheeldon, D. R., Wallwork, J. and English, T. A. H. (1983). Late cardiac function after heart transplantation. *J. Am. Coll. Cardiol.*, **1**, 721

14. Savin, W. M., Gordon, E., Green, S., Haskell, W., Kantrowitz, N., Lundberg, M., Melvin, K., Sonnelson, R., Verschagin, K. and Schroeder, J. S. (1983). Comparison of exercise training effects in cardiac denervated and innervated humans. *J. Am. Coll. Cardiol.*, **1**, 722

15. Savin, W. M., Schroeder, J. S. and Haskell, W. L. (1982). Response of cardiac transplant recipients to static and dynamic exercise: review. *Heart Transplant.*, **1**, 72

16. Savin, W. M., Haskell, W. L., Schroeder, J. S. and Stinson, E. B. (1980). Cardiorespiratory responses of cardiac transplant patients to graded symptom-limited exercise. *Circulation*, **62**, 55

17. Kivowitz, C., Parmley, W. W., Donoso, R., Marcus, H., Ganz, W. and Swan, H. J. C. (1971). Effects of isometric exercise on cardiac performance. The grip test. *Circulation*, **44**, 994

18. Helfant, R. H., De Villa, M. A. and Meister, S. G. (1971). Effect of sustained isometric handgrip exercise on left ventricular performance. *Circulation*, **44**, 982

19. Savin, W. M., Alderman, E. L., Haskell, W. L., Schroeder, J. S., Ingels, N. B., Daughters, G. T. and Stinson, E. B. (1980). Left ventricular response to isometric exercise in patients with denervated and innervated hearts. *Circulation*, **61**, 897

20. Haskell, W. L., Savin, W. M., Schroeder, J. S., Alderman, E. A., Ingels, N. B., Daughters, G. T. and Stinson, E. B. (1981). Cardiovascular responses to handgrip isometric exercise in patients following cardiac transplantation. *Circ. Res.*, **48** (Suppl. 1), 156

21. Donald, D. E. and Samueloff, S. L. (1966). Exercise tachycardia not due to blood-borne agents in canine cardiac denervation. *Am. J. Physiol.*, **211**, 703

22. Bexton, R., Milne, J., Cory-Pearce, R., English, T. A. H. and Camm, A. J. (1983). Effect of beta-blockade on the exercise response following cardiac transplantation. *J. Am. Coll. Cardiol.*, **1**, 722

23. Barnard, C. N. and Beck, W. (1972). The physiology of the transplanted heart. In Wells, C., Kyle, J. and Dunphy, J. E. (eds.) *Scientific Foundations of Surgery*. 2nd Edn. (London: Heinemann Medical)

24. Starling, E. H. (1918). *The Linacre Lecture on the Law of the Heart, 1915*. (London: Longmans Green)

25. Frank, O. (1959). On the dynamics of cardiac muscle. (Translated by Chapman, C. B. and Wasserman, E.). *Am. Heart J.*, **58**, 282, 467

26. Sarnoff, S. J. and Berglund, E. (1954). Ventricular function. I. Starling's law of the heart studied by means of simultaneous right and left ventricular function curves in the dog. *Circulation*, **9**, 706

27. Donald, D. E. and Shepherd, J. T. (1965). Supersensitivity to L. norepinephrine of the denervated sinoatrial node. *Am. J. Physiol.*, **208**, 255

28. Ebert, P. A. (1968). The effects of norepinephrine infusion on the denervated heart. *J. Cardio-vasc. Surg.*, **29**, 414

29. Donald, D. E. and Shepherd, J. T. (1964). Initial cardiovascular adjustment to exercise in dogs with chronic cardiac denervation. *Am. J. Physiol.*, **207**, 1325

30. Beck, W. and Gersh, B. J. (1976). Left ventricular bypass using a cardiac allograft: haemo-dynamic studies. *Am. J. Cardiol.*, **37**, 1007

31. Losman, J. G., Barnard, C. N. and Bartley, T. D. (1977). Haemodynamic evaluation of left ventricular bypass with a homologous cardiac graft. *J. Thorac. Cardiovasc. Surg.*, **74**, 695

32. Melvin, K. R., Pollick, C., Hunt, S. A., McDougall, R., Goris, M. L., Oyer, P. E., Popp, R. L. and Stinson, E. B. (1982). Cardiovascular physiology in a case of heterotopic cardiac transplantation. *Am. J. Cardiol.*, **49**, 1301

33. Kennelly, B. M., Piller, L. W., Tarjan, P. P., Losman, J. G., Barnard, C. N. and Beck, W. (1978). Use of a double atrial triggered standby pacemaker system for a patient with a biventricular bypass heterotopic cardiac homograft. *Am. J. Cardiol.*, **41**, 341

34. Cooper, D. K. C. (1984). Orthotopic and heterotopic transplantation of the heart—the Cape Town experience. *Ann. R. Coll. Surg.*, **66**, 228

35. Bexton, R. S., Nathan, A. W., Hellestrand, K. J., Cory-Pearce, R., Spurrell, R. A. J., English, T. A. H. and Camm, A. J. (1983). Electrophysiological abnormalities in the transplanted human heart. *Br. Heart J.*, **50**, 555

36. Bexton, R. S., Nathan, A. W., Hellestrand, K. J., Cory-Pearce, R., Spurrell, R. A. J., English, T. A. H. and Camm, A. J. (1984). The electrophysiologic characteristics of the transplanted human heart. *Am. Heart J.*, **107**, 1

37. Berke, D. K., Graham, A. F., Schroeder, J. S. and Harrison, D. C. (1978). Arrhythmias in the denervated transplanted human heart. *Circulation*, **47, 48** (Cardiovascular Surgery Suppl. III), 112

38. Schroeder, J. S., Berke, D. K., Graham, A. F., Rider, A. K. and Harrison, D. C. (1974). Arrhythmias after cardiac transplantation. *Am. J. Cardiol.*, **33**, 604

39. Goodman, D. J., Rossen, R. M., Cannom, D. S., Rider, A. K. and Harrison, D. C. (1975). Effect of digoxin on atrioventricular conduction studies in patients with and without auto-nomic innervation. *Circulation*, **51**, 251

40. Goodman, D. J., Rossen, R. M., Ingham, R., Rider, A. K. and Harrison, D. C. (1975). Sinus node function in the denervated human heart. Effect of digitalis. *Br. Heart J.*, **37**, 612

41. Gillis, R. A., Raines, A., Sohn, Y. J., Levitt, B. and Standaert, F. G. (1972). Neuroexcitatory effects of digitalis and their role in the development of cardiac arrhythmias. *J. Pharmacol. Exp. Ther.*, **183**, 154

11
Pathology of Acute Rejection

INTRODUCTION

Experimental cardiac transplantation using various animals preceded the first human-to-human cardiac transplant in 1967. Such experimental work provided a sound basis for our understanding of the clinical and pathological features of cardiac rejection and their modification by immunosuppressive agents. Pioneering experimental work in animals was performed by Carrel and Guthrie[1], Mann et al.[2], Downie[3], Lower et al.[4], and Blumenstock et al.[5]. Cooper[6] has reviewed the many stages of the experimental development of cardiac transplantation which span this century, and Uys and Rose[7] list key references to the cardiac pathology of experimental cardiac transplantation in dogs, rats, rabbits and baboons. Thomson[8], in 1968, was the first to describe the pathology of a transplanted human heart, and this was followed shortly thereafter by the report of Lower et al.[9].

While irreversible severe acute rejection may sometimes lead to surgical removal of the donor heart and its examination by the pathologist, the usual day-to-day problem facing the pathologist, in centres where cardiac transplantation is performed, is that of the histological recognition of acute rejection in endomyocardial biopsies from the donor heart.

MACROSCOPIC APPEARANCES

Mild or moderate rejection may produce no naked eye alterations in the transplanted heart. However, it has been shown experimentally that such rejecting allografts have an increased organ mass[10, 11]. Hearts removed because of cessation of function following irreversible severe acute rejection (Figure 11.1), usually show extremely severe acute rejection changes, since the immunosuppression is often greatly reduced in the period between cessation of graft function and surgical excision of the graft. Such hearts commonly are dilated and have a harmorrhagic-looking, swollen, mottled myocardial cut surface.

Focal pale areas of myocardial necrosis contrast sharply with the plum-coloured, viable myocardium. The ventricles often contain abundant apical stasis thrombi. Occasionally, stasis thrombus in the donor aortic valve pockets may extend upwards to occlude the donor coronary arteries, resulting in total or subtotal necrosis of the graft.

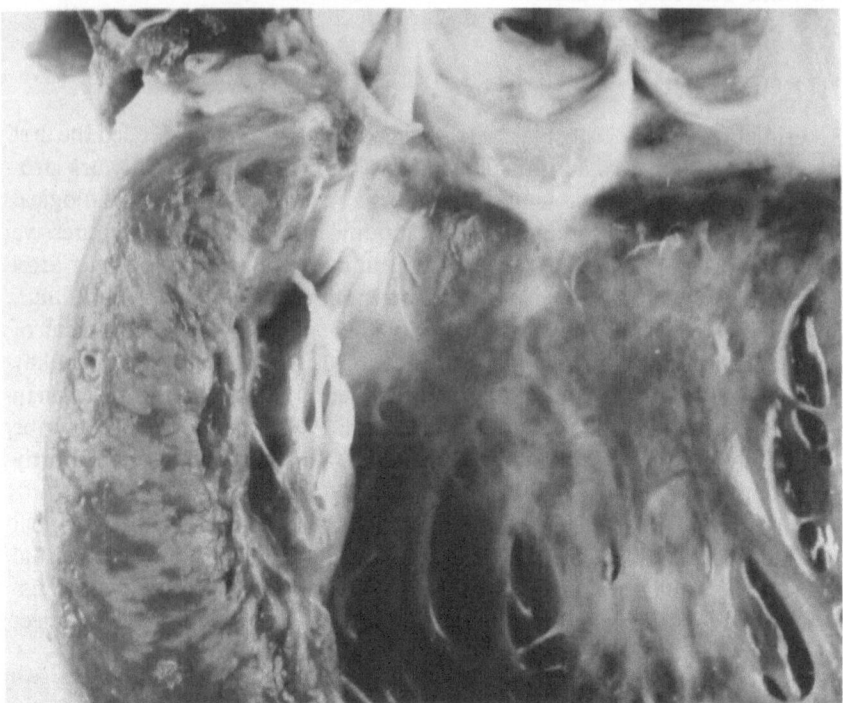

Figure 11.1　Close-up view of left ventricle of a donor heart showing severe acute rejection. Subendocardial haemorrhage is widely distributed and the myocardial cut surface shows pale areas of necrosis

LIGHT MICROSCOPIC APPEARANCES AND THE ROLE OF ENDOMYOCARDIAL BIOPSY IN THE DIAGNOSIS OF ACUTE CARDIAC REJECTION

The histopathology of acute rejection as seen in myocardial biopsies or in donor hearts removed surgically or at autopsy is similar. The only difference is with regard to severity, which may differ from patient to patient and from biopsy to biopsy. Biopsy material is obviously limited in amount and the pathologist has to detect rejection without having the multiple tissue sections which are available when the whole heart is examined. Criticism of endomyocardial biopsy has focused primarily on the possibility of sampling error and the subtlety of the histologic changes in diagnosing rejection[12, 13]. A study from our institution[14] attempted to validate the technique by examining 'biopsy' samples taken with a bioptome from formalin-fixed transplanted hearts from human transplant recipients and comparing these in a blind fashion with standard histologic sections taken from the same hearts. Using a scoring system to grade severity of acute rejection, agreement of results between the bioptome samples and routine sections was found in 86% of cases. More important was the fact that in 285 biopsy samples, only two false-negative results were obtained. Rejection involved both ventricles evenly.

Endomyocardial biopsy usually samples the septal wall of the right ventricle towards the apex. How many tissue samples should be submitted with each biopsy procedure? From the pathologist's point of view as many as the cardiologist performing the catheterization procedure is happy to take. In practice we usually receive an average of 3–4 endomyocardial samples per biopsy procedure. In our study referred to earlier, it was found that even as few as two endomyocardial samples revealed the presence of acute rejection[5]. Others consider that the myocardium is only adequately represented by a minimum of five endomyocardial samples per biopsy procedure[15]. Whilst the latter opinion was expressed regarding myocardial biopsy for suspected idiopathic cardiomyopathy, it is likely that the same principle should apply to rejection. If only one small endomyocardial sample is submitted, it is advisable for the examining pathologist to convey this information to the cardiac surgeon, since there is a possibility that significant rejection may be missed (false-negative biopsy). It will remain for the cardiac surgeon to decide, in the light of other clinical and laboratory parameters, whether an immediate or earlier than usual repeat biopsy is indicated.

Each endomyocardial sample is usually less than 3 mm in diameter and they are submitted to our laboratory in 5% buffered glutaraldehyde to facilitate subsequent ultrastructural examination of one of the fragments if this is deemed necessary. The fragments for assessment of rejection are transferred into 5% buffered formaldehyde in the laboratory and processed overnight for light microscopy in the routine manner. Paraffin-embedded sections are then stained by the haematoxylin-eosin, elastic van Gieson and Unna–Pappenheim methods. Such handling takes about 18 hours before the histological diagnosis is available. Frozen section is used only occasionally for the diagnosis of acute rejection. Electron microscopy and immunofluorescence microscopy play no diagnostic role in the recognition of rejection.

In patients receiving conventional immunosuppressive therapy

One of the earliest changes observed in acute rejection (Figure 11.2) is the development of interstitial oedema which is most prominent perivascularly and is less evident in the endocardium, which has a denser connective tissue component. The oedema is probably a result of microvascular damage. The vascular endothelium is that portion of the graft which first encounters both humoral antibodies and the host cells which are attracted into the graft.

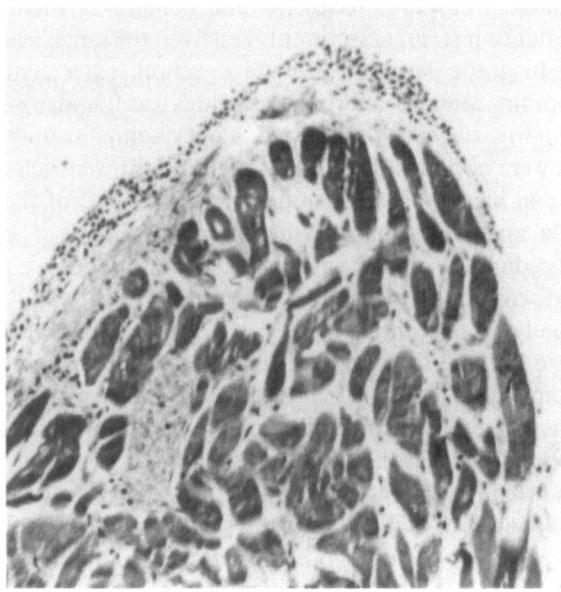

Figure 11.2   Early acute rejection. Mild interstitial oedema spares the endocardium, which contains an infiltrate of lymphoid cells. H & E × 135

Since the host cells reach the graft via the bloodstream, in the early stages of acute rejection the small blood vessels within the graft may be observed to contain increased numbers of mononuclear cells (Figure 11.3), and these cells may also be seen to be passing through the vessels' walls into the surrounding myocardium. The degree of interstitial oedema (Figure 11.4) does not always match the severity of the cellular infiltrate. The early infiltrating cells (Figure 11.5) consist mainly of non-activated lymphocytes and small unidentified mononuclear cells of lymphoid type, together with histiocytes and scanty neutrophils plus eosinophils. The cellular infiltration initially has a focal, mainly perivascular distribution. These cells soon develop a prominent cyto-plasmic pyroninophilia, as do the endothelial cells of the small blood vessels. Focal infiltrates of similar cells are also noted in the endomyocardium. Cardiac histiocytes (Anitschkow myocytes), presumably of donor heart origin, also appear activated and prominent. Vascular changes in the graft are observed at an early stage; the endothelial lining cells become swollen and oedema fluid accumulates in the intima (Figure 11.6). Sometimes this may lead to detachment of the endothelial cells.

If untreated, all of the above changes will progress and increase in intensity and be joined by other alterations associated with damage to the myofibres

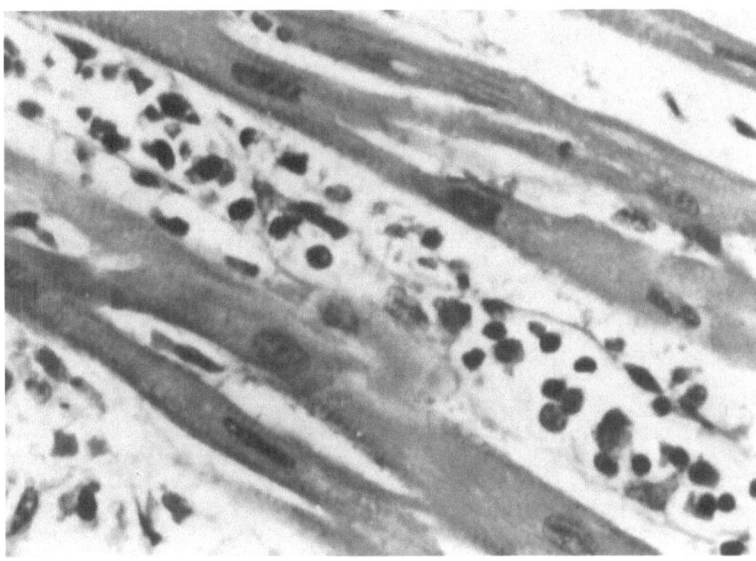

Figure 11.3 A capillary contains large numbers of mononuclear cells. Similar cells are present in the oedematous interstitium of this rejecting graft. H & E × 540

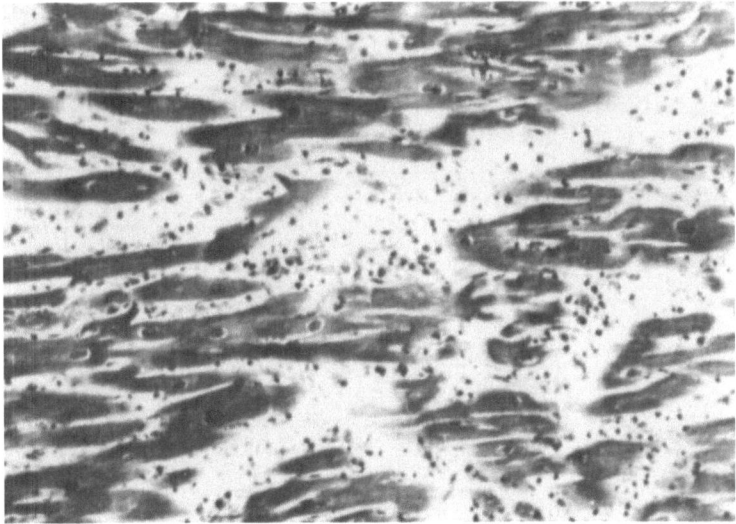

Figure 11.4 Prominent interstitial oedema accompanies a moderate mononuclear cellular infiltrate of acute rejection. H & E × 135

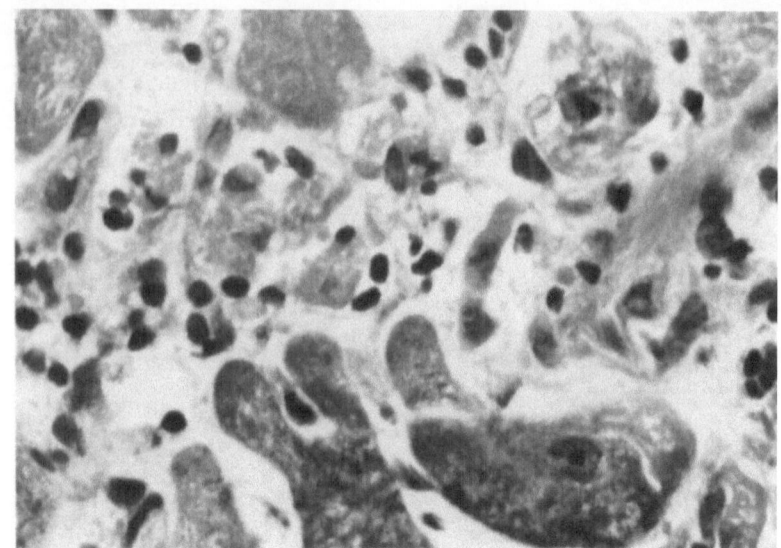

a

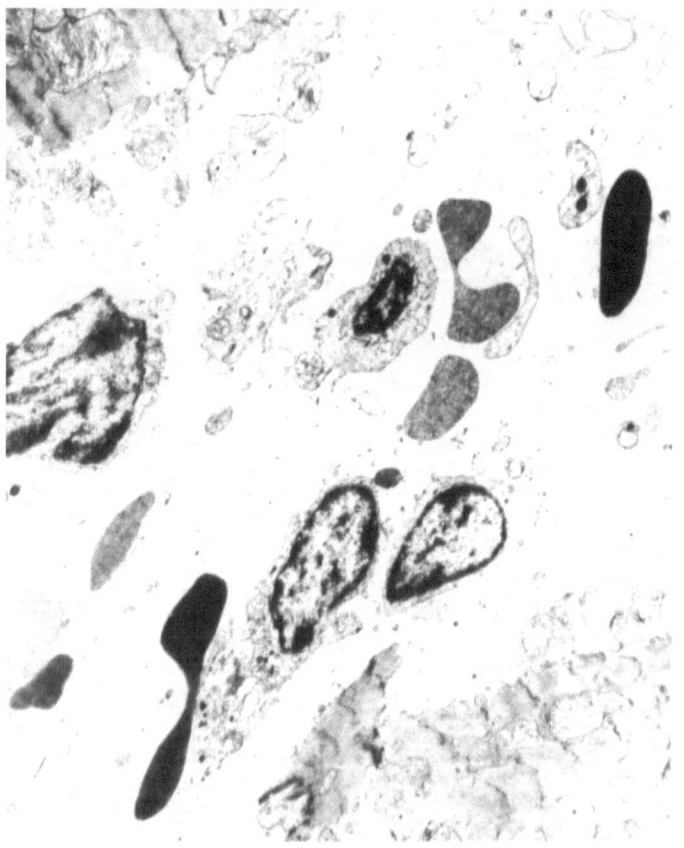

b

and the blood vessels. Thus, interstitial oedema becomes even more marked (Figure 11.4) and also separates bundles of myofibres, which previously had been in close apposition. Interstitial fibrin deposition also occurs, but fibrinolysis may render it inconspicuous microscopically[16]. With time, there is enlargement of the nuclei and cytoplasm of the lymphocytes, which now have the appearance of immunoblasts (Figure 11.7). Similar lymphoid series cells within blood vessels are admixed with proliferating endothelial and intimal cells and the lymphoid cells may also be seen within the media and the adventitia (Figure 11.6). This cellular accumulation, together with the intimal oedema and the sometimes encountered microvascular thrombi, leads to luminal narrowing.

Small vessel thrombi have been an inconspicuous feature of mild and moderate acute rejection in our human transplant material, but they have been encountered by others in canine cardiac allografts[17]. The occurrence of such thrombi in severe acute rejection in humans is not surprising, since there is evidence that rejection may activate the coagulation mechanism[18]. These microvascular changes, together with the cytotoxic effects of the infiltrating immunoblasts and humoral antibodies, combine to produce deleterious effects on the myocardium. Thus, the myofibres may show a range of appearances from normal through cytoplasmic swelling, lipid vacuolation and colliquative myocytolysis to coagulative necrosis (Figure 11.8). These changes may coexist in varying combinations. Myocytolysis is characterized by loss of cytoplasmic and nuclear detail, leaving an empty sarcolemmal sheath containing some lipofuscin granules as the tombstone of the vanished myofibre. Hearts with such areas of necrosis commonly also show interstitial haemorrhages due to disintegration of capillaries.

In severe acute rejection the intramyocardial coronary arteries, as well as some of the smaller epicardial branches of the major coronary arteries, may show fibrinoid necrosis (Figure 11.9) of a portion, or of the entire circumference of the artery. Occlusive thrombosis is a frequent accompaniment of this lesion. For some unknown reason the cardiac veins and the venules are seldom involved in the rejection changes described above[7]. In Chapter 16 we shall show how healing of acute rejection may lead to the constellation of myocardial and vascular changes in the donor heart which are referred to as chronic rejection.

We grade the severity of the rejection changes in the endomyocardial biopsies. A semiquantitative scoring system is used, which gives the clinician an easily understood guide as to the severity of the acute rejection changes present. The reproducibility of histological interpretation is enhanced since

Figure 11.5 a. Donor heart biopsy shows numbers of small lymphoid cells in relationship to degenerating myofibres. H & E × 540. **b.** The oedematous interstitium between two myofibres (top left and bottom right) contains activated lymphocytes and some free-lying erythrocytes. Lead citrate and uranyl acetate × 6000

we always use the same criteria to assess the biopsy specimens and give them scores, rather than basing the diagnosis of rejection on an overall impression of the specimens. In serial biopsies taken during an acute rejection episode it gives the clinician an easily interpretable guide as to the efficacy of increased immunosuppression. Lower histological scores should warrant less immuno-suppressive therapy than a severe rejection episode.

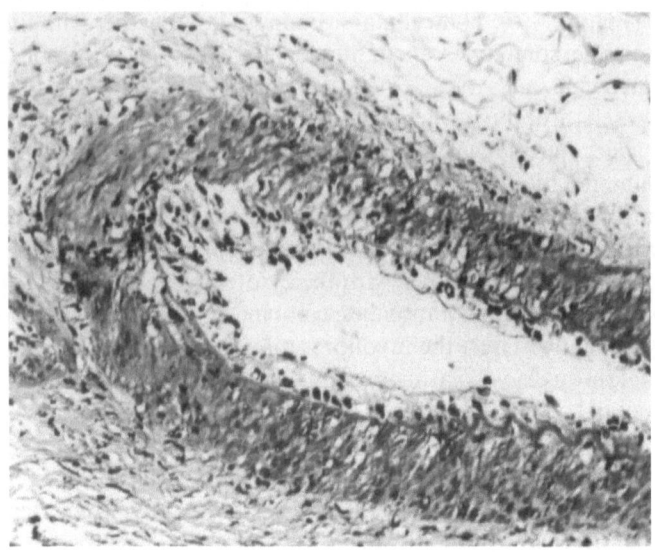

a

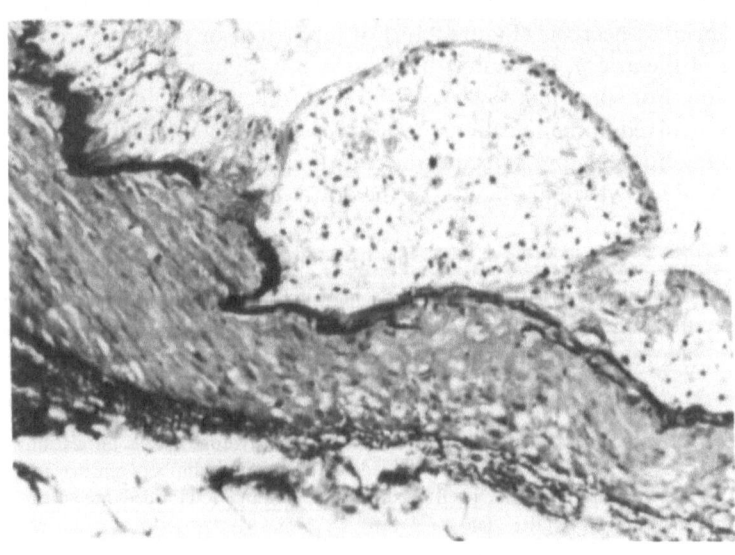

b

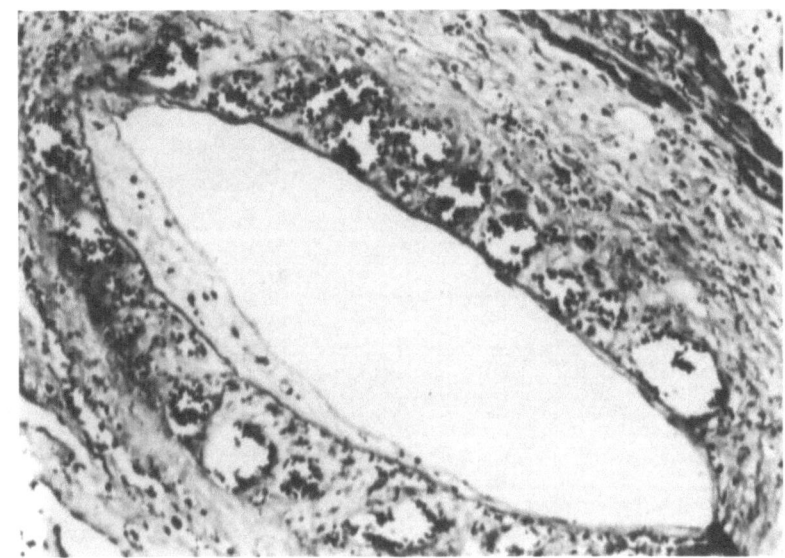

c

Figure 11.6 a. Acute rejection has caused subendothelial intimal oedema of this small coronary artery. Scanty mononuclear cells are present within the arterial wall. **b**. At times this oedema can be quite striking. **c**. Small coronary artery shows outer medial defects of the kind associated with an immune mediated arteritis. All H & E × 135

The histological scoring system used[19] independently assesses five histological criteria: (1) interstitial oedema, (2) interstitial mononuclear cellular infiltration, (3) cytoplasmic pyroninophilia of the mononuclear cells (the methyl-green pyronin stain identifies activated lymphocytes by staining the increased cytoplasmic RNA), (4) myofibre degeneration and (5) blood vessel alterations. Myofibre alterations include oedema, vacuolation, loss of sharp contour, indistinct cross-striations, colliquative myocytolysis, fragmentation and coagulative necrosis. Contraction banding of the myofibres, which is present in most biopsies, is regarded as a biopsy-induced artefact and is not scored. Blood vessel alterations include intimal cell proliferation or necrosis, medial cell loss and mononuclear cellular infiltration of the vessel wall.

The presence or absence of each of these five histological criteria is scored from 0 to 3 as follows: 0—absent or normal, 1—mild change, 2—moderate change, 3—severe change. The sum of these scores from the biopsy specimen is the final score and theoretically this may be as high as 15, though in clinical specimens scores above 7 are rarely encountered. In the experimental animal, when acute rejection is allowed to progress unimpeded, a score of 15 is not uncommon. In our experience, a final score of 0 implies that no rejection is present; 0.5–2 denotes mild acute rejection; 2.5–4 represents moderate acute rejection, and a score of greater than 4 indicates severe acute rejection.

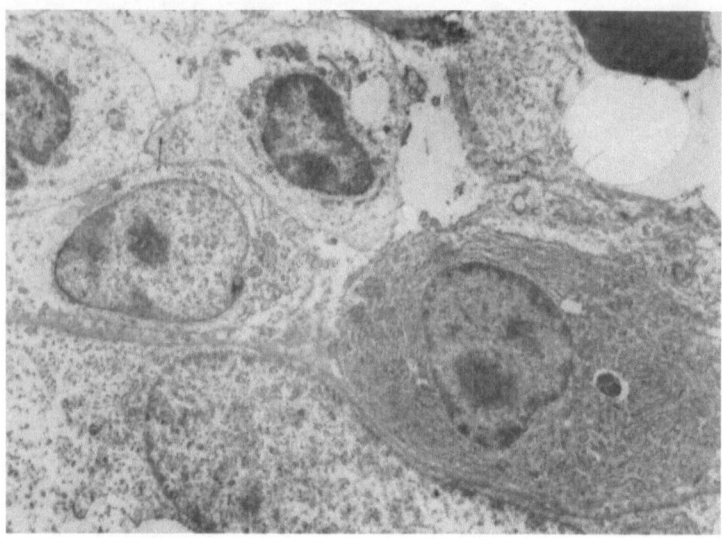

Figure 11.7   Acute rejection. A group of immunoblasts occupies the myocardial interstitium. One cell (lower right) has completed its transition into a plasma cell. Lead citrate and uranyl acetate × 3000

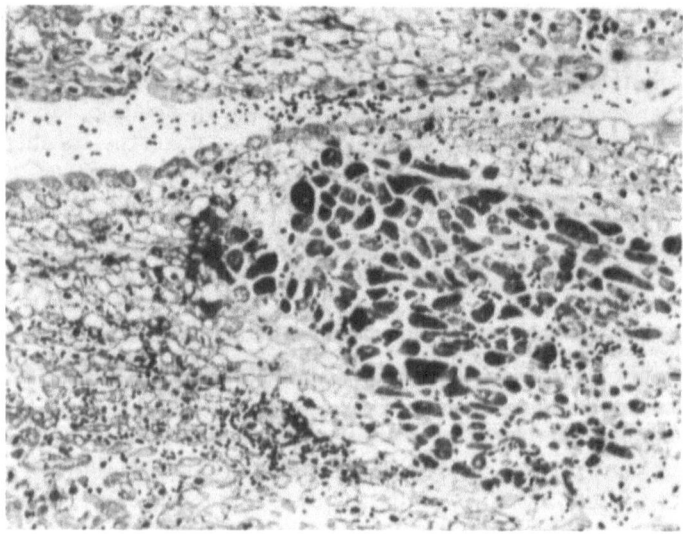

Figure 11.8   Severe acute rejection is associated with coagulative necrosis (dark-staining myofibres) and myocytolysis (empty sarcolemmal sheaths). H & E × 135

Examples of mild, moderate and severe rejection are given in Figures 11.10–11.12. Table 11.1 indicates the grades of acute rejection encountered in biopsies and in transplanted hearts at autopsy.

Resolving acute rejection (Figure 11.13) is encountered when augmented immunosuppression leads to abolishment of the acute rejection episode.

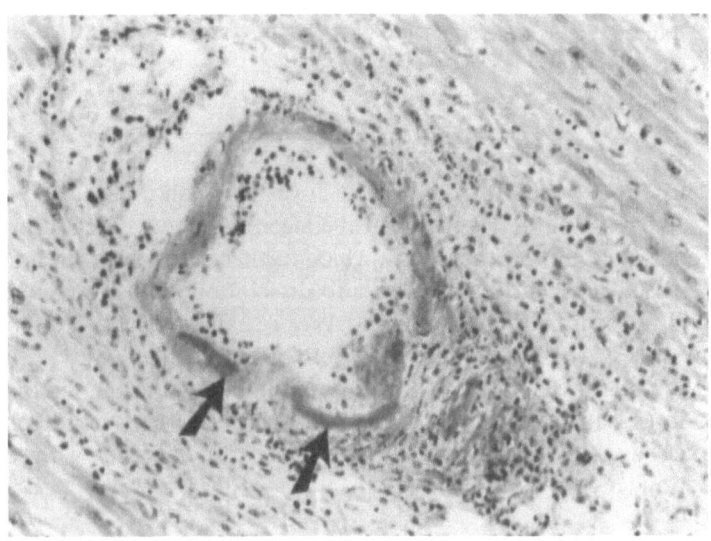

a

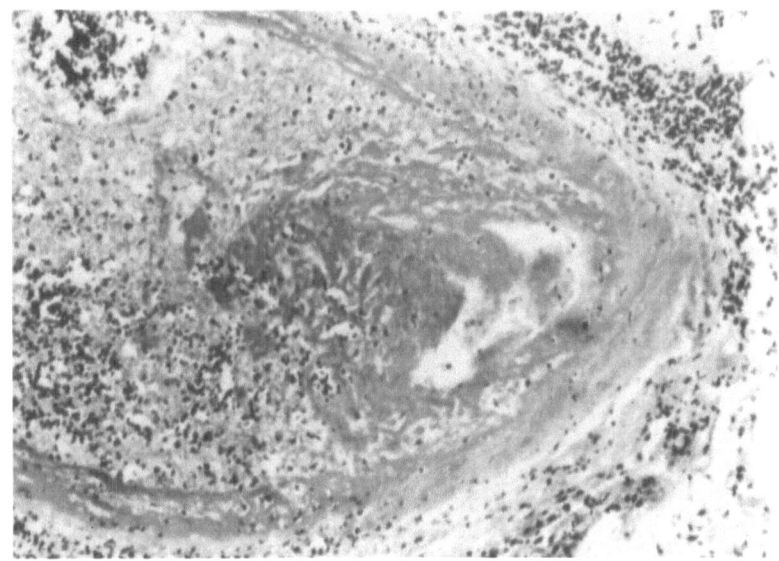

b

Figure 11.9 Severe acute rejection. **a**. Early fibrinoid necrosis (arrows) of wall of an intra-myocardial coronary artery. **b**. Advanced fibrinoid necrosis of a small coronary artery with superimposed thrombosis. Both H & E × 135

Table 11.1 Grades of acute rejection encountered in biopsies and in transplanted hearts at autopsy

Degrees of rejection (score)	Number of biopsies (%) (n = 157)	Number of autopsies (%) (n = 29)
No rejection (score 0)	20 (13)	15 (52)
Mild rejection (0.5–2.0)	57 (36)	8 (27)
Moderate rejection (2.5–4.0)	45 (29)	2 (7)
Severe rejection (> 4.0)	25 (16)	2 (7)
Inadequate biopsy	10 (6)	—
Necrotic graft	—	2 (7)

However, it takes several days or even 1–2 weeks for all evidence of acute rejection to be resolved. Since the clinical concern is as to whether rejection has been controlled, this is a period in which further biopsies are commonly taken. Increased steroidal therapy leads to dissolution of the mononuclear cellular infiltrate within a day or two. (As we shall see later, cyclosporin therapy has a less dramatic immediate effect on the cellular infiltrate.) The remaining lymphoid cells show minimal pyroninophilia and the removal of dead myofibres leads to early replacement fibrosis. The heart valves seldom show changes due to rejection and such alterations are only seen with severe acute rejection (Figure 11.14).

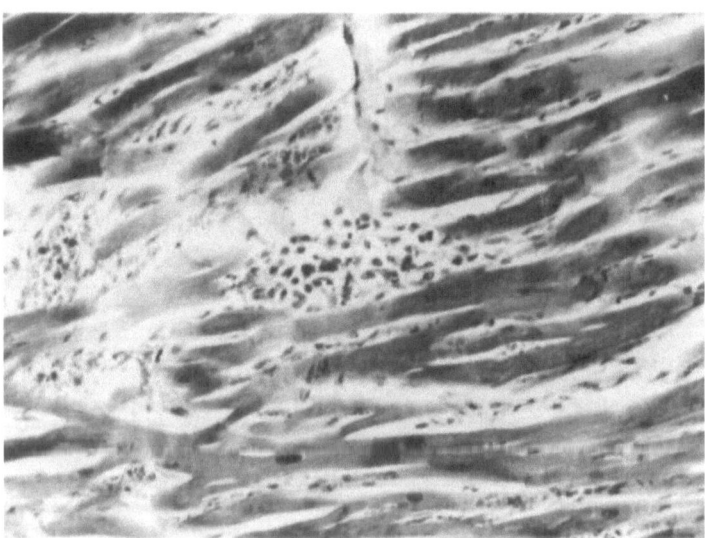

Figure 11.10 Mild acute rejection: scanty interstitial oedema and mononuclear cell infiltration. H & E × 135

In patients receiving cyclosporin A and steroids

The above-described histopathological changes of acute rejection are based upon our experience with cardiac transplants treated with an immunosuppressive regimen consisting of high-dose methylprednisolone, azathioprine and antithymocyte globulin. Since January 1983 the ten most recent heterotopic transplants have received the new immunosuppressive agent cyclosporin A[20]. Our personal experience with the effects of this drug on the morphology of acute rejection is limited.

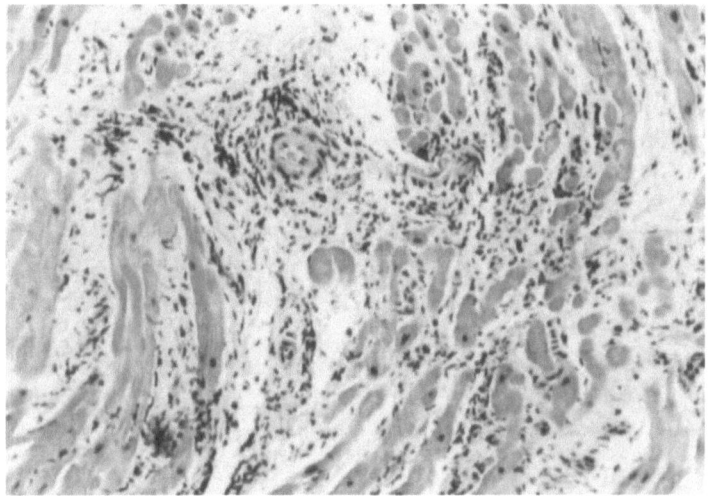

Figure 11.11 Moderate acute rejection: increased oedema and a more prominent cellular infiltrate are seen. H & E × 135

One important feature, which we have noted and which has also been observed by others[21,22], is the development of necrosis of myofibres in conjunction with what appears to be only a moderate degree of acute rejection. Billingham[23] reports that endomyocardial biopsies from cyclosporin-A treated cardiac recipients usually show a widely scattered, sparse infiltration of small mononuclear cells which do not indicate acute rejection. Mild lymphocytic infiltration in the absence of evidence of myocyte necrosis has been considered to necessitate only frequent biopsy surveillance[24]. Anti-rejection treatment has been withheld unless an increasingly severe infiltrate developed or active myocyte damage supervened. Early acute rejection is heralded by an increase of plump, pyroninophilic perivascular and interstitial mononuclear cells. Her experience is that acute rejection develops more slowly (e.g. over a week) and takes longer to resolve. The fine, intermyocyte fibrosis, which she regards as characteristic of cyclosporin treatment, has so far not been a notable feature in our patients. A coarser form of focal stromal collapse fibrosis following removal of necrotic myofibres has been observed in a few of our biopsies.

Oyer *et al.*[24] suggest that the rejection process in cyclosporin-A treated patients may be more focal than that seen in conventionally treated patients. They stress that at least three to five tissue samples from different areas of right ventricular endomyocardium should be obtained at each biopsy procedure in

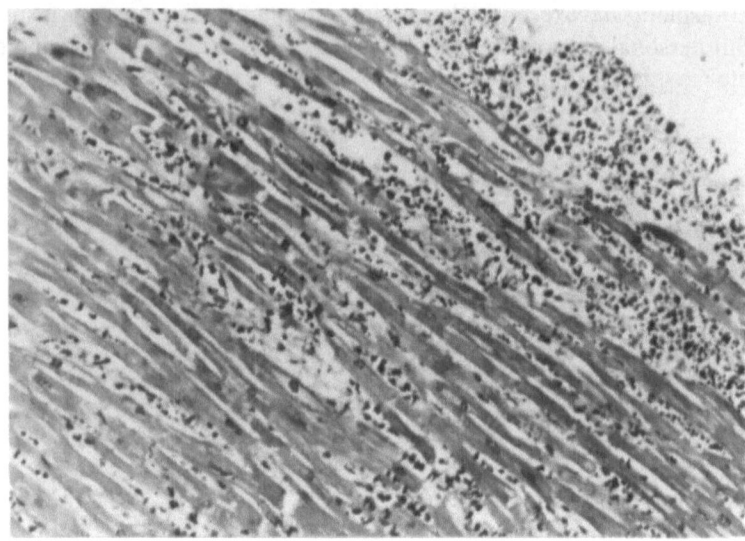

a

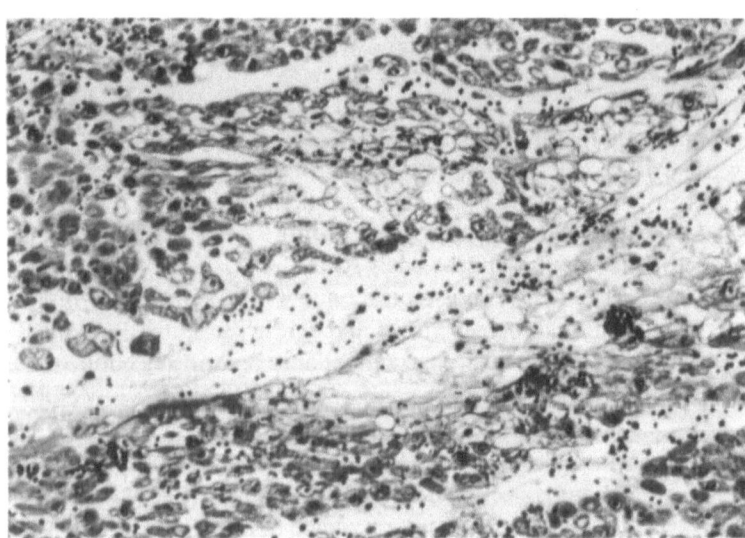

b

Figure 11.12 Severe acute rejection. **a**. Very numerous mononuclear cells are present. **b**. Myocytolysis is a prominent feature. This change is usually associated with occlusive arterial lesions. Both H & E × 135

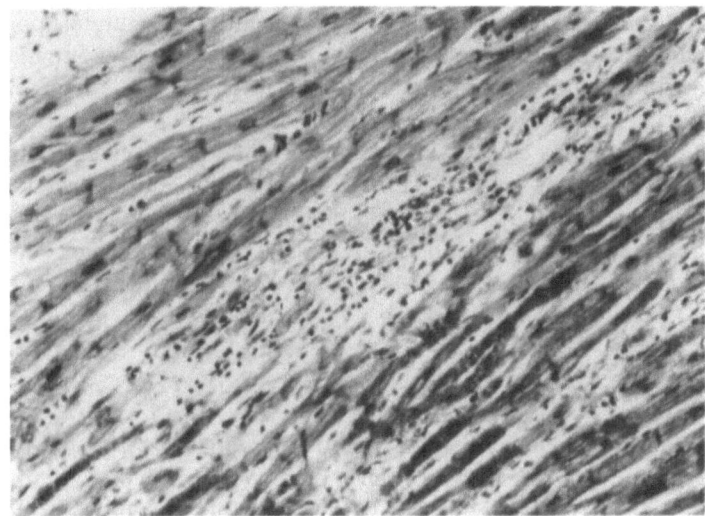

Figure 11.13 Resolving acute rejection shows few mononuclear cells and early stromal collapse fibrosis where some myofibres have been lost. H & E × 135

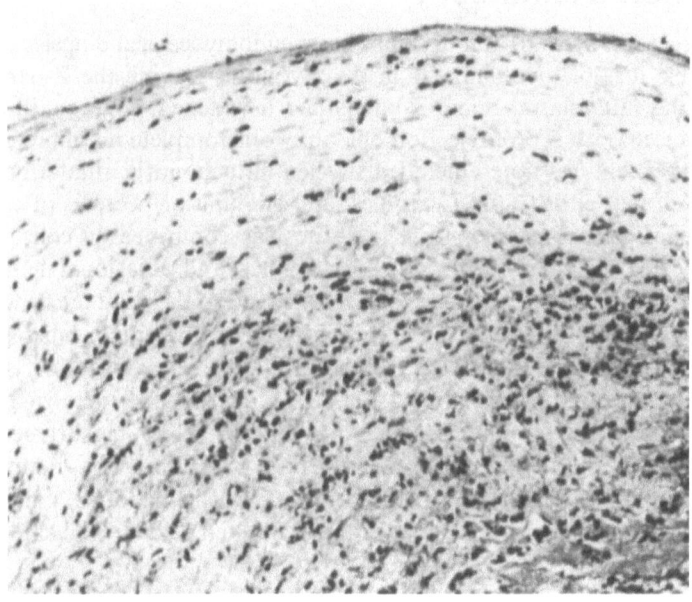

Figure 11.14 Mitral valve cusp of a patient with severe acute rejection contains numerous infiltrating lymphocytes. H & E × 150

order to gain an accurate overall impression of the status of the rejection process. Our experience is that even with conventional immunosuppression the rejection changes are not uniformly distributed throughout the myocardium and the endocardium, but endomyocardial biopsy is representative of the overall situation[14].

Additional features categorizing cyclosporin-modified acute rejection are that once established, acute rejection resolves slowly and myocyte damage may persist for a fortnight or more despite increased immunosuppression[21]. Severe acute rejection includes neutrophilic cells and haemorrhage plus myocyte necrosis as described for conventionally treated recipients.

IMMUNOFLUORESCENT STUDIES

Immunofluorescent studies on autopsy and biopsy material from transplanted human and animal hearts in which the immunoglobulins IgG, IgM, and IgA, and complement (C3) were sought, yielded unhelpful results by both direct immunofluorescence and the immunoperoxidase methods[7]. Only one surgically removed severely rejected heart showed moderate amounts of fibrinogen and C3 within the walls of some intramyocardial blood vessels.

ELECTRON MICROSCOPY

Ultrastructural examination of donor heart endomyocardial biopsies revealed a variable loss of myofilaments in the myofibres leaving the Z-bands free within the sarcoplasm. Some Z-bands had a widened, smudgy, ill-defined appearance. With severe rejection one observed complete myofibre destruction. Other features noted included swollen mitochondria, dilatation of the T-tubules, cytoplasmic lipid vacuoles, and swelling or necrosis of capillary endothelial cells. The interstitial infiltrate was confirmed as consisting of lymphocytes, activated lymphocytes, histiocytes, and occasional neutrophils and eosinophils. In the early stages of acute rejection there is a preponderance of mononuclear cells of undistinguished appearance. Later, activated lymphocytes are the predominant cell. In resolving acute rejection there is a predominance of mature-looking plasma cells which are characterized by the presence of numerous polyribosomes and cisternae of rough-surfaced endoplasmic reticulum. (Such cells stain weakly with the Unna–Pappenheim stain.) In biopsies of cardiac allografts implanted in baboons, unidentified mononuclear cells comprised 53% of the interstitial cellular infiltrate overall in acute rejection[10].

SPECIAL PROBLEMS REGARDING THE
LIGHT MICROSCOPIC DIAGNOSIS OF REJECTION

There are certain special problems that may be encountered in the interpretation of biopsies from donor hearts.

(1) Firstly, there is the adequacy of the endomyocardial sampling, which has been commented upon above. A not-infrequent situation which we encounter in regard to inadequate sampling is that one or more of the endomyocardial biopsies submitted by the cardiologist is composed solely of fibrin thrombus. The source of the thrombus is not always clear, and possible sites of origin include the biopsy catheter itself, endocardial thrombus, or thrombus at the vein entry site. Since the biopsies are all taken from a limited area at the apical portion of the right side of the interventricular septum, there is a possibility that the thrombus may even be derived from a previous biopsy site if serial biopsies have been taken.

(2) Another problem which is encountered from time to time is the sample composed solely of fibrous tissue. While such a finding raises the possibility of chronic rejection, our experience is that chronic rejection commonly spares the immediately subendocardial myofibres[19]. If the donor heart has a greatly reduced ejection fraction and the endomyocardial biopsy shows no sign of acute rejection, the possibility of chronic rejection should be borne in mind. In several biopsies we have been able to identify fibrous tissue as being portions of tricuspid valve chordae tendineae. Such biopsies appear to result in no significant valvular dysfunction.

(3) In one patient we made the initial diagnosis of infection of both the donor and the recipient hearts by *Toxoplasma gondii* (Figure 11.15) on endomyocardial biopsies. Electron microscopy and serology served to confirm the diagnosis[25].

Toxoplasmosis of the donor heart may interfere with the recognition of acute rejection in graft biopsy specimens. The interstitial mononuclear cell infiltrate that follows release of the organisms from infected myofibres is very similar to that seen in acute rejection. This causes difficulty both in detecting cardiac rejection and in assessing its severity. Pyroninophilia is not helpful in distinguishing the two conditions. The cellular infiltrate in toxoplasmosis is said to be of a more mixed type and includes lymphocytes, plasma cells, histiocytes and occasional eosinophils. In acute rejection, the cellular infiltrate at first consists almost entirely of activated lymphocytes[26]. Later, transformation into plasma cells occurs. Histiocytes may become activated, but they usually do not comprise a prominent part of the cellular infiltration in acute rejection. Despite these theoretical differences, we know of no certain way of diagnosing acute rejection in the presence of an active cardiac infection by *Toxoplasma*. Since our patient had a heterotopic transplant, the recipient heart served as a control for chemotherapy and for deciding whether a mononuclear cell infiltrate of the donor heart was likely to be due to rejection or toxoplasmosis. Other infections too, e.g. cytomegalic inclusion disease and coccidioidomycosis, may be detected by endo-myocardial biopsy.

(4) The paucity of human donor hearts available for transplantation has led to the concept of distant heart procurement, whereby the excised donor heart may be stored and transported in a cardioplegic solution in ice or by using a portable hypothermic perfusion system[27,28]. The major problem is the prevention of myocardial damage in the donor heart prior to implantation. Morphologically such myocardial damage may be seen as coagulative necrosis of myofibres or as a reperfusion type of myocardial infarction characterized by numerous contraction bands (coagulative myocytolysis) and widespread interstitial haemorrhages.

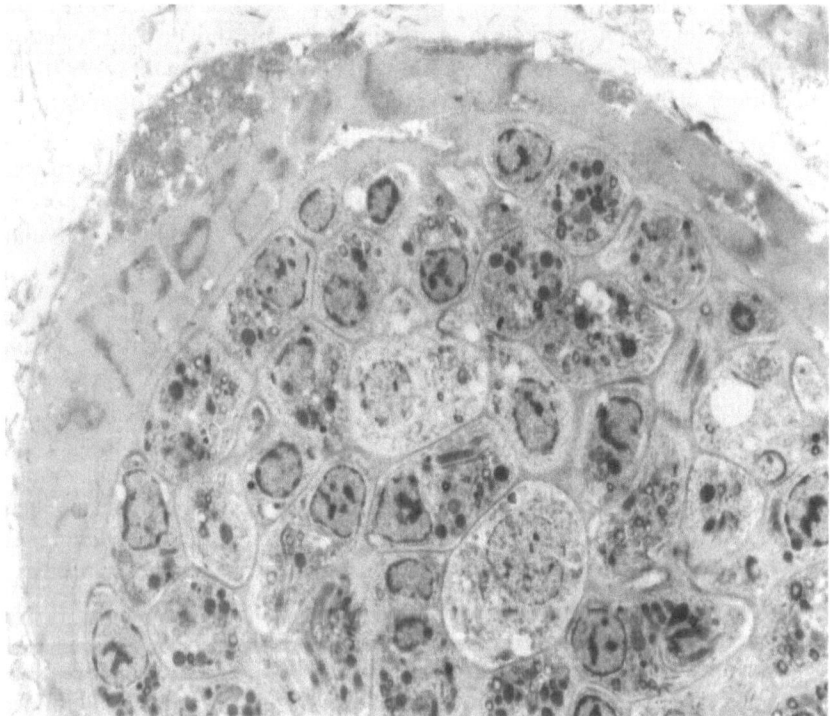

Figure 11.15   Donor heart biopsy shows numerous Toxoplasmas within a myofibre. Lead citrate and uranyl acetate × 10 800

At our institution a non-pulsatile perfusion apparatus has been developed in which circulation of the perfusate, as well as oxygenation and maintenance of acid-base balance, is provided by the flow of a mixture of 97% oxygen and 3% carbon dioxide. This perfusion system has been used successfully experimentally with cardiac allografts in baboons[29] and in several human cardiac transplants[30] (Chapter 5).

HYPERACUTE REJECTION

Hyperacute rejection may be encountered in patients with preformed, donor-specific antibodies or if the ABO blood groups are mismatched. Hyperacute rejection is predominantly encountered in the experimental situation where a graft is implanted across different species of animals. Such a graft, termed a xenograft, has occasionally been used in humans as a desperate attempt to save the life of a patient for whom no human donor is available. Two patients have received xenografts at our hospital in the hope that their own myocardium would recover its function or a donor heart may become available[7]. Histological features of note in hyperacute rejection include platelet aggregation, endothelial cell damage, fibrin deposition, capillary rupture, interstitial oedema, neutrophil emigration and ischaemic myocardial damage.

References

1. Carrel, A. and Guthrie, C. C. (1905). The transplantation of veins and organs. *Am. Med.*, **10**, 1101
2. Mann, F. C., Priestly, J. T., Markowitz, J. and Yater, W. M. (1933). Transplantation of the intact mammalian heart. *Arch. Surg.*, **26**, 219
3. Downie, H. G. (1953). Homotransplantation of the dog heart. *Arch. Surg.*, **66**, 624
4. Lower, R. R., Stofer, R. C. and Shumway, N. E. (1961). Homovital transplantation of the heart. *J. Thorac. Cardiovasc. Surg.*, **41**, 196
5. Blumenstock, D. A., Hechtman, H. B., Collins, J. A., Jaretzki, A., Hosbein, J. D., Zing, W. and Powers, J. H. (1963). Prolonged survival of orthotopic homotransplants of the heart in animals treated with methotrexate. *J. Thorac. Cardiovasc. Surg.*, **46**, 616
6. Cooper, D. K. C. (1968). Experimental development of cardiac transplantation. *Br. Med. J.*, **4**, 194
7. Uys, C. J. and Rose, A. G. (1983). The pathology of cardiac transplantation. In Silver, M. D. (ed.) *Cardiovascular Pathology*. Vol. 2, p. 1329. (New York: Churchill Livingstone)
8. Thomson, J. G. (1968). Heart transplantation in man—necropsy findings. *Br. Med. J.*, **2**, 511
9. Lower, R. R., Lontos, H. A., Kosek, J. C., Sewell, D. H. and Graham, W. H. (1968). Experiences in heart transplantation. Technic, physiology and rejection. *Am. J. Cardiol.*, **22**, 766
10. Rose, A. G., Uys, C. J., Losman, J. G. and Barnard, C. N. (1979). Morphological changes in 49 Chacma baboon cardiac allografts. *S. Afr. Med. J.*, **56**, 880
11. Nowygrod, R., Spotnitz, H. M., Dubroff, J. M., Hardy, M. A. and Reemsta, K. (1983). Organ mass: an indicator of heart transplant rejection. *Transplant. Proc.*, **15**, 1225

12. Thomas, F. T. and Lower, R. R. (1978). Heart transplantation—1978. *Surg. Clin. N. Am.*, **58**, 335

13. Copeland, J. G. and Stinson, E. B. (1979). Human heart transplantation. *Curr. Probl. Cardiol.*, **4**, 1

14. Rose, A. G., Uys, C. J., Losman, J. G. and Barnard, C. N. (1978). Evaluation of endomyocardial biopsy in the diagnosis of cardiac rejection. A study using bioptome samples of formalin-fixed tissue. *Transplantation*, **26**, 10

15. Baandrup, U., Florio, R. A., Roters, F. and Olsen, E. G. J. (1981). Electron microscopic investigation of endomyocardial biopsy samples in hypertrophy and cardiomyopathy. A semi-quantitative study in 48 patients. *Circulation*, **63**, 1289

16. Losman, J. G., Rose, A. G. and Barnard, C. N. (1977). Myocardial fibrinolytic activity in allogeneic cardiac rejection. *Transplantation*, **23**, 414

17. Kosek, K. C., Chartrand, C., Hurley, E. J. and Lower, R. R. (1969). Arteries in canine cardiac homografts. Ultrastructure during acute rejection. *Lab. Invest.*, **21**, 328

18. Lessof, M. (1978). Immunological reactions in heart disease. *Br. Heart J.*, **40**, 211

19. Cooper, D. K. C., Fraser, R. C., Rose, A. G., Ayzenberg, O., Oldfield, G. S., Hassoulas, J. N., Novitsky, D., Uys, C. J. and Barnard, C. N. (1982). Technique, complications, and clinical value of endomyocardial biopsy in patients with heterotopic heart transplants. *Thorax*, **37**, 727

20. Lanza, R. P., Cooper, D. K. C., Novitzky, D. and Barnard, C. N. (1983). Letter to the Editor: Survival after cardiac transplantation. *S. Afr. Med. J.*, **64**, 1007

21. Billingham, M. E. (1982). Diagnosis of cardiac rejection by endomyocardial biopsy. *Heart Transplant.*, **1**, 25

22. Griffith, B. P., Hardesty, R. L., Bahnson, H. T., Bernstein, R. L. and Starzl, T. E. (1983). Cardiac transplants with cyclosporin-A and low-dose prednisone: Histologic graduation of rejection. *Transplant. Proc.*, **15**, 1241

23. Billingham, M. E. (1983). The role of endomyocardial biopsy in the diagnosis and treatment of heart disease. In Silver, M. D. (ed.) *Cardiovascular Pathology*. p. 1205. (New York: Churchill Livingstone)

24. Oyer, P. E., Stinson, E. B., Reitz, B. A., Jamieson, S. W., Hunt, S. A., Schroeder, J. S., Billingham, M. E., Wallwork, J., Bieber, C. P., Baumgartner, W. A., Gamberg, P. L., Miller, J. L. and Shumway, N. E. (1982). Preliminary results with cyclosporin-A in clinical cardiac transplantation. In White, D. J. G. (ed.) *Cyclosporin-A*. p. 461. (Amsterdam: Elsevier Biomedical)

25. Rose, A. G., Uys, C. J., Novitzky, D., Cooper, D. K. C. and Barnard, C. N. (1983). Toxoplasmosis of donor and recipient hearts after heterotopic cardiac transplantation. *Arch. Pathol. Lab. Med.*, **107**, 368

26. Uys, C. J., Rose, A. G. and Barnard, C. N. (1979). The pathology of human cardiac transplantation: An assessment after 11 years' experience at Groote Schuur Hospital. *S. Afr. Med. J.*, **56**, 887

27. Wicomb, W. N., Boyd, S. T., Cooper, D. K. C., Rose, A. G. and Barnard, C. N. (1981). Ex vivo functional evaluation of the pig heart subjected to 24 hours' preservation by hypothermic perfusion. *S. Afr. Med. J.*, **60**, 245

28. Wicomb, W. N., Cooper, D. K. C., Hassoulas, J., Rose, A. G. and Barnard, C. N. (1982). Orthotopic transplantation of the baboon heart after 24 hours' preservation by continuous hypothermic perfusion with an oxygenated hyperosmolar solution. *J. Thorac. Cardiovasc. Surg.*, **83**, 133

29. Cooper, D. K. C., Wicomb, W. N., Rose, A. G. and Barnard, C. N. (1983). Orthotopic allotransplantation of the baboon heart following 24-hr. storage by a portable hypothermic perfusion system. *Cryobiology*, **20**, 385

30. Wicomb, W. N., Cooper, D. K. C., Novitzky, D. and Barnard, C. N. (1984). Cardiac transplantation following storage of the donor heart by a portable hypothermic perfusion system. *Ann. Thorac. Surg.*, **37**, 243

12
Diagnosis and Management of Acute Rejection

INTRODUCTION

At the present time it is impossible to predict whether or not any individual patient will experience episodes of acute rejection. There is no correlation between the number, frequency and severity of episodes of acute rejection and any other known factor. Certainly, in our experience, cyclosporin A (CYA) has led to a diminished incidence of severe acute rejection episodes.

Acute rejection is not a steady phenomenon but occurs in sporadic waves, episodes of severe acute rejection extending over a period of a few days or a week or two, alternating with periods of mild or even no rejection. These episodes of severe acute rejection diminish with time, the recipient's body appearing to adapt to the presence of the donor organ, and a state of partial tolerance being achieved. No centre involved in cardiac transplantation has yet, however, successfully weaned patients off immunosuppression altogether, even when several years have elapsed since the operation. It would appear that the possibility of an acute rejection episode is always present; this has been illustrated in one of our own patients who, after failing to take his own immunosuppressive medication regularly, developed a moderately severe acute rejection episode 5 years after transplantation.

DIAGNOSIS OF ACUTE REJECTION

The patient may feel completely well until the rejection episode has progressed for some days and donor heart function has deteriorated (sometimes irreversibly) to the point that cardiac failure occurs. The clinical diagnosis of acute rejection may prove more difficult in a patient with a heterotopic heart transplant, in whom the recipient heart may assist the cardiac output for a considerable period of time, delaying the onset of symptoms and signs of

177

cardiac failure. Severe, irreversible damage to the myocardium may occur before clinical features become manifest; for successful therapy to be initiated at an early stage, the diagnosis must therefore be made before clinical features of cardiac failure occur.

The search for a simple, non-invasive method of detecting acute rejection in its early stages has continued for a number of years, but to date has eluded workers, though the recent application of the technique of radionuclide scanning in our own unit may prove an answer to this problem.

Clinical features

Acute rejection is frequently totally asymptomatic, particularly in its early stages. In a patient with an orthotopic allograft, the clinical diagnosis of rejection relies mainly on symptoms and signs indicating cardiac failure, particularly of right ventricular failure due to the decreased compliance associated with cellular infiltration and oedema of the graft. In the heterotopic transplant, however, due to the support given by the patient's own right ventricle, evidence of right ventricular failure may not occur during rejection and, therefore, these symptoms and signs cannot be relied upon in the diagnosis of this complication.

The onset of features of cardiac failure, however, should always be considered to be due to acute rejection until proved otherwise. If acute rejection is confirmed, the treatment is primarily increased immunosuppression rather than anti-failure therapy.

Occasionally patients have complained of vague chest discomfort or have been feverish during an acute rejection episode, but, in our experience, these symptoms are unreliable. In the occasional patient with extremely severe acute rejection that is unresponsive to any medication, the patient may complain of malaise and develop a high fluctuating fever, which is presumably secondary to necrosis of myocardial tissue. These features of toxicity from myocardial necrosis, which persist until the donor heart has been excised, have been observed in one of our patients who acutely rejected his heart after 5 weeks; they were seen again following retransplantation when he rejected his heart after only 5 days, developing donor-specific antibodies in the process. In the majority of cases, however, the patient is totally unaware that he is undergoing a rejection episode, even if that episode leads to complete non-function of the donor heart.

Radiographic appearances

Radiographic evidence of rejection consists of progressive cardiomegaly, and occasionally the radiographic appearances of an exudate from the epicardium. Following orthotopic transplantation fluid exuding from the epicardium may show up as a pericardial effusion; after heterotopic transplantation it may present as a right-sided pleural effusion. In our experience, microscopic or biochemical examination of this fluid has not proved helpful in differentiating between an effusion resulting from underlying infection and one associated with acute rejection. The presence of a pericardial or pleural effusion should be considered suggestive of acute rejection until proved otherwise. A pleural effusion may, of course, suggest an underlying infective condition of the lung, which should also be aggressively sought. With satisfactory treatment of the acute rejection episode, these effusions will regress and disappear. Effusions, however, may be absent in patients with severe acute rejection, or may appear very late in the episode. Their appearance cannot therefore be used as a reliable diagnostic aid in the recognition of early rejection.

Electrocardiography

It has long been maintained that changes in the electrocardiogram (ECG), which can be monitored after orthotopic or heterotopic heart transplantation, may provide an indication that acute rejection is occurring[1-3]. Electrocardiographic evidence has been based primarily on a decrease in QRS voltage of the donor heart, but has also been said to include dysrhythmias, various degrees of heart block, occasional depression of ST segments, and a shift of axis[4,5]. A QRS complex voltage fall exceeding 20% has long been considered indicative of acute rejection. Many other conditions can, however, influence donor heart ECG voltage, noticeably the presence of pericardial or pleural fluid, generalized weight gain with oedema formation, pulmonary consolidation, pneumothorax and systemic infection[4,5].

Following heterotopic heart transplantation, the recipient's own heart is still present, and ECG data can be obtained from both hearts (Figure 12.1). Rejection should affect the ECG of the donor heart alone, but most other factors should influence the ECG of both hearts. A fall in donor heart ECG voltage alone, therefore, should be strongly suspicious of rejection, whereas a fall in the voltages of both hearts should be more suggestive of some other factor affecting both organs. Our clinical impression, however, has been that the ECG is not a reliable indicator of acute rejection.

To examine its reliability, we carried out a detailed study correlating changes in ECG with those seen on histological examination of endomyocardial biopsy of the donor heart in patients immunosuppressed with azathioprine, methylprednisolone and antithymocyte globulin[6]. There was no statistically significant correlation between any of the ECG changes believed to reflect acute rejection and the histopathological features seen on biopsy. A 20% decrease in QRS amplitude was accompanied by a large number of negative biopsy reports; positive biopsy findings were frequently associated with no significant change in ECG voltage. The ECG would, therefore, appear to be an unreliable predictor of early acute rejection in patients with heterotopic heart transplants.

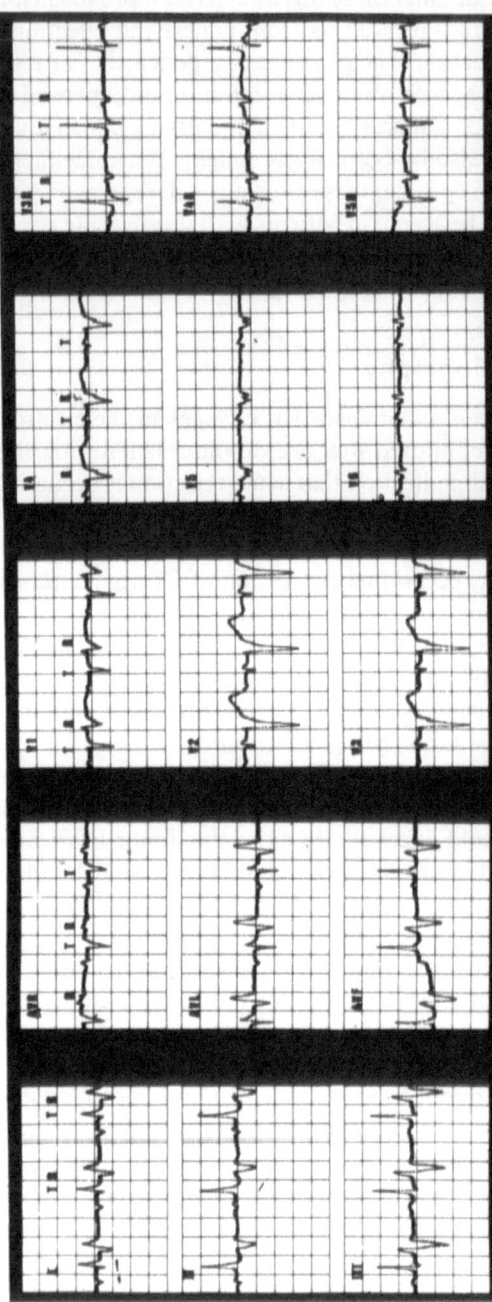

Figure 12.1 Electrocardiogram from a patient with a heterotopic heart transplant showing recipient (R) and transplant (T) heart complexes

This study is supported by numerous observations in animals which would suggest that the QRS voltage fluctuates grossly from day to day, and that it is only very late during an acute rejection episode that a persistent fall in voltage occurs, preceding cessation of function by only 24–72 hours[7-9]. Similarly, in normal individuals, there is a wide daily variation in the QRS complex amplitude; Losman and his colleagues have demonstrated that it ranges from as much as $+64\%$ to -63% of the mean over 76 hours[10]. Our own detailed observations of patients with heterotopic heart transplants would confirm wide fluctuation in the QRS amplitude of both donor and recipient hearts[6].

Several groups who felt the ECG was helpful in the diagnosis of acute rejection when azathioprine, corticosteroids and antithymocyte globulin were administered as the immunosuppressive agents, do not feel this to be the case when immunosuppression is induced with CYA[11,12]. Myocardial oedema, which is common during rejection episodes in patients on 'conventional' immunosuppression, and which may account for the fall in ECG voltage, is less obvious in patients receiving CYA; this observation has been put forward as a reason why the reliability of the ECG no longer holds in CYA-treated patients. Our own detailed study would suggest, however, that the ECG has never been reliable.

Haematological and immunological monitoring

A steady and progressive rise in the white blood cell count (WBC), or in the total lymphocyte count, or, particularly, in the rosetting T cell fraction of the lymphocytes, can, on occasion, indicate that a rejection episode is occurring. A rise in the T cell fraction has been considered a particularly helpful blood test and was used as a routine by the Stanford group in patients receiving conventional immunosuppression[13,14].

In our experience, however, none of these parameters is entirely reliable. We have seen total WBCs of more than 20 000 cells/mm³ in the first post-transplant month totally unrelated to either infection or acute rejection. Presumably this increase in WBC is related to the body's response to the presence of foreign tissue, but it does not necessarily indicate that severe acute rejection is occurring. A source of infection must obviously be excluded in such patients. Viral infection, of course, may result in a lymphocytosis alone.

The Stanford group has reported an analysis of data derived from systematic T cell monitoring that has shown that circulating T cell levels are markedly and uniformly reduced within 5 days of transplantation in cardiac recipients who received rabbit antithymocyte globulin (RATG), such that the T cells account for less than 10% of the total population of peripheral blood lymphocytes. Furthermore, a close correlation has been established between the time of subsequent significant elevation of the circulating T cell fraction from its depressed level and the time of onset of histologically detectable rejection, with T cell elevation preceding histological criteria by 1–3 days[13].

Fluctuations in the number of circulating T cells would appear, therefore, to reflect an earlier phase of the host immune response to the cardiac allograft than that provided by endomyocardial biopsy.

In the Stanford experience, circulating T cell levels tend to rise toward normal some 6 weeks after transplantation, despite continued therapy with ATG, irrespective of the presence or absence of graft rejection. During the first 6 weeks, however, this group has reported good correlation between the T cell count and the onset of acute rejection, with a false-negative rate of only 4% and a false-positive rate of 13%. They have also shown that patients who clear rabbit globulin rapidly from their serum develop more episodes of early acute rejection, which tend to be more severe, and have a significantly lower 1-year survival rate than those who clear rabbit globulin more slowly[13, 14].

Our own experience with regard to the reliability of the circulating T cell counts as an indicator of acute rejection has not been as conclusive as that at Stanford. Though we would agree that an increase in the circulating T cells might suggest the onset of an acute rejection episode, this has by no means always been the case. We have also seen acute rejection occur in the absence of a significant rise in the T cell fraction. As cyclosporin A does not depress the number of circulating T lymphocytes, monitoring of the T cell fraction has not been put forward as a valuable indicator of acute rejection in patients receiving this drug.

The development of monoclonal antibody and fluorescent labelling of peripheral blood lymphocyte subsets has recently refined standard T cell monitoring[15]. Several groups have reported that kidney grafts were rejected primarily in patients with T helper/suppressor (H/S) ratios < 1.3 (normal H/S ratio is 2.0), and that patients with ratios > 1.3 did not experience rejection[16, 17]. Other investigators, however, have had conflicting experience with T cell subset monitoring in kidney transplant patients[18]. In the University of Pittsburgh series of heart transplants the H/S ratio in myocardial biopsies also did not correlate with rejection[19].

There are some reports suggesting that serum and urinary β-2-microglobulin levels are useful for the diagnosis of acute kidney graft rejection[20, 21], and may be a useful adjunct in predicting and diagnosing acute heart transplant rejection[22]. β-2-microglobulin levels, however, may increase due to factors other than graft rejection (e.g. nephrotoxic antibodies and viral infections) and may vary if samples are not collected consistently or if the radioimmunoassay is not performed in a consistent fashion[22].

Indium III-labelled leukocytes have been shown to provide a sensitive early assay of cardiac allograft rejection in rats[23]. The labelled leukocytes progressively infiltrated rejecting cardiac grafts days before rejection was first detected 'clinically' by heart beat palpation. Isotopic count and scanning techniques allowed detection of rejection 3–4 days before weakening of the heart beat. Further evaluation of this technique is necessary, of course, before its clinical usefulness in humans can be assessed.

Arterial pulse wave monitoring

In patients with a heterotopic transplant, a comparison of the respective donor and recipient pulse waves, when measured on an external pulse trace taken over the femoral or carotid artery, has proved helpful in diagnosing acute rejection on many occasions (Figure 12.2)[24,25]. It is possibly the most reliable indicator of deteriorating donor heart function other than radionuclide scanning or endomyocardial biopsy. Clearly, it is an investigation that is not available in patients with orthotopic transplants.

The absolute height of the donor pulse wave is of no significance, but the comparative heights of the two pulse waves demonstrate the relative contributions of the two hearts. In a severe acute rejection episode, when donor myocardial function is impaired by cellular infiltration, oedema, and myofibre damage, the donor wave diminishes in height and the recipient increases. We have used this simple and quick test extensively in monitoring for acute rejection and have found it reliable in the majority of patients. False positives and false negatives can, however, be obtained on occasion.

Endomyocardial biopsy

Percutaneous transvenous or transarterial biopsy of right and left ventricles with a specially designed forceps, thus obtaining fragments of endocardium for histological examination, was first described by Sakakibara and Konno in 1962[26], and, 10 years later, was introduced as a clinical tool in heart transplantation by Caves and his colleagues[27]. Since 1976 it has been used increasingly at Groote Schuur Hospital in the management of patients undergoing heart transplantation. It is our policy to perform donor heart biopsy at approximately weekly intervals during the first month after transplantation, with decreasing frequency during subsequent months. Biopsy is also performed whenever a rejection episode is suspected, and to assess the efficacy of a course of antirejection therapy.

The percutaneous supraclavicular approach to either right or left subclavian vein is our approach of choice, though the infraclavicular route has been used in a number of patients. The procedure takes 15–30 minutes and is performed in the cardiac catheterization laboratory. The technique in both orthotopic[27,28] and heterotopic[29] transplant patients has been described elsewhere (Figure 12.3). It is a relatively safe invasive procedure with few significant technical problems. In our own centre, approximately 94% of biopsy procedures provide tissue samples adequate for meaningful histopathological assessment[29]. Repeated biopsy on any one patient can be undertaken without complication. The technique is not without a small risk, however, and pneumothorax and rupture of the right ventricle with resulting haemorrhage have occurred. The introduction of infection would also appear to be a potential hazard, particularly when technical problems necessitate introduction of the

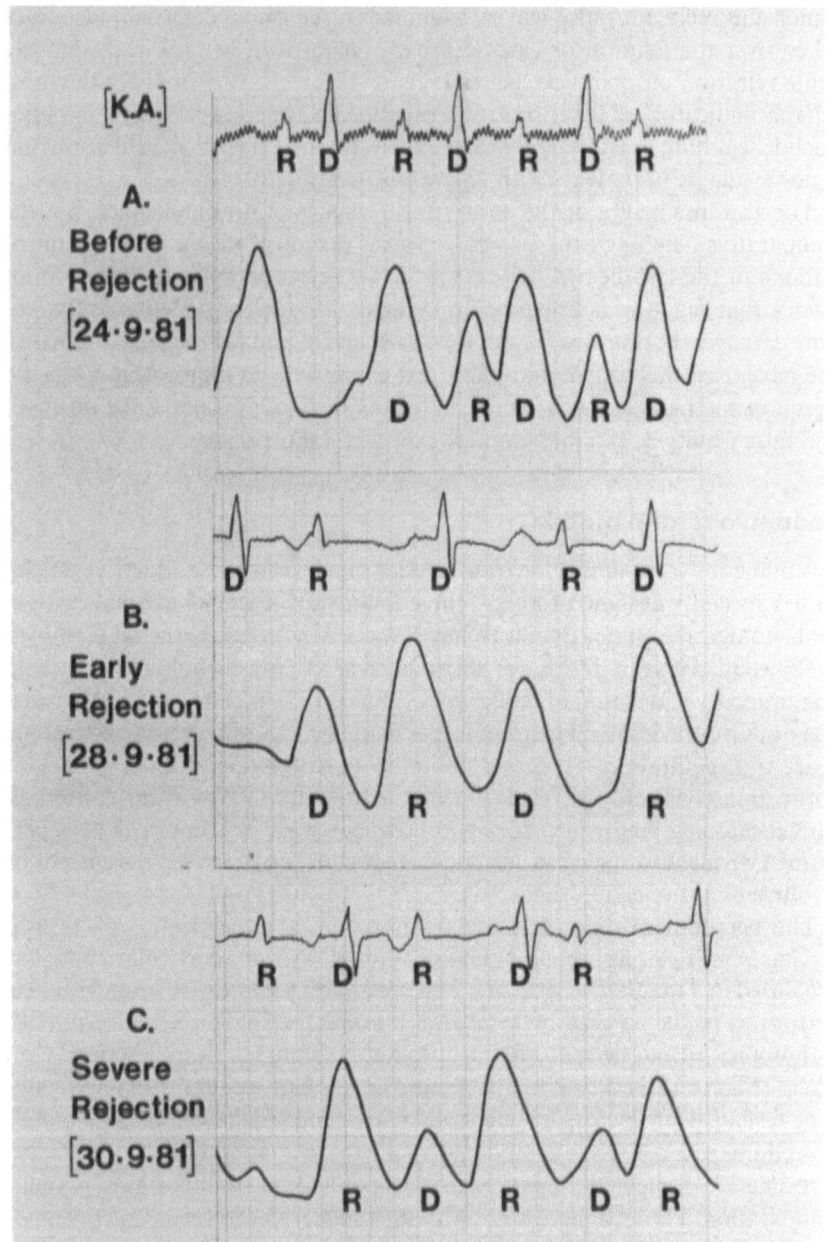

Figure 12.2   Recordings of electrocardiogram (ECG) (above) and arterial pulse waves (taken over femoral artery) (below) showing changes occurring during an acute rejection episode. (R = recipient; D = donor)

catheter at the groin[29]. Pulmonary or systemic embolism from dislodgement of mural thrombus, which may result from decreased myocardial contractions due to rejection, are also potential complications. The complication rate at our own centre is approximately 4%, though this includes very minor transient complications such as nerve paresis (e.g. brachial plexus or recurrent laryngeal) induced by infiltration of local anaesthetic. The morbidity of the procedure, however, is said to be lower than that for liver or renal biopsy[30].

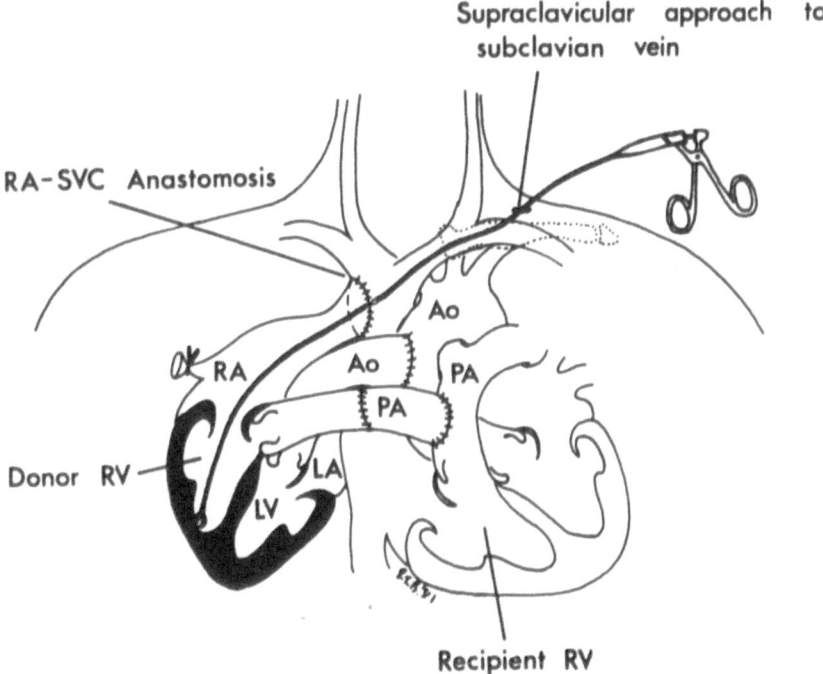

Supraclavicular approach to subclavian vein

RA−SVC Anastomosis

Ao

RA   Ao   PA

PA

Donor RV   LA

LV

Recipient RV

Figure 12.3 Diagram illustrating the passage of a bioptome into the donor right ventricle for endomyocardial biopsy in a patient with a heterotopic heart transplant. (SVC = superior vena cava; RA = right atrium; RV = right ventricle; PA = pulmonary artery; LA = left atrium; LV =. left ventricle; AO = aorta)

Assessment of rejection is based on light microscopy. At our own institution, we have attempted to grade the histopathological changes seen, the aim being to give the clinician a guide to the severity of rejection and to the efficacy of antirejection therapy[29]. The reproducibility of histological interpretation is enhanced since the same criteria are assessed each time and given a score, rather than the diagnosis of rejection being based on an overall impression of the biopsy. This scoring system has been detailed elsewhere (Chapter 11).

The clinical value of histological assessment has been shown to be considerable in approximately 95% of cases in which an adequate biopsy is obtained, either confirming acute rejection, when it was suspected on other grounds, or demonstrating it when hitherto unsuspected; a biopsy negative for rejection is of value as it prevents the needless continuation of a high-dose immuno-suppressive regimen. Occasional or even repeated biopsies have been shown to be misleading due to difficulty in obtaining adequate tissue, observer error, incorrect interpretation of the histopathological features, or inadequate clini-cal follow-up in suspicious cases (Table 12.1).

Table 12.1   Clinical value of histopathological assessment of 147 adequate endomyo-cardial biopsies in patients with heterotopic heart transplants

	Number of biopsies	%
Confirmed clinically suspected rejection	25	17
Denied clinically suspected rejection	15	10
Demonstrated clinically unsuspected rejection	25	17
Confirmed clinical absence of significant rejection	47	32
Demonstrated expected response to increased therapy	27	19
Inadequately interpreted	5	3
Misleading	3	2
Total	147	100

Radionuclide scanning

Acute rejection leads to cellular infiltration and oedema of the myocardium, together with damage of the myofibres, resulting in thickening of the ventricu-lar walls, reduction in ventricular cavity volume and impairment of myo-cardial function. In patients treated with CYA rather than azathioprine, myocardial oedema is much less prominent, and therefore ventricular wall thickening is less obvious. Cellular infiltration is present, however, resulting in a loss of compliance. Radionuclide scanning measures these left ventricular changes in volume and function.

In our unit radionuclide scanning of the donor left ventricle with tech-netium-99m labelled red cells has been used to monitor acute rejection after both heterotopic and orthotopic heart transplantation, and has been compared with histopathological evidence of rejection obtained from endomyocardial biopsy. The technique of multigated blood pool scanning and calculation of left ventricular volumes has been detailed[31]. Ejection fraction, end-diastolic, end-systolic, and stroke volumes were calculated on each occasion. Change in stroke volume showed a high correlation with histopathological evidence of rejection ($p < 0.001$); changes in end-diastolic and end-systolic left ventricular volumes showed a less high degree of correlation, and change in ejection fraction no correlation[32]. Cardiac output showed a significant correlation, but this was based entirely on the change in stroke volume, as change in heart rate showed no correlation with rejection. This study is still progressing, but preliminary work has shown a highly significant multiple correlation between radionuclide scanning parameters, using the significant correlates of stroke, end-diastolic, and end-systolic volumes, and endomyocardial biopsy[31].

Prediction of acute rejection by radionuclide scanning has several advantages over endomyocardial biopsy.

(1) The technique is non-invasive, and therefore the risks of any invasive procedure, such as the introduction of infection, are avoided.

(2) Apart from the initial investigation to calculate the attenuation factor (which adjusts for body wall thickness), radionuclide scanning can be performed in the patient's room; transfer of the patient to the catheterization laboratory is not necessary.

(3) An endomyocardial biopsy requires processing, staining, and examination before an opinion on the histopathological features can be given, a process which in our institution takes approximately 24 hours. An answer by radionuclide techniques is obtained within 1 hour. Treatment can therefore be initiated immediately in patients who are found to be undergoing acute rejection.

(4) Though it would appear that the myocardium is generally uniformly affected by acute rejection[30, 33], a biopsy may be relatively non-representative. Radionuclide techniques provide information on the status of the entire left ventricle.

(5) Interpretation of the histopathological picture of an endomyocardial biopsy remains a subjective procedure and is dependent on the experience and expertise of the pathologist concerned. The estimation of the degree of acute rejection obtained from the radionuclide scan is not dependent on human opinion or human error.

(6) Though a biopsy can be repeated at frequent intervals, the procedure is not without a certain discomfort to the patient and the risk of complication must surely be increased. Radionuclide studies can be repeated daily, or at more frequent intervals if indicated, with minimal risk and discomfort to the patient.

At the present time we continue to perform endomyocardial biopsy and radionuclide scanning on the same occasion as a clinical research programme. We believe, however, that if further clinical experience with this technique confirms its excellent correlation with endomyocardial biopsy and with the clinical progress of the patient, it may eventually replace the invasive procedure of biopsy, and the several other less reliable methods of predicting acute rejection, in patients with cardiac transplants.

Echocardiography

Preliminary results using two-dimensional echocardiography as an indicator of both rat and human heart transplant rejection have been encouraging[34]. Using this method, left ventricular mass increased with reversible rejection episodes without significant concurrent change in ejection fraction or end-diastolic volume. These results suggest that this non-invasive technique may prove to be a useful method for detecting early cardiac allograft rejection.

MANAGEMENT OF AN ACUTE REJECTION EPISODE

The first decision that has to be made is whether the acute rejection episode is severe enough to warrant extra immunosuppressive therapy. In our experience it is relatively rare when administrating 'conventional' immunosuppressive therapy to the patient to find absolutely no features of acute rejection on endomyocardial biopsy (i.e. a histopathological score of zero) or on radionuclide scanning. Since the introduction of CYA the complete absence of rejection has been noted more frequently. Such a score would even suggest that the patient might be over-immunosuppressed, and we would take steps to reduce the dosage of the drugs being administered. Evidence of mild acute rejection (scores of 0.5 to 2.0) is common, and our policy has been to give little or no extra therapy to such patients. Severe acute rejection (scores of 4.5 or more) clearly requires a course of increased therapy.

The difficult decisions are presented by patients seen to be suffering from moderately severe acute rejection (scores of 2.5 to 4.0). The decisions of whether to treat or not, and how much therapy to give, are based on several factors, in particular the patient's clinical course since transplantation. If previous biopsies or scans have confirmed no significant rejection (scores of 0, 0.5, or 1.0), but there has been a sudden increase to 3.5 or 4.0, then a full course of extra therapy would seem to be indicated. When the increase is to scores of only 2.5 or 3.0, a considerably attenuated course of extra therapy might be all that is required.

Careful monitoring of the patient is required, however, with a further biopsy or scan within 2–4 days, to ensure that the rejection episode is subsiding. It is in precisely these cases where radionuclide scanning has proved so valuable, in that the course of the rejection episode can be monitored daily or twice daily without risk or inconvenience to the patient.

Once it has been decided that extra therapy is indicated, the exact treatment of an acute rejection episode depends to a certain extent on the maintenance therapy being administered to the patient. With the introduction of CYA, our management of acute rejection episodes has been modified.

1. When maintenance immunosuppression is with azathioprine and corticosteroids

The standard treatment in such patients is the administration of 1 g 'pulses' of intravenous methylprednisolone sodium succinate given over 30–60 minutes on a daily basis, or occasionally at 12-hourly intervals, for 3 or more days, depending on the severity of the rejection episode and the response to therapy. We have been prepared to give a total dose of up to approximately 10–15 g (together with other therapy) in any one course, but thereafter have been inclined to abandon the donor heart if severe rejection has persisted, as we believe that the increasing risk of infection outweighs the possible benefit of further steroid therapy in such cases. Such occasions are fortunately relatively rare. In nearly all cases a course of increased therapy extending for 2 weeks will reverse an acute rejection episode, if treatment is begun early during that episode. If treatment is delayed by failure to diagnose the rejection episode until it is advanced, then irreversible damage might already have caused severe loss of function of the donor heart, and further therapy will probably not salvage the situation entirely.

By the standards of many renal transplant units, a total dosage of 15 g of methylprednisolone during a single course of antirejection therapy is extremely high. In patients with cardiac allografts, however, allograft survival has the highest priority, as these patients do not have an equivalent of renal dialysis to support them should the graft be totally rejected.

Whether increased corticosteroid therapy should be given intravenously or orally, and whether single doses of the magnitude of 1 g are essential, remains in question[35]. There is some evidence that much smaller daily doses would suffice in successfully reversing an acute rejection episode.

It is repeated, prolonged episodes of acute rejection, rather than a single episode, which suggest that, whatever therapy is proffered, the patient is eventually likely to lose adequate myocardial function. In patients with heterotopic transplants, on occasions the donor heart can be abandoned and the patient survive on his own heart. The decision to withhold further therapy in a patient with an orthotopic transplant is clearly more difficult, unless a suitable second donor becomes available.

Azathioprine dosage, which should already be at the maximum tolerated dose as judged by features of bone marrow and hepatic toxicity, should be maintained and not increased further; we would aim to maintain the total WBC in the range of 2500–5000 cells/mm^3.

If the rosetting T-lymphocytes are not already maintained at 50–150 cells/mm^3, then in severe rejection episodes, especially those which are not readily reversed with intravenous methylprednisolone, a short course of rabbit or equine antithymocyte globulin (ATG) is also administered. This should be administered daily or twice daily along the lines already outlined in Chapter 9. The length of the course will be determined by the response, as judged by the

T cell count, and by further endomyocardial biopsy or radionuclide scanning at frequent intervals.

In patients in whom an acute rejection episode is proving difficult to treat successfully, and in whom there is evidence of immune clearance of rabbit globulin, the Stanford group has on occasion used ATG prepared in an alternate species in the hope that this would have lower serum clearance rates and would therefore be more effective. ATG prepared in goats has been utilized in a small number of patients with resolution of the rejection process in the majority of cases[36]. There would appear to be no obvious reason why the more readily available equine ATG should not be used in such cases.

Refinement of antilymphocyte preparation is likely in the near future. Already, acute rejection episodes in patients with renal transplants have been successfully reversed by the administration of OKT3 monoclonal antibody (reactive with all mature peripheral blood T cells)[37]. The possibility of manipulating specific T cell subsets under clinical conditions is clearly imminent.

When there is histological evidence of a major cellular element to the rejection episode, it was our policy to administer a 3–4-day course of actinomycin D at 200 µg/day intravenously, unless bone marrow activity was already unduly depressed; we have found actinomycin D to add little to the other therapy available, however, and have now discontinued its use.

The response to increased therapy is then monitored by repeating the endomyocardial biopsy or radionuclide scan. This is usually carried out 2–4 days after the initiation of the course of extra therapy, depending on the initial severity of the episode. If evidence of severe acute rejection remains, then the course of therapy is continued. If improvement has occurred, then the dosage of these drugs may be reduced or discontinued. Biopsy or scan must be repeated within a further 2–4 days to ensure that the rejection episode continues in remission, and that relapse has not occurred following reduction of therapy.

In five of our patients, acute rejection was accompanied by a sustained rise in total WBC above the therapeutic range, uncontrolled by increasing doses of azathioprine (< 7 mg/kg per day) even when given intravenously. The total WBC was sustained at 7–10 000 cells/mm³, despite maintenance of the T cell count within the therapeutic range by RATG. The acute rejection episode proved difficult to control by the usual therapy outlined above. In three of these patients, azathioprine was replaced by cyclophosphamide (approximately 1.5–2.5 mg/kg per day); in the remaining two, small doses of cyclophosphamide (approximately 0.5–1 mg/kg per day) were added to the original drug regimen, azathioprine being continued. In all cases the administration of cyclophosphamide was followed by reduction in total WBC to therapeutic levels, and by control of the acute rejection episode. The therapeutic oral dose of cyclophosphamide is less than that of azathioprine; in our experience, doses of more than 2 mg/kg per day are rarely required.

In one patient, who experienced repeated moderately severe rejection episodes whilst receiving azathioprine, a change to cyclophosphamide in a dosage of 50–100 mg/day resulted in no further acute rejection episodes over the following 3 years. Cyclophosphamide has proved, however, a difficult drug to manage, and is not without major complications, particularly in regard to bone marrow suppression. We have been forced to abandon its use in two patients as a result of this complication. It can, however, be valuable when administered as a short course in selected patients suffering severe acute rejection resistant to other therapy.

Heavy immunosuppression is frequently associated with the appearance of herpes simplex lesions in the mouth and pharynx. Small ulcers appear, particularly on the tongue and buccal mucosa. In our experience these rarely lead to systemic herpes viraemia, but are an indicator that the patient is now heavily immunosuppressed; their appearance has acted as a warning to us that the limits of immunosuppression are being reached. They can be uncomfortable or even painful for the patient, particularly when swallowing, and may limit dietary intake. Topical antiseptic and analgesic tablets or liquids provide symptomatic relief and will also help prevent secondary infection of these lesions, which spontaneously regress when the immunosuppression is reduced.

2. When maintenance immunosuppression is with cyclosporin A and corticosteroids

Although the frequency of acute rejection episodes occurring in patients receiving maintenance CYA would appear to be approximately the same as in those receiving conventional therapy, the severity of such episodes is diminished. This drug appears to be a significant advance in reducing the severity of acute rejection episodes. When an acute rejection episode occurs, however, we again administer intravenous 'pulses' of methylprednisolone as described above, though on occasions we would now give only 500 mg rather than 1 g. If blood levels of CYA remain in the therapeutic range we see no reason to increase the CYA dosage, in view of the risk of inducing renal failure or other drug-related complication. No other therapy is given at this stage.

The effect of methylprednisolone boluses is assessed by endomyocardial biopsy or radionuclide scanning within 2–4 days. If the acute rejection episode has regressed, then no additional treatment is necessary, but another biopsy or scan is performed some 2–4 days later to confirm this remission. If severe rejection continues, however, then the intravenous course of methylprednisolone should be continued and the dosage possibly increased. In addition, we would consider giving a short course of intravenous antithymocyte globulin. The T cell response would be carefully monitored and the dosage of RATG adjusted to maintain the absolute T cell count between 50 and 150 cells/mm^3. We have used RATG successfully to reverse severe rejection episodes in three patients; each course has extended over only 2–4 days. There seems little doubt that a *prolonged* course of RATG together with CYA is associated with an increased risk of the development of lymphoma[38], and should be avoided.

In four patients experiencing either severe or repeated or prolonged moderate acute rejection episodes, the total WBC remained high, and it was felt that moderate bone marrow suppression might be associated with remission of the acute rejection episode. Just as the addition of a short course of cyclophosphamide to patients receiving conventional immunosuppression has proved helpful in reducing the WBC and controlling rejection, the addition of azathioprine (in a low dosage of 0.5–2 mg/kg per day) to patients on maintenance CYA has also had a beneficial effect. The WBC has fallen and, in all four cases, the acute rejection episode has regressed.

Patients undergoing transplantation of the heart and both lungs at Stanford Medical Center received only CYA and azathioprine during the first 2–3 weeks, to allow satisfactory healing of the tracheal suture line before steroids are added to the regimen. These patients have done well, and the use of this combination of drugs in patients receiving heart transplants alone warrants further exploration.

The concomitant administration of relatively low doses of several drugs (for example, CYA, azathioprine, corticosteroids), either as maintenance therapy, or when acute rejection is continuing, may prove to be the most effective form of immunosuppressive therapy. The toxic effects of any one drug would thus be avoided or minimized. Experimental work in animals and observations in patients suggest, however, that there is a higher risk of malignant tumour formation in patients receiving combination therapy in high doses[38,39]. The dosage of each drug might prove the critical factor, and would have to be carefully controlled.

References

1. Lower, R. R., Dong, E. Jr. and Shumway, N. E. (1965). Suppression of rejection crises in the cardiac homograft. *Ann. Thorac. Surg.*, **1**, 645
2. Lower, R. R., Dong, E. Jr. and Glazener, F. S. (1966). Electrocardiograms of dogs with heart homografts. *Circulation*, **33**, 455
3. Stinson, E. B., Dong, E. Jr., Bieber, C. P., Schroeder, J. S. and Shumway, N. E. (1969). Cardiac transplantation in man. I. Early rejection. *J. Am. Med. Assoc.*, **207**, 2233
4. Baumgartner, W. A., Reitz, B. A., Oyer, P. E., Stinson, E. B. and Shumway, N. E. (1979). Cardiac homotransplantation. *Curr. Probl. Surg.*, **16**, 1
5. Jamieson, S. W., Reitz, B. A., Oyer, P. E., Bieber, C. P., Stinson, E. B. and Shumway, N. E. (1979). Current management of cardiac transplant recipients. *Br. Heart J.*, **42**, 703
6. Cooper, D. K. C., Charles, R. G., Rose, A. G., Fraser, R. C., Isaacs, S., Novitzky, D. and Barnard, C. N. (1985). An investigation into the reliability of the electrocardiogram in the recognition of acute rejection following heterotopic heart transplantation. *Heart Transplant.* (In press)
7. Semb, B. K. H., Abrahamson, A. M. and Barnard, C. N. (1971). Electrocardiographic changes during the unmodified rejection of heterotopic canine heart allografts. *Scand. J. Thorac. Cardiovasc. Surg.*, **5**, 120

8. Dear, M., Cooper, D. K. C. and Murtra, M. (1973). Electrocardiographic prediction of unmodified rejection in heterotopic canine cardiac allografts. *Cardiovasc. Res.*, **7**, 687

9. Losman, J. G., Rose, A. G. and Barnard, C. N. (1977). Myocardial fibrinolytic activity in allogenic cardiac rejection. *Transplantation*, **23**, 414

10. Losman, J. G., McDonald, J., Levine, H. D., Campbell, C. D. and Replogle, R. L. (1981). The variations of the electrocardiographic voltage during the day in normal adult subjects. *Heart Transplant.*, **1**, 39

11. Devineni, R., McKenzie, N., Kostuk, W. J., Heimbecker, R. O., Keown, P., Stiller, C. and Silver, M. D. (1983). Cyclosporine in cardiac transplantation: observations on immunologic monitoring, cardiac histology, and cardiac function. *Heart Transplant.*, **2**, 219

12. Griffith, B. P., Hardesty, R. L., Thompson, M. E., Dummer, J. S. and Bahnson, H. T. (1983). Cardiac transplantation with cyclosporine: the Pittsburgh experience. *Heart Transplant.*, **2**, 251

13. Bieber, C. P., Griepp, R. B., Oyer, P. E., David, L. A. and Stinson, E. B. (1977). Relationship of rabbit ATG serum clearance rate to circulating T cell level, rejection onset, and survival in cardiac transplantation. *Transplant. Proc.*, **9**, 1031

14. Oyer, P. E., Stinson, E. B., Bieber, C. P., Reitz, B. A., Raney, A. A., Baumgartner, W. A. and Shumway, N. E. (1979). Diagnosis and treatment of acute cardiac allograft rejection. *Transplant. Proc.*, **11**, 296

15. Kung, P. C., Goldstein, G., Reinherz, E. L. and Schlossman, S. F. (1979). Monoclonal antibodies defining distinctive human T cell surface antigens. *Science*, **206**, 347

16. Cosimi, A. B., Colvin, R. B., Burton, R. C., Rubin, R. H., Goldstein, G., Kung, P. C., Hansen, W. P., Delmonico, F. L. and Russell, P. S. (1981). Use of monoclonal antibodies to T cell subsets for immunological monitoring and treatment in recipients of renal allografts. *N. Engl. J. Med.*, **305**, 308

17. Ellis, T. M., Lee, H. M. and Mohanakumar, T. (1981). Alterations in human regulatory T lymphocyte subpopulation after renal allografting. *J. Immunol.*, **127**, 2199

18. Severyn, W., Flaa, C., Fuller, L., Kyriakides, G. K., Esquenazi, V. and Miller, J. (1982). The role of immunological monitoring in transplantation. *Heart Transplant.*, **1**, 222

19. Rabin, B. S. (1983). Immunologic aspects of human cardiac transplantation. *Heart Transplant.*, **2**, 188

20. Vincent, C. and Revillard, R. (1980). Serum levels and urinary excretion of beta 2 microglobulins in patients under hemodialysis or after renal transplantation. *Acta Clin. Belg.*, **35**, 31

21. Rosenbaum, R. W., Kately, J., Sanchez, T. V., Hirota, T. F. and Mayor, G. H. (1980). Beta-2 microglobulin: an early indicator of renal transplant survival and function. *Trans. Am. Soc. Artif. Intern. Org.*, **26**, 77

22. Goldman, M. H., Lippman, R., Landwehr, D., Szentpetery, S., Wolfgang, T., Lee, H. M., Hess, M., Mendez-Picon, G., Hastillo, A. and Lower, R. R. (1983). Beta 2 microglobulin and the diagnosis of cardiac transplant rejection. *Transplantation*, **36**, 209

23. Oluwole, S., Wang, T., Fawwaz, R., Satake, K., Nowygrod, R., Reemtsma, K. and Hardy, M. A. (1981). Use of indium-III-labelled cells in measurement of cellular dynamics of experimental cardiac allograft rejection. *Transplantation*, **31**, 51

24. Barnard, C. N., Barnard, M. S., Cooper, D. K. C., Curchio, C. A., Hassoulas, J., Novitzky, D. and Wolpowitz, A. (1981). The present status of heterotopic cardiac transplantation. *J. Thorac. Cardiovasc. Surg.*, **81**, 433

25. Cooper, D. K. C., Novitzky, D., Hassoulas, J. and Barnard, C. N. (1982). Transplantation of the heart. *Br. J. Clin. Pract.*, **36**, 337

26. Sakakibara, S. and Konno, S. (1962). Endomyocardial biopsy. *Japan. Heart J.*, **3**, 537–42

27. Caves, P. K., Stinson, E. B., Graham, A. F., Billingham, M. E., Grehl, T. M. and Shumway, N. E. (1973). Percutaneous transvenous endomyocardial biopsy. *J. Am. Med. Assoc.*, **225**, 288

28. Caves, P. K., Billingham, M. E., Stinson, E. B. and Shumway, N. E. (1974). Serial transvenous biopsy of the transplanted human heart—improved management of acute rejection
episodes. *Lancet*, **1**, 821
29. Cooper, D. K. C., Fraser, R. C., Rose, A. G., Ayzenberg, O., Oldfield, G. S., Hassoulas, J.,
Novitzky, D., Uys, C. J. and Barnard, C. N. (1982). Technique, complications, and clinical
value of endomyocardial biopsy in patients with heterotopic heart transplants. *Thorax*, **37**,
727
30. Mason, J. W., Billingham, M. E., Rider, A. K. and Harrison, D. C. (1977). Myocardial
biopsy. In Willerson, J. T. and Sanders, C. A. (eds.) *Clinical Cardiology*. pp. 606–13. (New
York: Grune & Stratton)
31. Novitzky, D., Boniaszczuk, J., Cooper, D. K. C., Isaacs, S., Rose, A. G., Smith, J. A.,
Uys, C. J., Barnard, C. N. and Fraser, R. C. (1984). Prediction of acute cardiac rejection
using radionuclide techniques. *S. Afr. Med. J.*, **65**, 5
32. Novitzky, D., Cooper, D. K. C., Boniaszczuk, J., Isaacs, S., Fraser, R. C., Commerford, P. J.,
Uys, C. J., Rose, A. G., Smith, J. A. and Barnard, C. N. (1985). The significance of left
ventricular volume measurement in cardiac transplants using radionuclide techniques. *Heart
Transplant.* (In press)
33. Rose, A. G., Uys, C. J., Losman, J. G. and Barnard, C. N. (1978). Evaluation of endomyocardial biopsy in the diagnosis of cardiac rejection. *Transplantation*, **26**, 10
34. Nowygrod, R., Spotnitz, H. M., Du Broff, J. M., Hardy, M. A. and Reemtsma, K. (1983).
Organ mass: an indicator of heart transplant rejection. *Transplant. Proc.*, **15**, 1225
35. Salaman, J. R. (1983). Steroids in organ transplantation. *Heart Transplant.*, **2**, 118
36. Bieber, C. P., Griepp, R. B., Oyer, P. E., Wong, J. and Stinson, E. B. (1976). Use of rabbit
antithymocyte globulin in cardiac transplantation. *Transplantation*, **22**, 478
37. Cosimi, A. B., Burton, R. C., Colvin, R. B., Golstein, G., Delmonico, F. L., La Quaglia, M. P.,
Tolkoff-Rubin, N., Rubin, R. H., Herrin, J. T. and Russell, P. S. (1981). Treatment of acute
renal allograft rejection with OKT3 monoclonal antibody. *Transplantation*, **32**, 535
38. Hunt, S. A. (1983). Complications of heart transplantation. *Heart Transplant.*, **3**, 70
39. Pennock, J. L., Reitz, B. A., Bieber, C. P., Jamieson, S. W., Raney, A. A., Oyer, P. E. and
Stinson, E. B. (1981). Cardiac allograft survival in cynomolgous monkeys treated with
cyclosporin-A in combination with conventional immune suppression. *Transplant. Proc.*, **13**,
390

13
Infectious Complications

INTRODUCTION

Infection remains a major cause of death and morbidity in patients under-going cardiac transplantation, especially in the first few months when immuno-suppression is at its highest[1-3]. Study of these infections provides an alarming but fascinating insight into the delicate relationship between the transplant recipient and the wide variety of organisms, both pathogens and opportunists, in our environment. Although bacteria are the most common causative organisms (59%), other aetiological agents such as viruses (21%), fungi (14%), and protozoa (5%), account for a proportion of infectious episodes[3]. In our own and other centres, these complications have prompted a critical assessment of conditions favouring infections, of means for preventing them, and of diagnostic approaches to identification of causative organisms.

In this chapter we discuss several of the principles applied in the management of these patients. These principles include: the importance of maintaining immunosuppression at minimal effective levels, and the desirability of introducing agents like cyclosporin which may have less effect on host defence mechanisms; the importance of early mobilization of the patient; the maintenance of surgical sterility in the transplant ward; careful surveillance for infection without waiting for the usual signs of disease; a more aggressive .diagnostic approach; isolation of possible pathogens before treatment is commenced; and the use of broad spectrum therapeutic regimens because of the frequency with which infections are caused by multiple organisms.

INCIDENCE, TYPE AND SITE OF INFECTION

At some stage more than half of transplant recipients suffer a major episode of infection. This occurred in 22 of 40 heart transplant patients (55%) reported from our own institution between 1974 and 1981[3]. The importance of these infectious episodes is reflected in the fact that infection accounted for 39% of

195

all deaths in this series, and for 59% of deaths occurring in the first year after transplantation. Organisms gain access by several portals and, because of impaired host status, may present in a variety of ways. The relative frequency of these forms of presentation, and the systems involved, are listed in Table 13.1.

Table 13.1 Site of presentation of non-fatal infections after heterotopic cardiac transplantation at Groote Schuur Hospital (November 1974–October 1981)

Site	Presentation	Number of episodes (%)	Number of patients
Blood	septicaemia	1 (4)	1
Lung	pneumonia/lung abscess/empyema	7 (27)	6
Skin/subcutaneous tissue	rash/cellulitis/abscesses	7 (27)	6
Bone	osteitis/arthritis	3 (12)	2
GI tract	diarrhoea	3 (12)	3
Endocardium	septicaemia/embolic brain abscess	2 (7)	2
Myocardium	cardiac failure/myocarditis	1 (4)	1
Brain/meninges	encephalitis/meningitis	1 (4)	1
Cervix	vaginal discharge	1 (4)	1
Total		26 (100)	

Source: Cooper et al.[3]

Rubin et al.[4] have described a pattern of infection occurring in the renal transplant patient (Figure 13.1). A similar profile may be applied to the cardiac transplant patient.

In the first postoperative month, opportunistic (fungal, nocardial and protozoal) infections are extremely rare. The major causes of infection are bacterial and usually involve the wound, the lungs or, rarely, the urinary tract; these infections are readily treated with antibiotics. Non-bacterial infections provide a greater problem in diagnosis and treatment. The period 1–6 months after transplantation is the critical period for the recipient in terms of risk of life-threatening infection[4]. During this period immunosuppression reaches its peak, cytomegalovirus (CMV) and herpes simplex virus infections appear, and opportunistic infections become more common.

In the late post-transplantation period (more than 6 months after transplantation) chronic infection occurs, usually of viral aetiology, in particular cytomegalovirus and hepatitis. Cryptococcal infections also present during this period. Those diseases common in the community at the time must also be expected, e.g. tuberculosis or influenza.

Tables 13.2 and 13.3 summarize the fatal and non-fatal infections occurring in a sample of transplanted patients who received conventional immunosuppression (azathioprine, methylprednisolone and rabbit antithymocyte globulin) in our own hospital between 1974 and 1981[3]. Cyclosporin A was introduced into our unit in March 1983, and to date has been used in 10

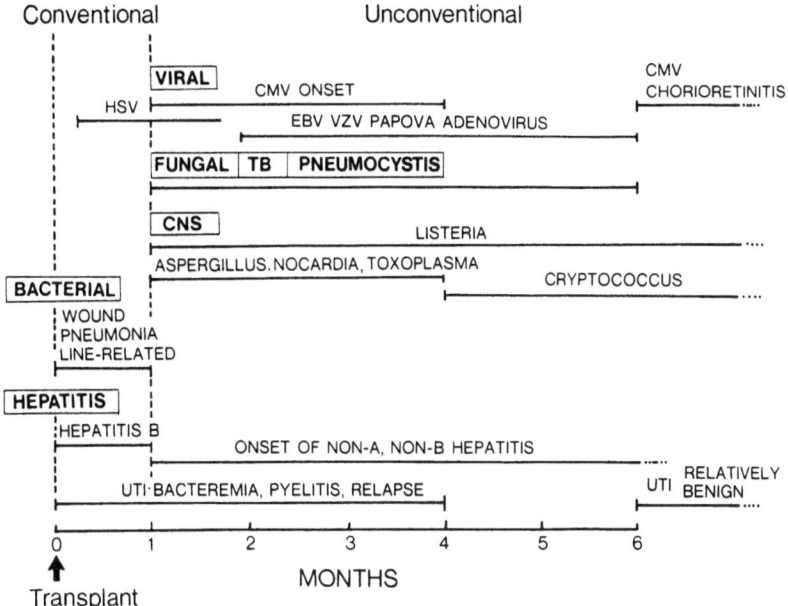

Figure 13.1 Common sequence of types of infection encountered in transplant patients (after Rubin *et al.*[4]). CMV = cytomegalovirus; HSV = herpes simplex virus; EBV = Epstein–Barr virus; VZV = varicella zoster virus; TB = tuberculosis; CNS = central nervous system; UTI = urinary tract infection

patients. It is not clear whether the prevalence of infection or the pattern of infecting organisms, or both, is altered by use of this drug. In renal transplant patients, fewer episodes of septicaemia, abscesses, and infections with cyto-megalovirus have been reported, while the prevalence of other viral infections, local fungal infections and urinary tract, skin and wound infections remains unaltered[5].

In our 10 patients, with a maximum follow-up period of 1 year, the follow-ing infectious complications arose: two developed mycobacterial infections of the lung; three, oral herpes simplex virus infections; one, pharyngitis caused by CMV; one, presumed viral bronchitis; and one had recurrent urinary tract infections caused by *Escherichia coli*. One patient, whose care had been trans-ferred to physicians abroad, died after 8 months of what was considered to be a fulminant bacterial septicaemia, though no confirmatory organisms were cultured.

FACTORS WHICH PREDISPOSE TO INFECTION

In the transplant patient the basis for enhanced susceptibility to infection is exceedingly complex, and appears more so as new data become available.

Nevertheless, it is important to attempt to identify individual elements of the weakened host defences, as at least some of these may be strengthened by specific preventative or therapeutic measures, without disturbing the immuno-suppression essential for graft survival. Aspects of host defences and mechanisms which are disrupted are listed in Tables 13.4, 13.5 and 13.6

Immunosuppression following cardiac transplantation is generally more intense than with other organ transplants, and consequently is associated with a higher incidence of infection[6]. Immunosuppression may be specific or non-specific. The majority is *non-specific* and readily achieved by one or more of a number of drugs and other agents. While non-specific immunosuppression is

Table 13.2 Fatal infections after heterotopic cardiac transplantation at Groote Schuur Hospital (November 1974–October 1981)

	Site of origin	Organisms cultured or isolated	Clinical course	Time of death (days after transplantation)
Bacterial (4 patients)	?Leg	Leg: *Clostridium perfringens*	?Following endomyo-cardial biopsy performed through femoral vein; gas gangrene right leg; amputation	76
	Lungs	Sputum: *Staphylococcus aureus* *Klebsiella pneumoniae* Blood: *Pseudomonas aeruginosa* *Escherichia coli*	(Retransplant) Adult respiratory distress syndrome; tracheostomy; pneumonia; septicaemia	24
	GI tract	Stools and blood: Salmonella group B Blood: (*Serratia marcescens*) (*E. coli*) (*Enterobacter* sp.)	Diarrhoea; lung abscess; broncho-pleural fistula; empyema	64
	Lungs	*E. coli* *Enterobacter* sp. *Peptococcus*	(Retransplant) Pneumonia	93
Fungal (4 patients)	Lungs	*Aspergillus fumigatus*	Pneumonia; dissemination	74
	Lungs	*Aspergillus* sp.	Pneumonia; dissemination	234
	Lungs	*Petriellidium boydii*	Pneumonia; dissemination	233
	Lungs	*A. fumigatus*	Pneumonia; dissemination	527
Viral (3 patients)	?Blood	Cytomegalovirus	Cytomegaloviraemia	61
	?Blood	?Herpes simplex	Infection of oesophagus, tongue and skin; encephalitis	220
	Lungs	Unidentified	Pneumonia	35

The significance of organism in parentheses remains uncertain
Source: Cooper *et al.*[3]

Table 13.3 Non-fatal infections after heterotopic cardiac transplantation at Groote Schuur Hospital (November 1974–October 1981)

	Site of origin	Organisms cultured or isolated	Months after transplantation	Clinical course
Bacterial (15 patients)	Blood	Acinetobacter sp.	3	Septicaemia. Resolved with treatment (RWT)
	Endocardium	Staphylococcus aureus	18	Infection on prosthetic valve; prosthesis removed; resolved
	Endocardium	Salmonella dublin. Bacillus cereus	25	Septicaemia; embolic brain abscess; infected saddle embolus (RWT)
	Lungs	Haemophilus influenzae	6	Pneumonia (RWT)
	Lungs	H. influenzae	12	Pneumonia (RWT)
	Lungs	Streptococcus pneumoniae	3	Pneumonia (RWT)
	Lungs	No organism identified	37	Pneumonia (RWT)
	Sternum	Staph. aureus (+ 7 other organisms)	1	Nine surgical drainage procedures; chronic discharging sinus for 36 months; resolved
	Sternum	Multiple organisms (10)	1	Three surgical drainage procedures; resolved
	GI tract	Shigella dysenteriae	1	(RWT)
	GI tract	Salmonella sp.	8	(RWT)
	GI tract	Salmonella sp.	1	(RWT)
	Subcutaneous tissue (leg)	Citrobacter sp.	5	Extensive abscesses of both legs; surgically drained; resolved
	Subcutaneous tissue (perineum)	E. coli	9	Perineal abscess following sigmoidoscopy and barium enema; surgically drained; resolved
	Subcutaneous tissue (perineum)	Non-haemolytic streptococcus	54	Perineal abscess; surgically drained; resolved
Mycobacterial (3 patients)	Lungs	M. kansasii	9	Chronic low grade pneumonia, treated but remained unresolved. Died at 14 months from disseminated Kaposi's sarcoma
	Lungs	M. tuberculosis	20	Chronic low grade pneumonia; refused treatment; died at 24 months from cerebral embolus
	Bone	M. haemophilum	48	Chronic discharging sinuses at left wrist, left thigh and left lower leg; low grade purulent infective arthritis left knee; not treated systemically; died at 54 months from chronic rejection (RWT)
Fungal (1 patient)	Meninges	Cryptococcus neoformans	56	(RWT)
Viral (5 patients)	Face and scalp	Herpes zoster (clinical diagnosis)	36	Resolved
	Chest wall	Herpes zoster (clinical diagnosis)	9	Resolved
	Chest wall	Herpes zoster (clinical diagnosis)	35	Resolved
	Ear	Herpes simplex (identified in isolate)	60	Resolved
	Cervix	Herpes, unidentified (clinical diagnosis)	18	Resolved
Protozoal (2 patients)	Myocardium	Toxoplasma gondii	3	Seen on endomyocardial biopsy; ?transferred from donor; clinically asymptomatic. (RWT)
	Lungs	Pneumocystis carinii	51	(RWT)

RWT = resolved with treatment   Source Cooper et al.[3]

effective in preventing rejection, when profound it is associated with an unacceptably high incidence of infection, particularly in the first 3 months after transplantation when drug therapy is heaviest. With time, however, adaptation permits reduction of therapy, with an associated lower risk of infection[7]. This accounts for the low incidence of fatal infections after the first year. At all stages, a compromise has to be accepted between the possibility of rejection and suppression of resistance to infection. In practice this is difficult

Table 13.4   Factors increasing the risk of infection in transplant patients

(1) Non-specific immunosuppression
    (a) *Iatrogenic:*
    Pharmacological agents
      glucocorticoids
      antimetabolites (e.g. azathioprine)
      cyclosporin A
      alkylating agents (e.g. cyclophosphamide)
    Biological agents
      antilymphocyte globulin
      (thoracic duct fistula)
      (plasmapheresis)
    Ionizing radiation
    (b) *Natural:*
    Debility from prolonged cardiac disease (poor nutrition and increased catabolism)
(2) Breach of surface barriers by:
      Central venous catheters/venous lines
      Chest drains
      Urinary catheter
      Endotracheal intubation and mechanical ventilation/tracheostomy
      Invasive procedures (e.g. endomyocardial biopsy)
(3) Increased exposure to micro-organisms
    Prolonged hospital stay
(4) Incorporation of prosthetic material (e.g. Dacron) (heterotopic transplantation)
(5) Neuropsychiatric disorders/non-compliance on the part of the patient

Table 13.5   Microbial infections associated with impaired T-lymphocyte function

BACTERIA	FUNGI
Brucella spp.	*Aspergillus* spp.
Listeria monocytogenes	*Candida* spp.
Mycobacteria spp.	*Cryptococcus neoformans*
Nocardia spp.	*Phycomycetes* spp.
Salmonella spp.	*Histoplasma capsulatum*
VIRUSES	PROTOZOA
Cytomegalovirus (CMV)	*Toxoplasma gondii*
Herpes simplex	*Pneumocystis carinii*
Vaccinia	
Varicella zoster	
Measles	

to achieve because of individual susceptibilities to immunosuppressive drugs, the need to be guided by tests confirming rejection, and the lack of uniform virulence of different classes of organisms. Even when severe infection occurs, prevention of graft rejection remains the priority (unlike the situation following renal transplantation, where immunosuppression may be reduced or even discontinued until the infection is controlled).

Table 13.6 Microbial infections associated with a shift in immunoglobulin type and poor opsonization

Streptococcus pneumoniae	*Streptococcus pyogenes* (group A)
Haemophilus influenzae	*Klebsiella pneumoniae*

Ideally, antirejection therapy should leave host resistance intact. The highest degree of specificity likely to be achieved by drugs is one which interacts specifically and exclusively with the subpopulations of proliferating T cells responsible for graft rejection (i.e. helper and killer T-lymphocytes). Even these drugs, however, would suppress the immunoproliferative response to pathogens. *Specific* immunosuppression, defined as treatment which directly or indirectly selectively suppresses the action of the lymphocyte clones responsible for rejection (i.e. antigen specific and directed at the histocompatibility antigens of the graft donor) will probably only be achieved by biological agents[8]. Until this is achieved, the threat of infection will remain.

A further consideration in the prevention of infections is the human factor. Patients who comply poorly with medical instructions and advice experience a higher incidence of infection[3,9]. In some instances, non-compliance is transient and associated with mild depressive disorders. These need to be recognized and treated, though it must be borne in mind that depression may be the first symptom of chronic illness, e.g. the development of tuberculous infection.

PREVENTION OF INFECTION

Literature relating to preventative and control measures in the transplant patient is often confusing and controversial, and it is difficult to distinguish those measures that are of proven efficacy from the many advocated on the basis of intuition or empiricism. Proof of efficacy is obtained only from properly designed clinical trials in homogenous groups of patients exposed to similar risk[10]. Furthermore, because infection in the transplant patient arises in a variety of circumstances, introduction of a single hygienic measure cannot be expected to bring about more than a modest reduction in infection rate, worthwhile though this may be[10]. A large number of hygienic precautions has to be considered for inclusion in any infection control programme. To submit more than a few of these to formal controlled trials is impractical. Because of the laborious nature of clinical trials and the numbers of patients needed, clinicians are at times forced to accept conclusions based on laboratory evidence alone, or derived from imperfectly controlled clinical studies and from situations not strictly comparable to the circumstances under consideration.

With these reservations in mind, the following components have been included in the care of our heart transplant patients. For each there is at least some supportive evidence.

The transplant unit

All transplant patients are nursed in a specially designed unit, occupying a separate floor of the hospital, despite the controversy surrounding the use of such isolation[11]. Separate nursing personnel care for the transplant patient; where possible, senior nursing staff are appointed on a permanent basis, and are specially trained in the care of such patients. The unit has three specialized single rooms equipped with intensive care facilities for the immediate postoperative care of the patients. There is air-conditioning (approximately 12 changes of air per hour) and terminal absolute filters in each room. Reliance is placed on ambient humidity in these areas, rather than upon artificial steam injection. The air is cooled by passage over refrigerated coils and any condensate is drained away immediately. Spot checks are carried out on the plant by members of the Department of Medical Microbiology. The nursing station is equipped with gauges, indicating humidity, temperature, and the pressure gradient across the main air filter to each room, which are checked at regular intervals. All room finishes are designed to facilitate easy cleaning. Buckets are autoclaved between use; mops are disinfected in a freshly prepared solution of organic chlorine.

Entry to the unit is by a change area only. All personnel entering the unit wear a gown, cap, mask and overshoes, measures found to be very effective in keeping unwanted persons out of the area. Personnel and visitors with sore throats or septic lesions are excluded from the area. All bedpans, urinals, urine measuring cylinders and jugs are autoclaved on a regular basis in a sterilizing unit adjacent to the ward, all respiratory support equipment is delivered to the unit from a central pasteurizing/ethylene oxide gas sterilizing facility, and respiratory tubing and humidifiers are changed daily.

The patient

Strict attention is given to the location and elimination of all sources of infection prior to transplantation, though routine bacteriological screening of the patient is not undertaken. Preference is given to the careful daily monitoring of the patient for clinical signs and symptoms of infection, appropriate specimens being taken at the first indication.

As prophylaxis at the time of transplantation, the recipient is given 1 g of cephalosporin (cephamandole) intravenously before operation, and 1 g 6-hourly for 48 hours after surgery. No other antimicrobial agents are used unless indicated, and then only with laboratory guidance.

Infection introduced through an intravenous line, although reported in the literature, has not been a problem in our patients. This may relate to the strict aseptic care given to the infusion lines, but their relatively short stay in the patient is probably more important. Lines are inserted under sterile conditions, and the cutaneous sites of entry redressed and monitored daily for infection.

The following principles of management are employed routinely to reduce the incidence of pulmonary infections. The duration of postoperative intermittent positive pressure mechanical ventilation is kept to a minimum (usually less than 24 hours). To avoid necrosis of nasal mucosa and sinusitis, orotracheal intubation is preferred to nasotracheal. Tracheostomy is avoided unless absolutely essential, since the stoma is a common site of infection and predisposes to pneumonia. Postoperative physiotherapy includes liberal use of intermittent positive pressure breathing with a pressure-cycled respirator for 15–20 minutes 4–6-hourly to prevent atelectasis. Early mobilization is encouraged to minimize the possibility of hypostatic pneumonia, an important cause of death in the early orthotopically transplanted patients in the Cape Town series.

It is uncertain which of these measures adopted in our unit have a bearing on the infection rate. Probably it is the skill and experience of the surgeon and the dedication and care of the nursing staff who attend to details of management that are most important.

PRESENTING FEATURES OF INFECTION

The most alarming aspects of infection in the immunocompromised patient are their rapidity of onset and evolution, the paucity of physical signs, atypical presentation, and the wide variety of organisms to be considered. (One such example was a 31-year-old male recipient who on the fourth post-transplant day developed progressive breathlessness and pulmonary opacification on chest radiograph compatible with pulmonary oedema, and who was found to have acid-fast bacilli in bronchial brushings obtained by fibreoptic bronchoscopy. There was no evidence of current or past tuberculosis at the time of surgery. Fever and leucocytosis were absent, as is frequently the case; patients may even be asymptomatic.) Herpetic or fungal mouth lesions, the presence of a cough, which is almost always dry in the initial phases of chest infection, are common and sometimes herald the onset of more serious infection.

Pulmonary infections

The lung is by far the most common site of presentation of infection in the transplant patient. However, the distinction between primary and secondary involvement of the lung in septicaemic dissemination of organisms is not always possible, since pleura, meninges, kidneys, joints and other sites may be involved early. Moreover, the pathogenic sequence of invasion, consolidation, and resolution by resorption or cavitation, that is usually seen in an infected lung, is variable in the immunocompromised patient. Radiographic features of consolidation may be minor even with overwhelming pneumonia and septicaemia, probably as a result of a poor leucocyte response. Cavitation often appears early, and rupture through to the pleural space, causing empyema, is not uncommon. This progression from tissue consolidation to cavitation with empyema formation has been observed in two patients in our own series. In one patient this followed diarrhoea caused by Salmonella Group B, and in the other was caused by *Streptococcus milleri* septicaemia.

Forms of bacterial pneumonia generally encountered in non-immunocompromised patients accounted for 24% of all infections in our series (Tables 13.2 and 13.3). This incidence is lower than that of the Stanford series (45%)[6], but may reflect a different approach to the diagnosis of disseminating infection. These pneumonias may be divided along conventional lines into bacterial, mycobacterial, fungal and viral. Cases of uncomplicated *Haemophilus influenzae* and *Streptococcus pneumoniae* pneumonia respond to conventional antibiotics. Bacterial pneumonias carry a worse prognosis when they occur in the presence of an endotracheal or tracheostomy tube, in association with adult respiratory distress syndrome, and/or respiratory failure requiring ventilatory support. Organisms such as *Staphylococcus aureus*, *Klebsiella pneumoniae*, *Pseudomonas aeruginosa*, *E. coli*, *Enterobacter* species and *Peptococci* have been encountered in this setting, with fatal consequences (Table 13.2).

Diagnostic approach to pulmonary infections

Investigations undertaken for suspected infection depend on the system involved. These have been reviewed by Armstrong[12] and Bartlett[13].

(1) *Blood cultures*. These are performed in all cases since, when positive, they provide confirmation of the relevant organism. To avoid spurious positive results they are carried out according to a strict aseptic protocol involving full surgical preparation of the skin.

(2) *Chest radiography*. Chest radiography is performed daily during the initial weeks after transplantation, and thereafter at each follow-up visit. Careful review of previous radiographs is essential to avoid missing subtle changes in the lung fields which give warning of developing infection. Any unexplained radiographic abnormality, especially in the presence of symptoms (dyspnoea, cough, fever, malaise) or leucocytosis, is investigated. Our

approach to the patient with an abnormality on chest radiograph is aggressive and urgent, with emphasis on obtaining bacteriological confirmation *prior* to commencement of antibiotics, because of the poor yield from transbronchial procedures if performed after treatment is commenced.

Several methods for achieving a *bacteriological diagnosis* of lung infection are available, ranging in invasiveness from sputum examination to open lung biopsy. Each has its own sensitivity, specificity and complication rate determined from series incorporating both non-immunocompromised and immunocompromised patients (reviewed recently by Matthay and Moritz[14]). Series comprising heart transplant recipients alone have been too small to permit meaningful conclusions.

(3) *Sputum examination*. Sputum, when available, is sent for Gram stain, and Ziehl–Neelsen stain and culture, but its diagnostic usefulness is limited by frequent contamination by commensal organisms originating in the upper respiratory tract or mouth. The presence of pus cells in sputum increases the suspicion of an organism being relevant, but at most this finding serves as a guide. Identification of mycobacteria is almost always significant, but cryptococcus or aspergillus detected in this way are merely indications for further investigation. Candida and herpes simplex virus isolated from sputum usually reflect oral infections, and seldom require more than local treatment[12].

In order of invasiveness, alternative procedures are percutaneous transtracheal aspiration, percutaneous needle aspiration of the lung, fibreoptic bronchoscopy with brushing (with sheathed or unsheathed brushes), transbronchial biopsies and limited lavage of bronchial tree, and open lung biopsy. The advantages and disadvantages of these procedures are outlined in Table 13.7.

(4) *Transtracheal aspiration*. Transtracheal aspiration specimens are more reliable than sputa, but negative results occur when infection is located peripherally and is not in communication with the bronchial tree[15]. In our experience it has a low diagnostic yield, except in patients with extensive pneumonia. For smaller lesions, local sampling as offered by needle aspiration and fibreoptic bronchoscopy is preferred.

(5) *Ultrafine needle aspiration*. Because of its comparative safety, ultrafine needle aspiration (with a 24 or 25 gauge needle) has replaced conventional needle aspiration of the lung, but is contraindicated in patients on anticoagulants with a low prothrombin index or with overt bleeding disorders[16]. It is particularly useful for peripheral lesions, and when diagnostic pleural aspiration is also indicated. It carries the highest sensitivity and specificity of all procedures, but a marginally higher complication rate than fibreoptic bronchoscopy[16]. The procedure is, however, well tolerated, and preferred by patients, and has been used to good effect in several patients at our institution.

(6) *Fibreoptic bronchoscopy*. The alternative procedures to ultrafine needle aspiration are performed through a flexible fibreoptic bronchoscope. These

Table 13.7 Advantages and disadvantages of methods used to diagnose pulmonary infections

Method	Advantages	Disadvantages/complications
(1) Sputum examination and culture	Easy	Irrelevant organisms obtained
(2) Transtracheal aspiration	Easy; performed in ward (False-negative 1%) (False-positive 21%)[14]	Subcutaneous emphysema 0.5% Haemorrhage 0.2% Paratracheal infection 0.2%
(3) Ultrafine (G 24–25) needle aspiration	Sensitivity 83% Specificity 100% (Value of −ve result 70%) (Value of +ve result 100%)[15]	Patient must be moved to fluoroscopy facility Pneumothorax 8% (requiring intercostal drainage 4%)[15]
(4) Needle aspiration (G 16–20)	As for 3 (above)[13]	Pneumothorax 30% Haemoptysis 10%[13]
(5) Fibreoptic bronchoscopy		
(a) Brush	High yield	Patient discomfort Hypoxia Irrelevant organisms obtained 52%
(b) PTC brush	Lower yield; specificity higher	Limited sample
(c) Biopsy	Useful for pneumocystis and tuberculous granulomata	Haemoptysis 1% Pneumothorax 1%[16]
(d) Limited lavage	Increases yield	None
(6) Open lung biopsy	Specificity	Risk of morbidity/mortality Not suitable for repeated examination

are favoured when the process is extensive or diffuse and when transbronchial biopsy is indicated, e.g. for suspected *Pneumocystis carinii* infection. Bronchoscopy is performed under local anaesthetic through the nasopharynx and, for this reason, although it provides a higher bacterial yield than needle biopsy, approximately half the isolates obtained are upper respiratory tract flora. The use of brushes protected by double telescoping catheters (PTC brush), which are plugged distally to prevent contamination of the specimen with organisms from the bronchoscope, overcomes this disadvantage, and provides a smaller but more reliable yield[17]. Since each of these brushes can be used to sample in only one location, we also routinely employ an unsheathed brush to sample from many other sites. When brushes are removed, smears are made directly on to sterile glass slides, and the brush immersed in a sterile test tube containing 2 ml sterile saline. The specimens are conveyed immediately to the bacteriology laboratory for staining, microscopy and culture. Any organism detected on both brushes or the sheathed brush alone is considered potentially pathogenic. Results from unsheathed brushes alone are interpreted with caution.

A review of published results of fibrebronchoscopic procedures in immunocompromised patients indicates that transbronchial biopsy alone provides a specific diagnosis in 41% of cases, bronchial brushing alone in 27%, and combined brush and biopsy in 52%[14]. Similar results were obtained in immunocompromised patients studied at Groote Schuur Hospital[18]. A notable difference between these two series was the lower incidence of complications in our own series. In the former series, the incidences of haemorrhage (of greater than 25 ml) and of pneumothorax were each 7%, whereas in our series the combined incidence of these complications in 809 bronchoscopies was less than 1%. The reason for this difference is not apparent, but the figures indicate the relative safety of the procedure. The problem of initiating a lower respiratory tract infection from nasopharyngeal organisms introduced during bronchoscopy[19,20] has not been encountered in our patients, possibly because the majority are placed on short-term broad-spectrum antibiotics after the procedure.

Ultrafine needle aspiration and fibreoptic bronchoscopy are used as complementary procedures to be employed when the other has failed to confirm the diagnosis. When necessary they may be performed repeatedly during resolution of the infective lesion.

The results of 15 consecutive fibreoptic bronchoscopies performed on heart transplant recipients at Groote Schuur Hospital between July 1979 and December 1983 for investigation of suspected infection are presented in Table 13.8. These results illustrate the improved yield when more than one form of specimen is taken (i.e. brush and biopsy specimens), and highlight the importance of withholding treatment until detailed bacteriological investigation has been attempted. Bronchoscopy failed to be diagnostic in all patients who had received or were receiving antibiotics at the time of the procedure (except in those with tuberculosis and pneumocystis, which broad-spectrum antibiotics would not be expected to clear). The diagnostic value of bronchoscopy in this group of cardiac transplant patients was significantly lower than that in a larger group of renal transplant recipients investigated concurrently, most of whom had not received antibiotics (72% positive yield (unpublished results)). The spontaneous resolution of occasional pulmonary shadows seen on the chest radiograph in heart transplant patients raises the possibility that some are non-infective in origin. They may represent small pulmonary infarcts following endomyocardial biopsy, or regions of atelectasis.

Arising from these considerations, our present policy is: (a) to withhold all antibiotic treatment until bacterial investigations have been completed, (b) to routinely include with fibreoptic bronchoscopy use of a double sheathed brush, a standard brush, limited bronchial lavage for bacteriology and virology and transbronchial biopsy for culture and histology, and (c) to utilize fluoroscopic screening with fibreoptic bronchoscopy to improve localization of small lesions.

(7) *Open lung biopsy*. Open lung biopsy is reserved for patients in whom the above diagnostic procedures have failed to provide conclusive results. It is also rarely performed when there is failure of resolution despite what is considered appropriate treatment. (Open lung biopsy was indicated in one such patient at our centre with active pulmonary tuberculosis (diagnosed bronchoscopically), who failed to improve after 4 weeks of supervised four-drug therapy. Biopsy confirmed pulmonary tuberculosis; organisms were identified in the tissue sections, but could not be cultured. The patient subsequently recovered fully.) We have not employed open lung biopsy as readily as has been advocated for bone marrow transplant recipients[21].

(8) *Computerized axial tomography*. Computerized axial tomography (CAT) is a useful method of detecting localized pleural or extrapulmonary disease, and, following heterotopic heart transplantation, in demonstrating lesions of the right lower lobe whose presence on chest radiography may be obscured by the donor heart. In two of our patients, one with a tuberculous cavity and another with a lung abscess, lesions in this location were missed in the early stages. In the former, the CAT scan identified the site and facilitated aspiration of the abscess.

Septicaemia

Patients with septicaemia may complain of symptoms similar to those with pulmonary infections. When no obvious pulmonary involvement is present, a detailed search for other primary sources should be made. This includes inspection of the wound, urine and throat swab cultures, mouth washings (obtained by gargling) for virological study, examination of the ears for middle ear infection, of the optic fundi for choroiretinitis and tubercles and of the central nervous system (CNS) to exclude meningitis and intracranial

Table 13.8 Results of fibreoptic bronchoscopy in heart transplant recipients at Groote Schuur Hospital (1979–1983)

Indication (on chest radiograph)	Procedure			Outcome	Conclusion
	Brush	Transbronchial biopsy	Bronchial lavage		
(1) Segmental consolidation	−	ND	−	Resolved (on tetracycline)	Failed
(2) Small segmental consolidation	M.S.O.	ND	ND	Resolved spontaneously	Failed
(3) Cavity L. midzone	M.S.O.	ND	ND	Prior amoxycillin; resolved on cotrimoxazole	Failed
(4) Small segmental consolidation	−	ND	ND	Prior cephamandole; resolved without further treatment	Failed
(5) Bilateral basal consolidation	−	ND	ND	Prior cefoxitin; died *E. coli* (blood culture)	Failed
(6) Segmental consolidation	M.S.O.	ND	ND	Prior clindamycin; resolved on clindamycin and cefoxitin	Failed
(7) Small segmental consolidation	−	ND	ND	Prior cotrimoxazole and cephamandole; resolved without further treatment	Failed
(8) Segmental consolidation	*S. pneumoniae*	ND	ND	Resolved on erythromycin	Diagnostic
(9) Segmental consolidation	*M. kansasii*	ND	ND	UTNA also positive. Treated	Diagnostic
(10) Bilateral nodular infiltrate	*M. tuberculosis*	−	ND	Prior sulphatriad. Treated	Diagnostic
(11) Bilateral nodular infiltrate	−	*M. tuberculosis*	ND	Prior sulphatriad and daraprim. Treated	Diagnostic
(12) Bilateral nodular infiltrate	−	*P. carinii*	+	Prior ampicillin, tobramycin and metronidazole; resolved on treatment	Diagnostic
(13) Patchy lobar infiltrate	*M. tuberculosis*	+	−	Prior INH; resolved on treatment	Diagnostic
(14) Bilateral nodular infiltrate	*M. tuberculosis*	−	−	Four-drug TB therapy; resolved	Diagnostic
(15) Small segmental consolidation	−	ND	ND	Inactive scar, no treatment	Helpful

M.S.O. = mixed salivary organisms; UTNA = ultra-thin needle aspiration; ND = not done; − = negative result; + = positive result

abscess. Any suspicion of the latter conditions is an indication for lumbar puncture, particular care being paid to identifying cryptococci; examination of 10 ml of cerebrospinal fluid (CSF) is recommended for this purpose[22]. Urinary tract infections, although rare, are an important source of infection, and recurrent septicaemia may originate from renal carbuncles. Examination and culture of aspiration and trephine biopsies of bone marrow are occasionally used, particularly when confirmation of disseminated tuberculosis is required; the yield, however, is fairly low[23].

Serology

Serological tests play only a minor role in the investigation of the pyrexial patient with suspected septicaemia because of several shortcomings which seriously limit their usefulness[24]. These include:

(1) The difficulty of interpreting a positive titre unless the previous antibody status is known. For this reason, serum levels of CMV antibodies are estimated before transplantation; changes in antibody titres can then be readily appreciated. For other organisms, a delay of up to a fortnight in obtaining results is inevitable, and diagnoses can only be made with confidence retrospectively. In practice, therefore, if organisms like mycoplasma or legionella are suspected, the therapeutic regimen is adjusted to cover these organisms.

(2) Many immunocompromised patients fail to develop antibodies in response to infections. This has been observed in transplant recipients with fungal infections[24].

(3) Positive fungal antibody tests (e.g. immunodiffusion tests for aspergillus precipitins) do not distinguish between colonization and invasive forms of infection[24], and the diagnosis of new and possibly invasive infection can only be made if there has been recent sero-conversion.

Organisms commonly tested for serologically in our patients include *Mycoplasma pneumoniae*, *Legionella pneumophila*, cytomegalovirus, herpes simplex virus, upper respiratory tract viruses (influenza and adenoviruses) and hepatitis viruses. Occasionally the Paul Bunnell, Weil–Felix, Widal, and Brucella serological tests are requested.

More promising techniques are being developed for demonstrating the presence of microbial antigens or other products of micro-organisms in tissue fluids and serum. These include immunofluorescent staining for antigens of *L. pneumophila*[25], and demonstration of cryptococcal antigen in serum of patients with interstitial pulmonary disease[26].

Tests of limited usefulness for diagnosis of infection are the erythrocyte sedimentation rate (ESR) and the Limulus lysate test. This latter test is based on the ability of bacterial endotoxin (lipopolysaccharide) to cause extracts of the amoebocyte cell of *Limulus polyphemus* (the horseshoe crab) to coagulate. Although very sensitive *in vitro*, when applied to the diagnosis of human Gram-negative bacteraemia, fewer than two-thirds have positive tests, and false-positive tests are not infrequent. False-negative results may result from the presence in serum of antibodies to endotoxin or inhibitors[23].

Central nervous system infections

Three patterns of infection of the central nervous system have been described in renal transplant patients[27]:

(1) acute or subacute meningitis, almost invariably caused by *Listeria monocytogenes*,

(2) subacute or chronic meningitis, caused by *Cryptococcus neoformans* or *Mycobacterium tuberculosis*,

(3) focal brain infection giving rise to focal neurological signs, caused by Listeria species, *Toxoplasma gondii*, Candida species, *Nocardia asteroides*, and, most commonly, *Aspergillus fumigatus*[27].

Similar presentations have been seen in heart transplant recipients, both in a large Stanford series reported in 1981[22] and in our own patients. One patient in the former series had an abscess of bacterial origin (Klebsiella); one of our patients had viral encephalitis (probably herpetic)[3]. Occasionally rhinocerebritis caused by members of the class Zygomycetes (rhizopus and mucor) are encountered[22].

Meningitis may occur at any time following transplantation, but frequently follows a temporary increase in treatment for rejection[22]. Headache, lethargy, and fever are common; examining the CSF is usually helpful in establishing the diagnosis. In cryptococcal meningitis, pleocytosis may be modest, most cells being mononuclear; slight elevation of protein is found. Cerebrospinal fluid glucose is low (compared with paired blood level) and India-ink preparation and Gram stain show the budding yeasts. By contrast, in Listeria meningitis, pleocytosis is marked (both polymorphonuclear leucocytes and mononuclears), and although Gram stain may be negative, Listeria colonies grow out on culture. Cerebrospinal fluid protein and glucose show the same abnormalities as in cryptococcal disease[22].

PRINCIPLES OF THERAPY OF BACTERIAL AND MYCOBACTERIAL INFECTIONS

Prospects for successfully treating infections in immunocompromised patients are improving with the introduction of newer antibiotics and antiviral agents. Nevertheless, the outcome of treatment is still largely dependent upon the patient's own antimicrobial defence mechanisms[21]. Other important factors are the nature of the invading organism, the stage at which treatment is commenced, and the site of infection.

Bacterial infections

Since the first heart transplant was performed, important new antibiotics have been introduced into clinical practice which have influenced prescribing habits for transplant patients. Although it is impossible to provide statistical confirmation of the benefits of these newer agents, several of their advantages are self-evident.

The following is a summary of current antibiotic prescribing for heart transplant patients in our own hospital.

(1) The preferred policy is to give specific, rather than 'blind', treatment for causative organisms. The difficulty is that delay in treating a rapidly progressing infection, while investigations are performed, may be disastrous. A compromise is often necessary, with 'presumptive' or 'best guess' antimicrobial therapy being introduced immediately after initiation of microbiological investigations, but before results of cultures are available. Adjustments to therapy or its discontinuance are made subsequently as the results of laboratory tests become known

(2) The choice of antimicrobials is made in consultation with a microbiologist, particular attention being paid to *in vitro* sensitivity of organisms and the emergence of resistant hospital strains.

(3) Unless a specific antibiotic has already been indicated by the results of investigation, initial therapy usually comprises two agents, and sometimes a third depending on the clinical circumstances. The first two are an aminoglycoside paired with a β-lactam agent. The former may be tobramycin, gentamicin or amikacin. Tobramycin is favoured because of its greater antipseudomonal activity and its lesser nephrotoxicity[28]. The loading dose and maintenance doses are determined according to body surface area, and the therapy adjusted according to serum levels of aminoglycoside measured immediately before and 1 hour after each dose. There is a continuing debate as to whether the β-lactam agent should be a cephalosporin or an antipseudomonal penicillin, such as carbenicillin or piperacillin. In our patients, unlike recipients of bone marrow transplants, pseudomonal septicaemia, with its associated high mortality, is relatively rare[21]. For this reason, penicillin or a cephalosporin is the preferred second agent. Cefotaxime, a third-generation cephalosporin, has the advantage of broad-spectrum activity against both Gram-negative organisms and, to a lesser extent, staphylococci, and may be used alone or occasionally in combination with metronidazole

to cover anaerobes. This regimen avoids the risk of aminoglycoside-induced nephrotoxicity. When staphylococcal infection is proved or suspected, cloxacillin or fusidic acid are added to the regimen. Alternatively, clindamycin may replace the β-lactam agent.

(4) Treatment is continued until the patient has been afebrile for 72 hours, provided there are no local areas of infected tissue (pulmonary consolidation and abscesses must have cleared, urine cultures should be negative, etc.). A longer course of treatment is indicated if neutropenia or thrombocytopenia persist, and when patients are on high doses of corticosteroids and anti-inflammatory drugs which might be suppressing the pyrexia. Short courses of therapy (3–5 days) may be adequate for uncomplicated lower urinary tract infections and certain vascular and catheter-associated infections, provided the offending line is removed.

Mycobacterial infections

The incidence of mycobacterial infections in our own series is high, reflecting a high prevalence of tuberculosis in the general population. For this reason isoniazid (INH) prophylaxis (300 mg daily) for 6 months is now used in all transplant recipients who are noted to have evidence of healed primary tuberculous foci on chest radiographs before transplantation. Where previous postprimary or reactivation tuberculosis has occurred, the patient is covered with INH and ethambutol or triple drug therapy for at least 1 year after transplantation.

Both *M. tuberculosis* and mycobacteria other than tuberculosis (MOTT) infections have followed an indolent course in our patients and have been difficult to eradicate in spite of effective tuberculocidal drugs (rifampicin and INH) as part of four-drug combination therapy. They have not, however, been responsible for the death of any patient. Prolonged and intensive therapy is required for these infections[29].

CLINICAL FEATURES AND MANAGEMENT OF THE COMMONER OPPORTUNISTIC INFECTIONS

Viral infections

Members of the Herpesviridae are the viruses most frequently associated with serious disease in transplant patients. These include cytomegalovirus, varicella zoster, herpes simplex and Epstein–Barr viruses.

Cytomegalovirus (CMV). In common with other members of this family, this virus is widespread, is acquired during childhood, and lies latent in white blood cells and in the urogenital and other systems. The virus may be introduced into a non-immune recipient with the donor heart or, rarely, by blood transfusion[30]. In a series of heart transplant patients reported by Rand *et al.*[30], a group of patients who, prior to transplantation, had no CMV antibodies, had a higher incidence of death from pulmonary infection (pneumonia and lung abscess) than those with measurable antibody levels; the infections were caused by organisms other than fungi. CMV transmitted by blood transfusion was considered to be the cause of the increased mortality in this group.

Common clinical features of CMV infection (in order of frequency) are fever, leucopenia, thrombocytopenia, the presence of atypical mononuclear cells in the blood, abnormal liver function tests, lower respiratory tract infection, hepatic and splenic enlargement and, rarely, pericarditis, arthritis, polyneuritis, pancreatitis and encephalitis. Primary infections occur 5–7 weeks after transplantation, and reactivation after approximately 5–12 weeks[31].

Varicella zoster (VZ). VZ infection occurs in transplant patients ten times more frequently than in normal adults, though the majority of cases follow a relatively benign course[31].

Herpes simplex virus (HSV). HSV infections in the form of 'cold sores' of lips and oropharyngeal mucosa are very common during the first post-transplant month[31]. Rarely, they spread to involve the face, eye and alimentary tract, causing a fatal gastroenterocolitis. Clinical manifestations usually represent reactivation rather than primary infection. HSV infections, unless present in classical form, require laboratory confirmation by at least one or more of the following methods: (1) identification of the virus by immunological or other means, (2) isolation of the agent and (3) by serology.

HSV and VZ may be identified by electron microscopy (EM) or immunofluorescence, but culture is necessary for confirmation of EM results. CMV can be identified in urine, sputum or respiratory tract washings by EM and culture; immunofluorescence is unreliable. Evidence of HSV and CMV infection has been found in lung tissue from approximately 40% of heart transplant patients dying of unrelated causes[32]. Complement fixation tests, although used routinely for HSV, VZ and CMV, are not as rapid or useful as immunofluorescence, radioimmunoassay, or enzyme-linked immunosorbent assay. The latter identify specific IgM antibodies, which are essential for diagnosis in immunosuppressed patients, particularly where primary infections are suspected[31].

Most viral infections cannot be successfully treated. Interferon holds promise, but is not yet freely available for clinical trial. Acyclovir, an acyclic analogue of a natural nucleoside, is the most effective drug currently available for treatment of herpes infections. Used intravenously, it is useful both prophylactically and therapeutically against HSV[33], but information on its value in VZ and CMV infections is awaited. The most effective measure for life-threatening CMV infections is reduction of immunosuppression, but this is usually not possible in the heart transplant patient[31].

Fungal infections

In our patients, as in other series[34], fungal infections are not uncommon (14% of our cases[3]) and, when disseminated, are associated with a high mortality. Fungal infections may be due to reactivation of latent infection acquired from the environment prior to transplantation, or to new opportunistic infection acquired following transplantation. Blastomycosis and coccidiodomycosis, which arise by the former route, are not found in South Africa, but aspergillosis, cryptococcosis and candidiasis are common opportunists in our patients.

Aspergillosis. Species of the aspergillus fungus are associated with several categories of lung disease in non-compromised hosts (allergic bronchopulmonary aspergillosis and mycetomas), but do not generally invade unless impairment of immunocompetence occurs. Invasive aspergillosis usually manifests as pneumonia, less often as brain abscess and meningoencephalitis, and rarely as gastrointestinal or skin lesions. In the lungs, almost any type of infiltrate, ranging from a diffuse interstitial one to focal cavitatory lesions, may be seen. The tendency of the organisms to invade blood vessels may cause clotting and pulmonary infarction, and dispose to haematogenous dissemination. Sputum is positive (usually on culture only) in about one-third of patients with invasive pneumonia. Although false-positive results are common, the more often the sputum is positive, the greater is the likelihood that the result is relevant[34].

Aspergillus is also the commonest cause of meningoencephalitis and focal brain abscess in transplant patients. In the Stanford series this tended to occur early following transplantation[21]. The patients presented with disorientation and confusion, and progressed to coma. Some had hemiparesis, hemianopia, and dysphagia. Cerebrospinal fluid examination was generally unhelpful, showing a modest degree of pleocytosis and raised protein, but no organisms. The diagnosis may be made by direct needle aspiration of the intracranial lesion, but should be strongly suspected when aspergillus is isolated from coexistent lung lesions[21]. Computed tomography of the brain has shown minimal, non-specific, low-density lesions, which do not exhibit contrast enhancement[22].

Amphotericin B is the only proven effective treatment for invasive aspergillosis, but is of little use if given late or for CNS involvement. Intravenous therapy is given as indicated in Table 13.9.

Cryptococcosis. C. neoformans is an encapsulated yeast which gains access to the body via the respiratory tract. Isolation of cryptococcus from sputum or other specimen from the lungs of an immunocompromised patient is an indication for a careful search for pulmonary and extrapulmonary lesions caused by this organism[35, 36]. Investigations for extrapulmonary disease involve aspiration or biopsy of any suspicious skin or bone lesions, examination and culture of CSF, of at least three specimens of urine, of blood, and possibly bone marrow. The presence of extrapulmonary lesions carries a poor prognosis[35]. Where no pulmonary or extrapulmonary lesions are found, vigilance with repeated cultures of sputum may be sufficient, since saprophytic occurrence of *C. neoformans* in sputum is known to occur[35, 37].

Treatment of transplanted patients should comprise a combination of amphotericin B and 5-flucytosine (Table 13.9), even if the infection appears to be confined to the lung, since resistant organisms may emerge if flucytosine is used alone[37, 38].

Surgical resection of pulmonary lesions adds little to the success of treatment, except perhaps when lesions are large and persist after several weeks of therapy; by reducing the mass of organisms, resection may shorten the course of the infection and diminish the potential for recurrence[36, 37].

Candidiasis. Candidal infections of mucous membranes of mouth, pharynx, and oesophagus are common problems in patients who are debilitated, immunosuppressed and on broad-spectrum antibiotics. For this reason, all our transplant patients are given nystatin lozenges and suspension as prophylaxis (Table 13.9) from the time of operation until immunosuppression is reduced to low levels (usually during the second month). This may account for the absence of disseminated candidiasis in our series. Several cases of this infection, some fatal, have been reported from Stanford[6].

The diagnosis of disseminated candidiasis, particularly in immunocompromised patients, and the associated problem of when to commence systemic therapy present several difficulties[39]. As with aspergillosis, definitive confirmation of the diagnosis is made only by histopathological demonstration of organisms invading visceral tissues—lungs, brain, meninges, myocardium, kidneys, skin, bone and eye. Blood cultures are frequently negative even in the presence of visceral involvement, nor is candidaemia certain proof of dissemination. Indwelling venous catheters are a frequent source of candidaemia; removal of the catheters may be all that is necessary to correct this situation. Isolation of candida from urine usually reflects local urinary tract infection and, as an isolated finding, is an indication for local treatment alone.

The following features have been suggested as indicative of dissemination requiring systemic therapy: (1) identification of candida in three or more of the following sites—oral or urogenital mucosa, venous catheter tip, blood, urine or lung (via needle aspiration or sheathed brush), (2) the presence of peripheral embolic lesions, e.g. macronodular skin lesions (which can be biopsied for a rapid diagnosis) or endophthalmitis, (3) identification of candida in CSF or aspirates from bones or joints and (4) histological confirmation in biopsy specimens, e.g. lung, kidney or liver.

Petriellidosis. Infection by unusual organisms like *Petriellidium boydii* are occasionally encountered in cardiac transplant patients. This organism was found at necropsy in one patient in our series, the findings suggesting primary infection of the lungs with haematogenous dissemination to the brain, kidneys and skin[3, 32]. Disseminated petriellidosis has previously been described in patients on corticosteroids[40].

Table 13.9 Recommended therapeutic schedules of antifungal agents

Mode (site) of administration/agent	Schedule	Toxicity
Intravenous		
Amphotericin B	Test dose: 1 mg in 250 ml 5% dextrose over 2–4 hours. Initial dose 5 mg in 500 ml 5% dextrose over 4 hours. Increase by 5 mg up to 1 mg/kg per day. Then administer 1 mg/kg every other day (limit 60 mg/day) in 500–1000 ml 5% dextrose. If creatinine rises, reduce dose by 10–20 mg and/or increase interval between doses (to up to 3 days)	Chills, fever, hypotension, bronchospasm, phlebitis, nausea, vomiting, hypokalaemia, hypomagnesaemia, renal impairment, anaemia, hepatic toxicity
Miconazole	400–600 mg 6-hourly i.v.	Phlebitis, nausea, hepatic toxicity
Intraventricular (cerebral)		
Amphotericin B	First dose 0.05 mg. Then increase by 0.05–0.1 mg increments daily or twice daily up to 0.5 mg/day. Thereafter, 0.5 mg/day or alternate days	Headache, meningismus, seizures
Oral		
Nystatin	400 000–10 million units 4 times/day, mouth wash and swallow. Lozenge (suppository) 4 times/day	Mouth soreness, nausea
5-Flucytosine	150 mg/kg per day in four divided doses	Thrombocytopenia, pancytopenia (more common with renal failure); hepatitis
Bladder		
Amphotericin B	50 mg in 1000 ml of 5% dextrose; irrigate once or twice/day	Local irritation
Topical (skin)		
Nystatin	Apply 2–4 times/day	Local irritation and rash
Miconazole	Apply 2–4 times/day	Local irritation and rash

Nocardiosis

Nocardia species, bacteria with branched filamentous morphology, are often misclassified as fungi. *N. asteroides* accounts for at least 85% of pulmonary or disseminated nocardiosis[29]. The importance of diagnosis lies in the satisfactory response of the infection to therapy, even in immunocompromised hosts. In specimens obtained from lung, identification is achieved by recognition of morphology, and positive staining in Gram, Ziehl–Neelsen and methenamine-silver stained preparations. The diagnosis is confirmed by culture of nocardial colonies, which serves to distinguish them from actino-myces, with which they share morphological similarities. To confirm the diag-nosis, invasive procedures are usually necessary, because sputum is positive in less than 30% of cases[29].

In most cases, infection enters via the lungs, and since nocardia are not part of the normal human flora, a positive sputum culture is highly suggestive of active infection[29]. Although some cases are mild, the majority of patients with nocardiosis have symptomatic lung disease features. Nocardial lung lesions may be solitary nodules, localized pneumonitis, or single or multiple lung abscesses. About 25% of patients develop CNS involvement (usually a brain abscess), on occasions after the pulmonary lesion has healed.

The treatment of choice is sulphonamides (sulphadiazine 2–3 g 6-hourly), though cotrimoxazole, minocycline and combinations of ampicillin and eryth-romycin have also proved effective in subjects allergic to sulphonamides[29]. A combination of amikacin and sulphonamide has given good results in some patients. Treatment should be continued for at least 6–8 weeks.

Protozoal infections

Pneumocystis. Pneumonia caused by *Pneumocystis carinii* is characterized by prominent dyspnoea (91% of patients), fever (66%) and cough (50%), associ-ated with cyanosis (39%), basal or widespread pulmonary crackles (33%) and hepatomegaly (35%). The pneumonia is generally not, however, associated with sputum production and prominent signs of consolidation[41]. Diffuse bilateral infiltrates are seen on chest radiograph in almost all cases. Early diagnosis is important because of the profound disturbance of gas exchange and respiratory failure which ensues. The chances of recovery are greatly increased if ventilatory support can be avoided[42].

Drug therapy consists of a combination of sulphamethoxazole (100 mg/kg per day) and trimethoprim (20 mg/kg per day)[42]. In most cases a clinical response is observed within 4 days. Since approximately one-third of patients fail to respond to this therapy, progressive deterioration after 4 days is an indication for substituting pentamidine for the initial regimen[42].

Prophylaxis with low-dose combined therapy (sulphamethoxazole 20 mg/kg per day and trimethoprim 5 mg/kg per day) given orally in two divided doses has been advocated and has proved effective in several categories of immuno-suppressed patients[43]. This has not been given routinely in our patients as the incidence of infection with pneumocystis is low, and treatment is effective. Since pneumocystis infections frequently recur, however, prophylaxis is advisable for immunosuppressed patients who have previously been treated for pneumocystis infection[43].

Toxoplasmosis. The most serious consequences of infection with *Toxo-plasma gondii* are encephalitis, pneumonitis, myocarditis and chorioretinitis. The encephalitis is diffuse, but may occasionally be asymptomatic. Toxoplasma cysts and microglial nodules form, and abscess formation has also been described[22]. Aspirates from lesions (stained with Wright–Giemsa and haematoxylin and eosin stains) may show toxoplasma cysts and trophozoites, both extracellularly and inside inflammatory cells. Sulphadiazine and pyrimethamine therapy is successful in some patients.

Toxoplasmosis of both donor and recipient hearts was diagnosed by means of endomyocardial biopsy specimens after heterotopic cardiac transplantation in one of our patients[44]. It seemed likely that the infection was transferred with the donor heart. Drug therapy was successful in eradicating the infection.

FUTURE DEVELOPMENTS IN THE CONTROL OF INFECTION IN THE IMMUNOCOMPROMISED PATIENT

Although the transplant recipient is frequently invaded by exogenous microorganisms, many life-threatening infections appear to be endogenous in origin[21]. Much can be done to minimize potential exogenous sources of infection. The future of prevention and control of infection in the transplant patient, however, lies in the domain of enhancing the host's ability to resist the low-grade virulence of commensal and saprophytic organisms without endangering graft survival. Immunotherapy is one of several forms of treatment that may assist in this regard[45]. The use of antitoxin serum offers another exciting possibility, its action being to limit the effects of endotoxaemia caused by Gram-negative bacilli of gut origin[46]. An alternative approach to the control of infection is, of course, the development of highly specific immunosuppression that does not impair the patient's antimicrobial defence mechanisms.

References

1. Baumgartner, W. A., Reitz, B. A., Oyer, P. E., Stinson, E. B. and Shumway, N. E. (1979). Cardiac homotransplantation. *Curr. Probl. Surg.*, **16**, 1
2. Barnard, C. N., Barnard, M. S., Cooper, D. K. C., Curchio, C. A., Hassoulas, J., Novitzky, D. and Wolpowitz, A. (1981). The present status of heterotopic cardiac transplantation. *J. Thorac. Cardiovasc. Surg.*, **81**, 433
3. Cooper, D. K. C., Lanza, R. P., Oliver, S. P., Forder, A. A., Rose, A. G., Uys, C. J., Novitzky, D. and Barnard, C. N. (1983). Infectious complications following heterotopic heart transplantation. *Thorax*, **38**, 822
4. Rubin, R. H., Wolfson, J. S. and Cosimi, A. B. (1981). Infection in the renal transplant recipient. In Dixon, R. E. (ed.) *Nosocomial Infections*. p. 121. (Atlanta: Yorke Medical Books)
5. Canadian Multi-Center Transplant Study Group. (1983). A randomized clinical trial of cyclosporine in cadaveric renal transplantation. *N. Engl. Med. J.*, **309**, 809
6. Jamieson, S. W., Stinson, E. B. and Shumway, N. E. (1982). Cardiac transplantation. In Morris, P. J. (ed.) *Tissue Transplantation*. p. 147. (Edinburgh: Churchill Livingstone)
7. Baumgartner, W. A. (1983). Infection in cardiac transplantation. *Heart Transplant.*, **3**, 75

8. Fabre, J. W. (1982). Specific immunosuppression. In Morris, P. J. (ed.) *Tissue Transplantation*. p. 80. (Edinburgh: Churchill Livingstone)

9. Cooper, D. K. C., Lanza, R. P., Nash, E. and Barnard, C. N. (1984). Non-compliance in heart transplant recipients: the Cape Town experience. *Heart Transplant*, **3**, 248

10. Parker, M. T. (1978). Microbiological facilities for the surveillance and control of the spread of infection in hospitals. In Daschner, F. (ed.) *Proven and Unproven Methods in Hospital Infection*. p. 35. (Stuttgart: Gustav Fischer)

11. Preston, G. A., Larson, E. L. and Stamm, W. E. (1981). The effect of private isolation rooms on patient care practices, colonization and infection in an intensive care unit. In Dixon, R. E. (ed.) *Nosocomial Infections*. p. 285. (Atlanta: Yorke Medical Books)

12. Armstrong, D. (1981). The diagnostic microbiology laboratory in the care of the immuno-suppressed patient. In Lorian, V. (ed.) *Significance of Medical Microbiology in Care of Patients*. p. 73. (Baltimore: Williams & Wilkins)

13. Bartlett, J. G. (1982). Making optimum use of the microbiology laboratory. *J. Am. Med. Assoc.*, **247**, 857, 1336, 1868

14. Matthay, R. A. and Moritz, E. D. (1981). Invasive procedures for diagnosing pulmonary infection. A critical review. *Clin. Chest Med.*, **2**, 3

15. Bartlett, J. G. (1977). Diagnostic accuracy of transtracheal aspiration: bacteriologic studies. *Am. Rev. Respir. Dis.*, **115**, 777

16. Zavala, D. C. and Schoell, J. E. (1981). Ultra-thin needle aspiration of the lung in infectious and malignant disease. *Am. Rev. Respir. Dis.*, **123**, 125

17. Wimberley, N., Faling, L. J. and Bartlett, J. G. (1979). A fibreoptic bronchoscopy technique to obtain uncontaminated airway secretions for bacterial culture. *Am. Rev. Respir. Dis.*, **119**, 337

18. Willcox, P. A., Benatar, S. R., Potgieter, P. D., Ferguson, A. D. and Bateman, E. D. (1981). Fibreoptic bronchoscopy—Groote Schuur Hospital experience. *S. Afr. Med. J.*, **60**, 651

19. Beyt, B. E., King, D. K. and Glew, R. H. (1977). Basal pneumonitis and septicaemia after fibreoptic bronchoscopy. *Chest*, **72**, 105

20. Robbins, H. and Goldman, A. L. (1977). Failure of a 'prophylactic' antimicrobial drug to prevent sepsis after fibreoptic bronchoscopy. *Am. Rev. Respir. Dis.*, **116**, 325

21. Meyers, J. D. and Thomas, E. D. (1981). Infection complicating bone marrow transplantation. In Rubin, R. H. and Young, L. S. (eds.) *Clinical Approach to Infection in the Compromised Host*. p. 507. (New York: Plenum)

22. Britt, R. H., Enzmann, D. R. and Remington, J. S. (1981). Intracranial infection in cardiac transplant recipients. *Ann. Neurol.*, **9**, 107

23. Young, L. S. (1981). Fever and septicaemia. In Rubin, R. H. and Young, L. S. (eds.) *Clinical Approach to Infection in the Compromised Host*. p. 75. (New York: Plenum)

24. Penn, R. L., Lambert, R. S. and George, R. B. (1983). Invasive fungal infections. The use of serologic tests in diagnosis and management. *Arch. Intern. Med.*, **143**, 1215

25. Rubin, R. H. and Greene, R. (1981). Etiology and management of the compromised patient with fever and pulmonary infiltrates. In Rubin, R. H. and Young, L. S. (eds.) *Clinical Approach to Infection in the Compromised Host*. p. 123. (New York: Plenum)

26. Fisher, B. D. and Armstrong, D. (1977). Cryptococcal interstitial pneumonia: value of antigen determination. *N. Engl. J. Med.*, **297**, 1440

27. Rubin, R. H. (1981). Infection in the renal transplant patient. In Rubin, R. H. and Young, L. S. (eds.) *Clinical Approach to Infection in the Compromised Host*. p. 553. (New York: Plenum)

28. Smith, C. R., Lipsky, J. J., Laskin, O. L., Hellmann, D. B., Mellits, E. D., Longstreth, S. and Lietman, P. S. (1980). Double-blind comparison of the nephrotoxicity of gentamicin and tobramycin. *N. Engl. J. Med.*, **302**, 1106

29. Simon, H. B. (1981). Mycobacterial and nocardial infections in the compromised host. In Rubin, R. H. and Young, L. S. (eds.) *Clinical Approach to Infection in the Compromised Host*. p. 229. (New York: Plenum)

30. Rand, K. H., Pollard, R. B. and Merigan, T. C. (1978). Increased pulmonary superinfections in cardiac transplant patients undergoing primary cytomegalovirus infection. *N. Engl. J. Med.*, **298**, 951

31. Tobin, J. O'H. (1983). Virus infections in the immunocompromised. In Waterson, A. P. (ed.) *Recent Advances in Clinical Virology*. No. 3, p. 1. (Edinburgh: Churchill Livingstone)

32. Uys, C. J., Rose, A. G. and Barnard, C. N. (1979). The pathology of human cardiac transplantation. *S. Afr. Med. J.*, **56**, 887

33. Alford, C. A. (1982). Acyclovir treatment of herpes virus infections in immunocompromised humans. *Am. J. Med.*, **73** (Suppl.), 225

34. Armstrong, D. (1981). Fungal infections in the compromised host. In Rubin, R. H. and Young, L. S. (eds.) *Clinical Approach to Infection in the Compromised Host.* p. 195. (New York: Plenum)

35. Kerkering, T. M., Duma, R. J. and Shadomy, S. (1981). The evolution of pulmonary cryptococcosis. Clinical implications from a study of 41 patients with and without compromising host factors. *Ann. Intern. Med.*, **94**, 611

36. Butler, W. T., Alling, D. W., Spickard, A. and Utz, J. P. (1964). Diagnostic and prognostic value of clinical and laboratory findings in cryptococcal meningitis. A follow-up study of 40 patients. *N. Engl. J. Med.*, **59**, 270

37. Hammerman, K. J., Powell, K. E., Christianson, C. S., Huggin, P. M., Larsh, H. W., Vivas, J. R. and Tosh, F. E. (1973). Pulmonary cryptococcosis: clinical forms and treatment. A Center for Disease Control co-operative mycoses study. *Am. Rev. Respir. Dis.*, **108**, 1116

38. Medoff, G. and Kobayashi, G. S. (1980). Strategies in the treatment of systemic fungal infections. *N. Engl. J. Med.*, **302**, 145

39. Edwards, J. E., Lehrer, R. I., Stiehm, E. R., Fischer, T. J. and Young, L. S. (1978). Severe candidal infections. Clinical perspective, immune defence mechanisms, and current concepts of therapy. *Ann. Intern. Med.*, **89**, 91

40. Walker, D. H., Adamee, T. and Krigman, M. (1978). Disseminated petriellidosis (Allescheriosis). *Arch. Pathol. Lab. Med.*, **102**, 158

41. Walzer, P. D., Perl, D. P., Krogstad, D. J., Rawson, P. G. and Schultz, M. G. (1974). *Pneumocystis carinii* pneumonia in the United States: epidemiologic, diagnostic and clinical features. *Ann. Intern. Med.*, **80**, 83

42. Winston, D. J., Lau, W. K., Gale, R. P. and Young, L. S. (1980). Trimethoprim-sulphamethoxazole for the treatment of *Pneumocystis carinii* pneumonia. *Ann. Intern. Med.*, **92**, 762

43. Hughes, W. T., Kuhn, S., Chaudhary, S., Feldman, S., Vertosa, M., Aur, R. J. A., Pratt, C. and George, S. L. (1977). Successful chemoprophylaxis for *Pneumocystis carinii* pneumonitis. *N. Engl. J. Med.,* **297**, 1419

44. Rose, A. G., Uys, C. J., Novitzky, D., Cooper, D. K. C. and Barnard, C. N. (1983). Toxoplasmosis of donor and recipient hearts after heterotopic cardiac transplantation. *Arch. Pathol. Lab. Med.*, **197**, 368

45. Jones, R. J. (1981). Vaccines and antisera against Gram-negative bacilli. *J. Hosp. Infect.*, **2**, 105

46. Gaffin, S. L. (1982). Control of septic shock — present day concept. *S. Afr. J. Hosp. Med.*, **8**, 4

14
Malignant Neoplasia in the Immunocompromised Patient

INTRODUCTION

Immunosuppressed recipients of human donor organ grafts have an increased incidence of neoplasia[1]. The incidence of *de novo* malignant tumours at major transplant centres in the USA, Europe and Australia varies from 1% to 16% (mean of 4%), an incidence on average approximately 100 times greater than that of the matched general population[2]. Most of the observed experience has been in recipients of renal allografts, and there are relatively few data regarding recipients of cardiac allografts.

High rates of neoplasia have been found in the latter patients, who often receive more immunosuppression than patients with kidney grafts. In a recent review of the Stanford series of cardiac allograft recipients, 19 tumours (Table 14.1) were observed in 148 patients (12.8%) at risk 3 months or longer after transplantation[3]*. During the same interval three malignant neoplasms

Table 14.1 Malignant neoplasms occurring in 148 3-month heart transplant survivors at Stanford University*

Type	Number
Squamous cell carcinoma	8
Adenocarcinoma of the colon	1
Lymphomas	10
Central nervous system	(4)
Lung	(2)
Soft tissue	(2)
Systemic	(2)

*From Pennock *et al.*[3]

---

* As of December 1983 there was a total of 30 malignancies (18 lymphomas, nine squamous cell carcinomas, two adenocarcinomas, one leukaemia, and one basal cell carcinoma) in 287 patients (10.5%) at Stanford (personal communication from Dr Stuart Jamieson).

223

developed in 30 patients at our own institute who survived with a functioning cardiac allograft for at least 3 months, an incidence of 10%[4].

MALIGNANT TUMOURS OCCURRING AFTER CARDIAC AND RENAL TRANSPLANTATION AT GROOTE SCHUUR HOSPITAL

Tumours have developed in three (10%) cardiac allograft recipients and in seven (4.2%) renal allograft recipients (Table 14.2)[4,5]. The age at transplantation, type of tumour, time of diagnosis after transplantation, treatment, and outcome for each patient are given in Table 14.3. There was a greater than twofold increase in the overall incidence of neoplasia in the cardiac recipients when compared with the kidney recipients, and almost a sixfold increase in the incidence of visceral neoplasia ($p < 0.02$, χ^2).

Table 14.2 Incidence of malignant neoplasms in heart and kidney transplant recipients at Groote Schuur Hospital, Cape Town

Donor organ	3-month survivors	Kaposi's sarcoma	Skin carcinoma	Other malignant neoplasms	Number (%) of survivors with malignant neoplasms
Heart	30	1	0	2	3/30 (10%)
Kidney	167	2	3*	21†	7/167 (4.2%)

*Two squamous cell and one basal cell carcinomas
†One undifferentiated thyroid carcinoma and one intraductal biliary carcinoma

The average age of the ten patients developing tumours was 41, and that of those who did not was 36 years. The average duration of immunosuppression of the ten patients prior to diagnosis of the malignant tumours was 34 months. The shortest periods after transplantation during which tumours developed were 10, 16 and 18 months, these all being Kaposi's sarcomas.

Heart transplants

Adenocarcinoma of the stomach was diagnosed in a patient 19 months after orthotopic cardiac transplantation; he died 2 months later with abdominal and liver metastases. A cerebellar microglioma developed in a second patient, confirmed by biopsy 61 months after heterotopic cardiac transplantation. The tumour responded to cranial radiotherapy, and the patient continues in remission 18 months later with only slight residual neurological dysfunction. Kaposi's sarcoma developed in a black recipient 10 months after heterotopic cardiac allografting; the tumours were localized mainly in the trunk. Immunosuppression was reduced in an effort to curtail the proliferation and dissemination of the tumours, but the patient died 4 months later with widespread dissemination of the neoplasm.

Kidney transplants

Kaposi's sarcoma also developed in two of the kidney transplant recipients. Both were of mixed racial background (i.e. Cape Coloured). One of these patients died as a result of dissemination of the tumour 19 months after diagnosis, despite chemotherapy, and complete withdrawal of immunosuppressive therapy. The other patient had tumours localized to the lower limbs that responded well to radiotherapy and withdrawal of immunosuppressive therapy, with complete regression of the neoplasms. Two of the kidney allograft patients developed squamous cell carcinoma and one recurrent basal cell carcinoma of the skin. These lesions all developed on sun-exposed skin areas and responded well to local radiotherapy or excision. In another patient who died from septicaemia, a localized sclerosing undifferentiated carcinoma of the thyroid was found at autopsy. The final kidney recipient died from an intraductal biliary carcinoma.

POSSIBLE AETIOLOGICAL FACTORS

Impairment of immunosurveillance

The high incidence of malignant tumours in transplant recipients is almost certainly due to the heavy immunosuppression they receive. The more intensive immunosuppression of cardiac recipients may account for the significantly higher incidence of tumours found in our cardiac patients when compared with our renal patients. This immunosuppression may lead to impairment of surveillance mechanisms for neoplastic mutant cells[6-8]. Transformed cells arising by somatic mutation or viral infestation, which have the potential to become malignant, are more likely to escape elimination by the patient, because of the attenuated efficacy of immunosurveillance.

Direct action of immunosuppressive agents

Direct or potentiating actions of rabbit antithymocyte globulin (RATG) or other immunosuppressive agents may be causal; the Stanford cardiac transplantation group has reported the occurrence of tumour at the site of multiple RATG intramuscular injections in two patients[9]. RATG causes immunosuppression by eliminating specific types of lymphocytes implicated in immune reactions and may directly lead to proliferation, by failing to stimulate a suggested feedback mechanism, predisposing the lymphoreticular system to neoplasia[10]. When used in conjunction with chemical carcinogens or oncogenic viruses, antilymphocyte globulin has been shown to have a potentiating effect on cancer development[11-14].

Although no direct oncogenic effect has been demonstrated, azathioprine is known to cause chromosome breaks and nuclear abnormalities in both

Table 14.3   Clinical details of malignant neoplasms occurring in heart and kidney transplant recipients at Groote Schuur Hospital, Cape Town

Donor organ	Age at transplantation	Type of tumour	Months of immuno-suppression	Treatment	Outcome
Heart	52	Gastric adenocarcinoma	19	Palliative	Died
Heart	51	Kaposi's sarcoma	10	Palliative	Died
Heart	32	Cerebellar microglioma	61	Radiotherapy	No recurrence
Kidney	26	Sclerosing undifferentiated thyroid carcinoma	30	—	Discovered at autopsy
Kidney	34	Intraductal biliary carcinoma	62	Palliative	Died
Kidney	42	Squamous cell carcinoma, skin	44	Excision	No recurrence
Kidney	43	Basal cell carcinoma, skin	49	Radiotherapy	No recurrence
Kidney	44	Squamous cell carcinoma, skin	92	Excision	No recurrence
Kidney	44	Kaposi's sarcoma	16	Chemotherapy + withdrawal of IS	Died
Kidney	45	Kaposi's sarcoma	18	Radiotherapy + withdrawal of IS	No recurrence

IS = immunosuppression

animals and man[15], and has been shown to potentiate the actions of onco-genic stimuli[16].

The higher incidence of malignant neoplasia in cardiac transplant recipients may be related to a heavier immunosuppressive regimen. The maintenance immunosuppressive regimen used in renal transplant recipients at Groote Schuur Hospital has varied considerably but, before the introduction of cyclo-sporin A (CYA) in 1983, consisted of methylprednisolone sodium succinate 86 mg/day, reducing by 2 mg/day until 32 mg/day was reached at approxi-mately 1 month; thereafter, reductions were slow until an eventual mainten-ance dosage of 8 mg/day was achieved, usually during the second year. Azathioprine administration was maintained between 0.7 and 2.1 mg/kg per day. Dosages of these drugs were not, therefore, different from those used in the cardiac transplant recipients. Although equine antilymphocyte globulin (EALG) and RATG have been used on occasions in the renal transplant recipients, they have not formed a regular and substantial component of the immunosuppressive regimen as in the cardiac transplant recipients. This would seem to represent the major difference in immunosuppressive therapy between the two groups of patients.

This additional immunosuppression may account for the increased inci-dence of malignancy in the cardiac recipients.

In addition, episodes of acute rejection are almost certainly treated more vigorously in patients with cardiac allografts, even when heterotopic, as there is no artificial support system comparable to dialysis to maintain the life of the patient should total donor organ failure occur. Prolonged courses of anti-rejection therapy, consisting of intravenous methylprednisolone and large daily doses of EALG or RATG, have been given to a number of the cardiac patients. Our renal transplant surgical colleagues have been more ready to abandon the donor kidney when the patient was at risk from the compli-cations of heavy immunosuppressive therapy.

Chronic antigenic stimulation

Prolonged antigenic stimulation of the lymphoreticular system by the donor heart itself may be important in the development of neoplasia[17, 18]. It has been suggested that partial immunosuppression results in failure to stimulate a feedback system which normally controls immune reactions, and may allow viral activation and proliferation with subsequent tumour formation[10].

It is well known that certain viruses can cause neoplastic change[19]. Since immunosuppressed patients are highly susceptible to viral infection, it certainly seems possible that they might also be especially prone to viral oncogenesis. Oncogenic viruses have been thought to play an important aetiological role in the development of lymphomas, cancers of the skin and other types of malig-nancy commonly encountered in transplant patients[20].

TYPES OF NEOPLASIA FOUND IN TRANSPLANT PATIENTS

The types of malignant tumours occurring at our own institution may be contrasted with the types occurring in transplant patients throughout the world (Table 14.4).

Table 14.4   Incidence of malignant tumours in transplant patients worldwide*

Type of tumour	World experience		
	Number	%	
Skin cancers	725	38	
Lymphomas	325	17	
reticulum cell sarcoma	160		8
Kaposi's sarcoma	64		3
Hodgkin's disease	10		1
other lymphomas	91		5
Primary carcinomas	685	36	
uterus	134		7
lung	92		5
head and neck	76		4
(thyroid)	(29)		(2)
(other)	(47)		(2)
colon and rectum	70		4
breast	60		3
kidney	48		3
vulva and perineum	45		2
urinary bladder	32		2
liver and bile ducts	27		1
stomach	25		1
ovary	22		1
testis	19		1
pancreas	18		1
prostate gland	17		1
Metastatic carcinomas (primary site unknown)	46	2	
Leukaemias	47	2	
Soft tissue sarcomas	27	1	
Brain neoplasms (excluding lymphomas)	13	1	
Miscellaneous tumours	29	2	
Total	1897		

* Based on data collected by the Cincinnati (formerly Denver) Transplant Tumor Registry up to August 1983—courtesy I. Penn

Skin cancer

Skin tumours are the most frequently encountered neoplasms in transplant recipients, accounting for 38% of the neoplasms worldwide and 30% of the neoplasms at our own institution. The incidence of skin cancer has been found to vary with the amount of exposure to the oncogenic effects of sunlight[2]. In parts of the world with relatively little sunshine, the incidence is approximately 4–7 times greater than that in the matched general population; in regions with high sunshine exposure the incidence rises to almost 21 times greater than the already high incidence found among the general population of these areas. In one Australian series, where there was high sunshine exposure, skin tumours accounted for 87 (80%) of 109 neoplasms[21].

These cancers also differ qualitatively from those encountered in the general public[22]. Although basal cell carcinoma usually far outnumbers squamous cell carcinoma, this relationship is reversed after transplantation (51% squamous vs. 28% basal worldwide, and two squamous vs. one basal at our own centre). Transplant patients in whom these lesions occur are approximately 30 years younger than individuals in the public at large who develop similar malignancies.

The vast majority of the skin malignancies occurring worldwide after transplantation are low-grade, and only 8% show lymph node metastases when first diagnosed[2]. Five per cent of the patients die from metastases (two-thirds from squamous cell carcinoma and one-third from malignant melanoma); although malignant melanomas occur very rarely they are very aggressive and cause death in nearly 40% of the cases.

In the sunnier climates, transplant recipients should be instructed to avoid excessive sun exposure or to protect the exposed skin areas with clothing and sunscreening lotions and creams. All suspicious lesions on the skin and lips should be biopsied and, if malignant, widely excised. Radiotherapy and cryosurgery can also be useful. In the presence of metastases from squamous cell carcinoma, block dissection of draining lymph nodes may be required. Although in some renal transplant patients withdrawal of immunosuppressive therapy is occasionally recommended, this, of course, is not an option available in the case of the cardiac transplant patient. Immunosuppression may be reduced, but when systemic metastases are present, the prognosis remains grave, even if chemotherapy is instituted. Topical application of 5-fluorouracil or other chemotherapeutic agents is useful in the management of multiple superficial carcinomas.

Lymphoma

Excluding skin cancers, lymphomas occur at the highest frequency in transplant recipients, comprising 17% of all neoplasms worldwide. This contrasts with the incidence of lymphoma in the general population where it represents only 3–4% of all tumours[22].

A striking feature is the marked incidence of central nervous system (CNS) involvement; 40% show CNS involvement, compared with an incidence of only 28% in the general population[1]. In our own series the involvement of the brain by a microglioma—the only lymphoma other than Kaposi's sarcoma that occurred—is consistent with this observation. The weak immunological reactions of the CNS are thought to allow tumour cells to proliferate more readily than at other sites[23].

The predominant type of lymphoma is the reticulum cell carcinoma, which occurs in 49% of cases. Its incidence is approximately 350 times that found in the general population[1]. By contrast, Hodgkin's disease is a relative rarity in transplant recipients, accounting for only ten (3%) of the 325 lymphomas worldwide. This is in sharp contrast with its incidence in the general population of 18%[24]. The incidence of Hodgkin's disease in transplant recipients is therefore only one-sixth that in the general population, whereas non-Hodgkin lymphomas occur 28 times more often in transplant patients than in the remainder of the population[25].

This high incidence of lymphoma may reflect an abnormal immune response to the HLA antigens present on the transplanted tissue, since the neoplasms which occur usually show morphological features of antigen-activated lymphocytes[26]. Although the aetiology remains uncertain, oncogenic viruses are suspected of playing an important role. In four of 134 CYA-treated transplant patients, lymphoma occurred; Epstein–Barr virus (EBV) nuclear antigen was found in the tumour cells of one patient[27] and rising titres of antibody to EBV capsid antigen were present in three[28]. EBV, of course, has clearly been associated with Burkitt's lymphoma, and has been implicated in the pathogenesis of lymphoma in transplant recipients who did not receive CYA[19]. In the case of CYA-treated patients, and possibly others, it is thought that the cell-mediated T cell response to transformation and viral infection is inhibited by either primary infection or reactivation of latent virus[29]. The polyclonal proliferative B cell response is thought to allow development of monoclonal lymphomas. The lymphomas developing in patients immunosuppressed with CYA have thus far occurred relatively early after transplantation (approximately 6 months (Israel Penn, personal communication)).

In a recent review of 31 consecutive patients who received CYA after cardiac transplantation, five (17%) developed malignant lymphomas[30]. This is a higher incidence of lymphoma than the 2–13% reported in the literature for cardiac and renal allograft recipients on conventional immunosuppression[31], or than the 3% incidence in the combined CYA-treated liver and renal allograft patients at three different centres[32]. Whether this difference was due to higher doses of CYA or to the fact that the cardiac patients also received RATG is uncertain.

Central nervous system lymphoma should always be suspected whenever a transplant patient develops neurological symptoms. The treatment of lymphomas is currently evolving and may include reduction of immunosuppression and antiviral agents. Localized lesions are excised if possible or treated by radiotherapy. As illustrated by the patient in our own series, an excellent response may be obtained from radiotherapy for cerebral lymphoma. When lymphoma is systemic, treatment with antineoplastic agents is given; a reduction of immunosuppressive therapy is recommended, if this should prove possible.

Kaposi's sarcoma

Kaposi's sarcoma is an unusual malignancy which occurred in a striking three (30%) patients in our own series; this represents a significant increase over the 3% incidence in transplant patients worldwide ($p < 0.001$). Before the recent Acquired Immune Deficiency Syndrome (AIDS) epidemic, Kaposi's was seldom seen in America or Europe (0.06% of all malignant neoplasms in the Chicago area)[33].

Kaposi's sarcoma occurs relatively early after transplantation—in our own series, after an average period of 15 months (compared with 51 months for the other tumours ($p < 0.05$), and in the worldwide series after 17 months (compared with 56 months).

All three Kaposi's sarcomas in our own institution occurred in transplant recipients with African ancestry. One occurred in a patient from central Africa (Kenya) where, in the general population, Kaposi's sarcoma represents 9% of all malignant tumours[33]. That there was only a 3% chance of all three Kaposi's sarcoma developing in patients with African ancestry would suggest that black patients living in Africa who undergo transplantation may have a propensity for this complication to develop. The relative rarity of transplant operations in this group would explain why this association has not been reported at other transplant centres.

In non-transplant patients, a probable impairment of cellular immune mechanisms in the pathogenesis of the disease has been described[34]. There is also evidence that Kaposi's sarcoma may be caused by viral infection[35]. A genetic factor may well be important; apart from the high incidence in central African blacks referred to above, it has been shown that Kaposi's sarcoma occurs 400–500 times as often in patients with Jewish or Mediterranean origin compared with the matched population[36].

Kaposi's sarcoma should always be suspected when a patient develops red-blue macules or plaques in the skin or oropharyngeal mucosa, or when an apparently infected granuloma fails to heal normally[22].

Although the treatment of Kaposi's sarcoma is currently under review, a reduction in immunosuppression together with local radiotherapy to skin lesions is generally recommended. Again, while immunosuppressive therapy is often withdrawn in renal transplant recipients, this is not possible in cardiac transplant recipients.

Other tumours

Malignant tumours involving the colon and rectum, uterine cervix, prostate and bronchus do not show an increased incidence in transplant patients[2]. *In situ* carcinomas of the body of the uterus, however, develop 14 times as frequently in transplant patients as in the age-matched population[37].

Carcinomas of the vulva and perineum also show a much higher incidence in transplanted patients than in the population at large.

References

1. Penn, I. (1979). Tumour incidence in human allograft recipients. *Transplant. Proc.*, **11**, 1047
2. Penn, I. (1984). Neoplastic consequences of immunosuppression. In Dean, J. H., Munson, A. E. and Luster, M. (eds.) *Toxicology of the Immune System*. (New York: Raven Press) (In press)
3. Pennock, J. L., Oyer, P. E., Reitz, B. A., Jamieson, S. W., Bieber, C. P., Wallwork, J., Stinson, E. B. and Shumway, N. E. (1982). Cardiac transplantation in perspective for the future. *J. Thorac. Cardiovasc. Surg.*, **83**, 168
4. Lanza, R. P., Cooper, D. K. C., Cassidy, M. J. D. and Barnard, C. N. (1983). Malignant neoplasms occurring after cardiac transplantation. *J. Am. Med. Assoc.*, **249**, 1746
5. Cassidy, M. J. D., Disler, R. B. and Swanepoel, C. R. (1982). De novo malignant tumours in renal transplant recipients. *S. Afr. Med. J.*, **62**, 58
6. Burnet, F. M. (1967). Immunological aspects of malignant disease. *Lancet*, **1**, 1171
7. Keast, D. (1970). Immunosurveillance and cancer. *Lancet*, **2**, 710
8. Kersey, J. H., Spector, B. D. and God, R. A. (1973). Immunodeficiency and cancer. *Adv. Cancer Res.*, **18**, 211
9. Bieber, C. P., Hunt, S. A., Schwinn, D. A., Jamieson, S. W., Reitz, B. A., Oyer, P. E., Shumway, N. E. and Stinson, E. B. (1981). Complications in long-term survivors of cardiac transplantation. *Transplant. Proc.*, **13**, 207
10. Schwartz, R. S. and Beldotti, L. (1965). Malignant lymphomas following allogenic disease: Transition from an immunological to a neoplastic disorder. *Science*, **149**, 1511
11. Allison, A. S., Berman, L. D. and Levy, R. H. (1967). Increased tumour induction by adenovirus type 12 in thymectomized mice and mice treated with antilymphocyte serum. *Nature (Lond.)*, **215**, 185
12. Law, L. W., Ting, R. C. and Allison, A. C. (1968). Effects of antilymphocyte serum on induction of tumours and leukaemia by murine sarcoma virus. *Nature (Lond.)*, **220**, 611
13. Balner, H. and Dersjant, R. (1969). Increased oncogenic effect of methylcholanthrene after treatment with anti-lymphocyte serum. *Nature (Lond.)*, **224**, 376
14. Rabbatt, A. G. and Jeejeebhoy, H. F. (1970). Heterologous antilymphocyte serum (ALS) hastens the appearance of methylcholanthrene induced tumours in mice. *Transplantation*, **9**, 164
15. Jensen, M. K. (1967). Chromosomes studies in patients treated with azathioprine and amethopterin. *Acta Med. Scand.*, **182**, 445
16. Koranda, F. C., Loeffer, R. T., Koranda, D. M. and Penn, I. (1975). Accelerated induction of skin cancers by ultraviolet radiation in hairless mice treated with immunosuppressive agents. *Surg. Forum*, **26**, 145
17. Smithers, D. W. and Field, E. O. (1969). Immunosuppression and cancer. *Lancet*, **1**, 672
18. Walford, R. L. (1966). Increased incidence of lymphoma after infection of mice with cells differing at weak histocompatibility loci. *Science*, **152**, 78
19. Hanto, D., Frizzera, G., Gajl-Peczalska, K., Purtilo, D., Klein, G., Simmons, R. L. and Najarian, J. S. (1981). The Epstein–Barr virus (EBV) in the pathogenesis of post-transplant lymphoma. *Transplant. Proc.*, **13**, 756
20. Penn, I. (1977). Development of cancer as a complication of clinical transplantation. *Transplant. Proc.*, **9**, 1121
21. Sheil, A. G. R., Mahony, J. F., Horvath, J. S., Johnson, J. R., Tiller, D. J., Stewart, J. H. and May, J. (1981). Cancer following successful cadaveric donor renal transplantation. *Transplant. Proc.*, **13**, 733
22. Penn, I. (1982). Problems of cancer in organ transplantation. *Heart Transplant.*, **2**, 71

23. Schneck, S. A. and Penn, I. (1971). De novo brain tumours in renal transplant recipients. *Lancet*, **1**, 983

24. Penn, I. (1983). Lymphomas complicating organ transplantation. *Transplant. Proc.*, **15**, 2790

25.. Hoove, R. and Fraumeni, J. F. (1973). Risk of cancer in renal transplant recipients. *Lancet*, **2**, 55

26. Penn, I. (1978). Tumours arising in organ transplant recipients. In Klein, G. and Weinhouse, S. (eds.) *Advances in Cancer Research*. Vol. 28, p. 31. (New York: Academic Press)

27. Crawford, D. H., Thomas, J. A., Janossy, G., Sweny, P., Fernando, O. N., Moorhead, J. F. and Thompson, J. H. (1980). Epstein–Barr virus nuclear antigen positive lymphoma after cyclosporin A treatment in patients with renal allograft. *Lancet*, **1**, 1355

28. Nagington, J. and Gray, J. (1980). Cyclosporin A, immunosuppression, Epstein–Barr antibody, and lymphoma. *Lancet*, **1**, 536

29. Bird, A. G. and McLachlan, S. M. (1980). Cyclosporin A and Epstein–Barr virus. *Lancet*, **2**, 418

30. Oyer, P. E., Stinson, E. B., Jamieson, S. W., Hunt, S., Reitz, B. A., Bieber, C. P., Schroeder, J. S., Billingham, M. and Shumway, N. E. (1983). One year experience with cyclosporin A in clinical heart transplantation. *Heart Transplant.*, **1**, 285

31. Sheil, A. G. R. (1977). Cancer in renal allograft recipients in Australia and New Zealand. *Transplant. Proc.*, **9**, 1133

32. Humphrey, J. H., Hows, J. M. and Gordon-Smith, E. C. (1982). Cyclosporin A in human transplantation. *Immunol. Today*, **3**, 228

33. Rothman, S. (1962). Remarks on sex, age and racial distribution of Kaposi's sarcoma and possible pathological factors. *Acta Unio Int. Contra Cancrum*, **18**, 326

34. Master, S. P., Taylor, J. F. and Kyalwazi, S. K. (1970). Immunological studies in Kaposi's sarcoma in Uganda. *Br. Med. J.*, **1**, 600

35. Gottlieb, G. J., Ragaz, A., Vogel, J. V., Friedman-Kien, A., Rywlin, A. M., Weiner, E. A. and Ackerman, A. B. (1981). A preliminary communication on extensively disseminated Kaposi's sarcoma in young homosexual men. *Am. J. Dermatopathol.*, **3**, 111

36. Harwood, A. R., Osaba, D., Hofstader, S. L., Goldstein, M. B. M., Cardella, C. J., Holecek, M. J., Kunynetz, R. and Giammarco, R. A. (1979). Kaposi's sarcoma in recipients of renal transplants. *Am.. J. Med.*, **67**, 759

37. Forreco, R., Penn, I., Droegemveller, W., Greer, B. and Makowski, E. (1975). Gynecologic malignancies in immunosuppressed organ homograft recipients. *Obstet. Gynecol.*, **45**, 359

15
Psychiatric Aspects

INTRODUCTION

Cardiac transplantation emerged in 1967 as a dramatically new way of saving the life of a dying cardiac patient[1]. It was not so much the radical nature of the procedure that triggered the reactions, but the removal and replacement of an organ that is seen by some as a physiological pump and by others as the symbolic seat of love and loyalty.

Psychiatric experience in this field is indebted to contributions from two allied areas: firstly, the care of patients undergoing closed and open heart surgery, and secondly, experience obtained from involvement in renal and liver transplantation programmes. The psychiatric implications of closed and open heart surgery have been extensively documented[2,3]. Of particular relevance has been Kimball's identification of nuclear patterns of emotional reaction in patients assessed preoperatively; these patterns have been found to have predictive value. Out of the four groups that he identified, namely the adjusted, the symbiotic, the depressed, and those denying anxiety, it was the members of the latter two that caused concern. He reported that the depressed group had a high postoperative mortality rate, whilst those who denied anxiety had a high incidence of postoperative psychiatric complications[2].

The second area, psychiatric experience obtained from involvement in organ transplantation since the first kidney transplant was performed in 1950, has centred around the issues of selection criteria, organ incorporation versus rejection, postoperative psychosis, the complications of immunosuppressive medication, compliance and rehabilitation.

Psychiatric experience in heart transplantation over the past 15 years has been similar; recipients require psychosocial screening, develop early and late postoperative emotional or behavioural disturbances and have to adapt to incorporating a new life-giving organ. Heart transplant recipients also face the early challenges of organ rejection and systemic infections, in addition to the need to readjust to family relationships and employment later. It is in all these areas that psychiatric insights have helped transplant teams. Each of these aspects will be considered in greater detail.

The importance of the role of the psychiatrist is well illustrated by the observation at our own institution that no fewer than 26% of deaths or loss of allograft function were related in some part to non-compliance on the part of the patient[4], thus drawing attention to the psychological problems such patients face.

PATIENT SELECTION

'Patient selection is important because basic issues of social policy, the limits of medical responsibility, major ethical and legal considerations are encapsulated in the decision to choose or reject patients ...'[5].

In the early years of cardiac transplantation, mental deficiency and active psychosis were the only psychiatric grounds used to justify exclusion from a programme[6]. With improved survival and the subsequent expansion of transplantation the selection of suitable recipients has recently become an important issue. Most centres now have a committee of medical personnel who take medical, psychological and social criteria into account. A preliminary screening inevitably occurs prior to the actual referral, which reflects to some extent the reactions of the referring physician to the patient's personality and to the character of his or her family. Self-referrals for cardiac transplantation must be viewed with some caution since this may be indicative of exhibitionistic traits in patients seeking publicity. (The self-referral of donors, however, requires immediate psychiatric intervention, since this suggests suicide intent.)

The psychiatric assessment of patients who have been referred for transplantation includes an interview that reviews the patient's personal development, family background and history of psychiatric illness, as well as his or her attitudes to the illness, disability, death and transplantation. During this interview it is also of value to assess the patient's personality structure and the usual defence mechanisms used to handle anxiety, as well as motivation for recovery and potential for rehabilitation. Dreams are useful cues to reveal unspoken concerns. It is important to examine current mental functioning using a standardized method[7], which should include enquiry about depression, suicidal ideas and memory impairment, as well as assessment of intelligence, insight and capacity to make sound judgements, with special relevance to the giving of informed consent. Formal psychological testing may be of assistance[8].

Evidence of organic impairment may be found in patients with poor cerebral perfusion, but if these are associated with neurological deficits the impairment is likely to be permanent and due to cerebral arteriosclerosis. Where there are language barriers, competent and empathic interpreters who are familiar with the transplant regimen are invaluable.

Evidence of a disturbed personality, indicated by alcohol and drug dependence, an erratic work record, unstable interpersonal relationships, and anti-social behaviour, have been added in most programmes to the original exclusion criteria of mental deficiency and active psychosis. The quality of the patient's psychosocial support is of great importance and must also be taken into account[9, 10].

The nature of the heart disease in itself may be a cue to the patient's personality and his/her customary ways of adapting to stress. Since some candidates have a history of myocardial infarction (complicating coronary artery disease), they may well show features of the type A behaviour pattern described by Friedman and Rosenman[11]. Such individuals characteristically show ambitiousness, striving, overcommitment to work, time urgency and impatience[12]. They strive to be 'good' patients postoperatively and are highly motivated to survive. Another identifiable group comprises those with cardio-myopathy, which has been associated with shorter survival when linked to significant alcohol abuse and unstable work and relationship patterns[4]. Careful thought has to be given before a transplant operation is performed on such unpredictable individuals.

While patients with rheumatic or congenital heart disease, who have tolerated previous operative intervention, are likely to handle the stress of the transplantation procedure satisfactorily, they may have difficulty in relinquishing the sick role; rehabilitation then becomes a major exercise.

Factors that are predictive of a favourable outcome include a patient's ability to discuss the possibility of his or her own death as well as having a clear use for the time gained by longer survival and sound social support[13].

WAITING FOR A TRANSPLANT

Once a patient has been accepted for a programme, he or she has to await a donor heart. Patients referred from distant places may have to live temporarily near the hospital and are often supported by only one family member. This alien environment can be stressful, especially if the patient has to wait many weeks. Initial optimism may give way to anxiety, despair and even depression.

IMMEDIATE POSTOPERATIVE PERIOD

In the early days of cardiac transplantation many patients became psychologically disturbed during the initial postoperative period, just as they did in the early days of heart surgery[3]. These changes were attributed to the convergence of such factors as altered cerebral circulation, prolonged anaesthesia, overstimulation by the monitoring systems, the sensory deprivation of immobility, and the unfamiliar bland environment peopled by masked strangers.

The acute psychosis that can occur in this phase bears the features of both 'organic' and 'functional' disturbance; symptoms include reduced level of consciousness, hallucinations, paranoid delusions, disorientation for time and place, and mood disturbances such as depression or undue euphoria. Unconscious anxieties and fantasies about the transplanted heart may be voiced in this context[14].

More recent reports now indicate that there is little disturbance in the early postoperative period, which is possibly indicative of improved patient preparation prior to the procedure[8]. Although many patients are persistently euphoric at having survived the procedure and are delighted with their increased vital capacity and physical strength, this state of well-being can be threatened by episodes of organ rejection or infection that may trigger depression and anxiety. Boredom and social isolation may also take an emotional toll. The steroids required to combat organ rejection pose an additional hazard since they are known to produce depression and even psychosis[15]. Mild symptoms respond to a psychotherapeutic interview and programme modification, though regressed behaviour, irritability, paranoid fears, suicidal feelings and ideas must be sought and treated, if necessary with neuroleptic medication such as chlorpromazine or thioridazine. Antidepressives such as the tri- or tetracyclic agents, however, should only be administered with caution. It is well-documented that emotional factors can influence the immunological balance of the body, and that these changes may affect organ acceptance or rejection[16].

Regressed behaviour, which is often triggered by medical complications, responds to empathic and firm handling by staff. As dependency on the staff lessens, it becomes necessary for the patients to practise autonomy in taking control of some aspects of the treatment programme. Many patients are anxious about leaving the security of the hospital and require gradual weaning from the intensive care unit and, later, the ward environment. The spouse also needs reassurance and instruction. The psychiatrist, clinical psychologist or psychiatric social worker can help the surgical team understand the anxieties that inevitably occur during and after any hospitalization, particularly if the hospital stay has been for heart transplantation[17].

It is also very important to remember that disturbed behaviour, confusion and headaches, may actually have a neurological cause, such as an intracranial viral, bacterial or fungal infection, which occur more frequently in the immunologically compromised host. Epileptic fits, local pain, or paralysis are indications for immediate neurological investigation to rule out infarction or infection. Neoplasia may account for later neurological disturbance[18].

REHABILITATION

The successful transplant recipient has survived a unique life experience. Some survivors of cardiac arrest admit to thoughts of resurrection and fantasies of rebirth[19, 20]. An effective donor heart pumps new life through the body and the brain, bringing physical vigour, an enriched personality, improved memory and the promise of health. Cardiac resuscitation and cardiac surgery have introduced a new dimension in human experience; the patients both 'die' and are 'reborn' or 'resurrected'[21]. To quote Paul Coffey, a British heart transplant survivor, 'Following the transplant and being given a second chance of life one has time to think about what really matters'[22].

Integration of the new heart into the body image is effected in various ways. The organ has to be 'taken in' and become part of a healthy body representation. The heart is seen as a pump to the mechanically-minded patient, devoid of emotional significance, which can be replaced if worn out. At the other extreme, however, some recipients unmistakably identify with the sex and personality of the donor. Reactions to the organ influence compliance with medication. Complete integration of the organ into the body image involves dealing at some level with feelings of guilt and indebtedness for having received an organ at the cost of another's life[14, 23].

Recipients of donor hearts have to deal with fantasies about the donor. At the present time most recipients are men; most donors are also men, frequently young men who have sustained head injuries in road traffic accidents[5]. Louis Washkansky, the first heart transplant patient, however, received a heart from a female donor. He enquired 'Do you think ... that I might develop busts like a woman? ... or become chicken-hearted?'[24]. Other male recipients receiving hearts from female donors have also had this type of reaction.

The early transplant patients' fame nourished the rehabilitation process and ensured a 'survivor mission' reaction, which has frequently been useful in gaining their co-operation in carrying out research, for example, on the physiology of the denervated heart[25]. For subsequent survivors the rehabilitation process has been a less dramatic affair, with mundane issues such as housing, employment and restored marital relationships to be faced. While euphoria and improved self-esteem are found in many, the steroid facies make the recipients feel self-conscious, and not all are able to adapt to the new, bloated appearance. In some patients there are difficulties in concentration, emotional lability, and irritability[15], while in others features of mild organic brain impairment can be found[26]. Recipients may show a morbid interest in their surgical 'twins' who have received organs from the same donor (e.g. kidneys), and identify closely with them.

Follow-up has to be carefully planned. On the one hand, transfer to physicians or surgeons remote from the transplant centre, who have had little experience with transplantation programmes, engenders insecurity, and may jeopardize compliance with dietary instructions and medication—and hence survival. On the other hand, follow-up by the patients' own doctors lessens the overidentification with fellow transplant patients and grief at their death.

The return to the family means that there has to be a reorganization of the family system[8]. Wives often feel insecure in adapting to a more active spouse, and marital relations may be jeopardized by drug-induced impotence[27]. Marital and family counselling may be required. The risk of rejecting the transplanted heart initially inhibits long-term planning. Nevertheless, favourable reports of the effective rehabilitation of 91% of the patients who had survived more than 6 months after transplantation at Stanford, have spurred enthusiasm in transplant programmes[28,29]. Improved survival has ensured official and community support for continuation and expansion of these programmes.

TEAMWORK

Human organ transplantation is notable for its intensive interdisciplinary team work. It is a collaborative enterprise that requires the skills of surgeons, anaesthetists, physicians (renal, cardiac, pulmonary), microbiologists, immunologists, haematologists, neurologists, psychiatrists, social workers, nurses, radiographers, physiotherapists and occupational therapists, as well as the technicians who assemble the heart-lung machine, and carry out the many necessary immunological and biochemical assays[5]. Newcomers to the service, however, may find that the unique demands of the programme tax their professional equilibrium, especially if they have unrealistic expectations of their roles. Psychiatric assistance may be necessary for such individuals if team support is not enough. Frequent team meetings are valuable to allow members to express their feelings and ensure good communication and support.

ETHICAL ISSUES

Heart transplantation raises the cosmic issues of death, resurrection and immortality that transcend the mundane daily concerns of heart sounds, lymphocyte counts and blood cultures. A programme of this kind demands the best that an academic centre has to offer, and stretches the imagination in seeking how to extend productive lives. 'Heart transplantation remains a major undertaking on the part of both patient and transplant team, but offers carefully selected patients with advanced myocardial disease the possibility of a good quality of life for a number of years'[4].

Psychiatrists and social workers have played a useful role in renal, liver and heart transplantation programmes by assisting with selection and helping transplant teams handle the more complicated behavioural, emotional and family problems which regularly accompany major procedures that aim to prolong life. Donor families may also need support in coming to terms with their anger about delays in burial as well as with the finality of death that removal of the heart, in particular, confirms. These families often seek to find out the identity of the recipient, since the survival of the recipient gives their loss some meaning.

In addition, cardiac transplantation has opened up important ethical issues of selection, the finality of life, the definition of death, informed consent, and priorities in the allocation of scarce life-saving resources[30-32]. The giving and receiving of a body organ—a gift of enormous value—is the most significant aspect of human organ transplantation. It is not a private transaction between the donor and recipient, but rather takes place within a network of personal relationships that includes families, the medical team and society. Mauss[33] has described the gift relationship as a series of implied obligations—to give, to receive and to repay. In the context of cardiac transplantation it is life that is given up, received and renewed. Thus, donor, recipient and kin can become bound to one another emotionally and morally in ways that can be fettering as well as self-transcending. Organ transplantation has brought issues of gift exchange and social solidarity to the fore, and has shown how technical advances tend to outstrip contemporary psychological and social organization. Heart transplantation highlights the value medical science places on individual human life, and the progress that is possible through the application of science.

References

1. Barnard, C. N. (1967). A human cardiac transplant: an interim report of a successful operation performed at Groote Schuur Hospital, Cape Town. *S. Afr. Med. J.*, **41**, 1271
2. Kimball, C. P. (1969). Psychological responses to the experiences of open heart surgery. *Am. J. Psychiatry*, **126**, 348
3. Abram, H. P. (1971). Psychotic reactions after cardiac surgery—a critical review. In Castelnuovo-Tedesco, P. (ed.) *Psychiatric Aspects of Organ Transplantation*. pp. 70–78. (New York: Grune & Stratton)
4. Cooper, D. K. C., Lanza, R. P., Nash, E. S. and Barnard, C. N. (1984). Non-compliance in heart transplant recipients: the Cape Town experience. *Heart Transplant.*, **3**, 248
5. Fox, R. C. and Swazey, J. P. (1974). *The Courage to Fail.* p. 242. (Chicago: University of Chicago Press)
6. Christopherson, L. K. and Lunde, D. T. (1971). The selection of cardiac transplant recipients and their subsequent psychological adjustment. In Castelnuovo-Tedesco, P. (ed.) *Psychiatric Aspects of Organ Transplantation.* pp. 36–45. (New York: Grune & Stratton)
7. Institute of Psychiatry, London. (1973). *Notes on Eliciting and Recording Clinical Information.* (London: Oxford University Press)
8. Allender, J., Shisslak, C., Kaszniak, A. and Copeland, J. (1983). Stages of psychological adjustment associated with heart transplant. *Heart Transplant.*, **2**, 228
9. Baumgartner, W. A., Reitz, B. A., Oyer, P. E., Stinson, E. B. and Shumway, N. E. (1979). Cardiac homotransplantation. *Curr. Probl. Surg.*, **16**, 1
10. Pennock, J. L., Oyer, P. E., Reitz, B. A., Jamieson, S. W., Bieber, C. P., Wallwork, J., Stinson, E. B. and Shumway, N. E. (1982). Cardiac transplantation in perspective for the future. *J. Thorac. Cardiovasc. Surg.*, **83**, 168
11. Friedman, M. and Rosenman, R. H. (1959). Association of specific overt behaviour patterns with blood and cardiovascular findings: blood cholesterol level, blood clotting time, incidence of arcus senilis, and clinical coronary artery disease. *J. Am. Med. Assoc.*, **169**, 1286
12. Davies, M. H. (1982). Stress, personality and coronary artery disease. *S. Afr. J. Hosp. Med.*, **8**, 271

13. Kaplan, H. I., Freedman, A. and Sadock, B. (1980). *Comprehensive Textbook of Psychiatry.* III. Vol. 2. 3rd Edn., p. 2065. (Baltimore/London: Williams & Wilkins)
14. Castelnuovo-Tedesco, P. (1973). Organ transplant, body image, psychosis. *Psychoanal. Q.,* **42,** 349
15. Hall, R. C., Popkin, M. K., Stickney, S. K. and Gardner, E. R. (1979). Presentation of the steroid psychoses. *J. Ment. Nerv. Dis.,* **167,** 229
16. Freebury, D. R. (1974). The psychological implications of organ transplantation—a selective review. *Can. Psychiatr. Assoc. J.,* **19,** 593
17. Kraft, I. A. and Vick, J. (1971). The transplantation milieu, St Luke's Episcopal Hospital, 1968–1969. In Castelnuovo-Tedesco, P. (ed.) *Psychiatric Aspects of Organ Transplantation.* pp. 17–25. (New York: Grune & Stratton)
18. Hotson, J. R. and Pedley, T. A. (1976). The neurological complications of cardiac transplantation. *Brain,* **99,** 673
19. Blaiberg, P. (1969). *Looking at my Heart.* p. 120. (New York: Stein & Day)
20. Lunde, D. T. (1969). Psychiatric complications of heart transplants. *Am. J. Psychiatry,* **126,** 369
21. Blacher, R. S. (1983). Death, resurrection, and re-birth: observations in cardiac surgery. *Psychoanal. Q.,* **52,** 56
22. Dobson, L. (1983). Every day is a bonus for us. *Nursing Times,* **79,** 8
23. Basch, S. H. (1973). The intrapsychic integration of a new organ. *Psychoanal. Q.,* **42,** 364
24. Barnard, C. N. and Pepper, C. B. (1969). *One Life.* p. 322. (Cape Town: Howard Timmins)
25. Beck, W., Barnard, C. N. and Schrire, V. (1969). Heart rate after cardiac transplantation. *Circulation,* **40,** 437
26. Molish, H. B., Kraft, I. A. and Wiggins, P. Y. (1971). Psychodiagnostic evaluation of the heart transplant patient. In Castelnuovo-Tedesco, P. (ed.) *Psychiatric Aspects of Organ Transplantation.* pp. 46–57. (New York: Grune & Stratton)
27. Wolpowitz, A. and Barnard, C. N. (1978). Impotence after heart transplantation. *S. Afr. Med. J.,* **54,** 693
28. Christopherson, L. K., Griepp, R. B. and Stinson, E. B. (1976). Rehabilitation after cardiac transplantation. *J. Am. Med. Assoc.,* **236,** 2082
29. Gaudiani, V. A., Stinson, E. B., Alderman, E., Hunt, S. A., Schroeder, S. S., Perlroth, M. G., Bieber, C. P., Oyer, P. E., Reitz, B. A., Jamieson, S. W., Christopherson, L. K. and Shumway, N. E. (1981). Long-term survival and function after cardiac transplantation. *Ann. Surg.,* **194,** 381
30. Paton, A. (1981). Life and death: moral and ethical aspects of transplantation. In Castelnuovo-Tedesco, P. (ed.) *Psychiatric Aspects of Organ Transplantation.* pp. 161–168. (New York: Grune & Stratton)
31. Simmons, R. G., Klein, S. D. and Simmons, R. L. (1977). *Gift of Life: The Social and Psychological Impact of Organ Transplantation.* (New York: Wiley)
32. Oosthuizen, G. C. (ed.) (1972). *The Ethics of Tissue Transplantation.* (Cape Town: Howard Timmins)
33. Mauss, M. (1954). *The Gift: Forms and Functions of Exchange in Archaic Societies.* (Translated by Gunnison, I.) (Glencoe: Free Press)

16
Pathology of Chronic Rejection

INTRODUCTION

In the 15 years since the first human heart transplant was performed by Barnard in 1967[1], there has been significant progress in establishing this procedure as an acceptable method of treating irremediable cardiac failure. Survival times have progressively improved[2]. In the patients who die in the first few months after cardiac transplantation when immunosuppression is maximal, infection is a major cause of death[3,4]. Rejection is also an important factor which, if not primarily responsible for the patient's death, contributes significantly to it, even when overwhelming infection is present[5,6]. The pattern of acute cardiac rejection and the role of the endomyocardial biopsy in its diagnosis have been outlined in Chapter 11.

While the changes which characterize acute rejection may persist beyond the first few weeks post-transplantation and indeed may occur in patients who die years after transplantation[6], they are progressively replaced by a chronic rejection response which is dominated by an obliterative lesion of the large coronary radicles. A significant step towards human transplantation was a successful orthotopic transplant in the dog performed by Lower *et al.* in 1961[7]. This pioneering effort was followed in 1965 by accounts of observations on treated and untreated orthotopic transplants in dogs which had survival times up to 250 days[8]. In 1968 Lower and his colleagues were the first to draw attention to the proliferative and obliterative intimal changes of chronic vascular rejection in the epicardial coronary arteries of long-surviving canine transplants[9]. The first description of a human heart with these obliterative vascular changes of chronic rejection was in 1969 when Thomson[10] described the donor heart of a patient who had survived 19½ months after transplantation. Since then, with increasing survival times, this lesion has been recorded with increasing frequency[5,6,11–18].

MACROSCOPIC APPEARANCES

The donor heart with chronic rejection shows a variable spectrum of macro-scopic appearances. In our series of cases the anastomotic sites all showed signs of complete healing. The sutures were usually buried in connective tissue with smooth endocardial surfaces overlying the anastomoses. In none of the hearts were these the site of thrombus formation. Depending on the degree of chronic rejection, the ventricular myocardium in some appeared near normal while in others a varying extent of scarring occurred similar to healed infarc-tion. In yet others there was evidence of superimposed acute infarction (Figures 16.1, 16.2), particularly in heterotopic transplants which had ceased to function for some time before the patient's death or surgical extirpation of the heart.

In addition, the coronary arteries in many of the hearts were strikingly abnormal. The epicardial branches of the main coronary arteries were thickened and on transverse section showed marked reduction in lumen size. In addition many had a notable degree of lipid deposition in the vessel walls,

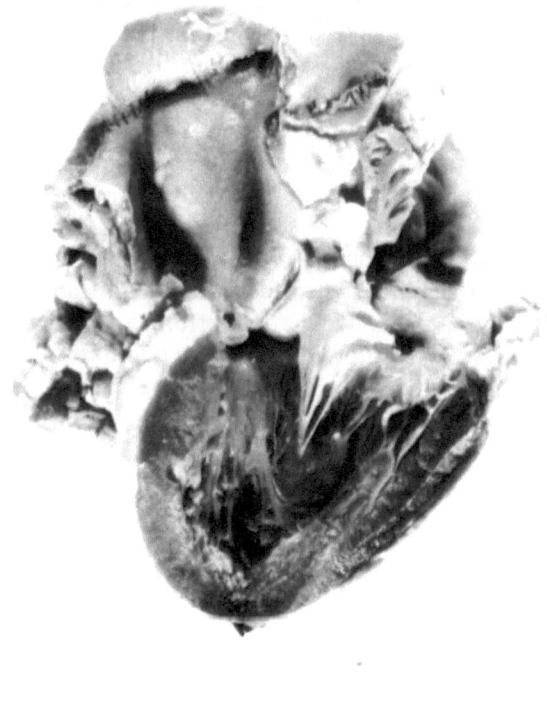

cm |0 | 187 70 | |5 | | | | |10

Figure 16.1 Orthotopic cardiac transplant performed for cardiomyopathy. Postoperative sur-vival 1.7 years. The patient died of diffuse carcinomatosis. This is the only long-surviving transplant in which the coronary arteries showed no evidence of chronic rejection (Figure 16.16)

with accompanying thrombotic occlusion of the lumina. In heterotopic transplants with chronic rejection, examined at autopsy, mural thrombus occupied a large proportion of both ventricular cavities of the donor hearts. The epicardial surfaces were fibrous and adherent to adjacent structures, while the pulmonary arteries, aorta and valves were usually macroscopically unremarkable.

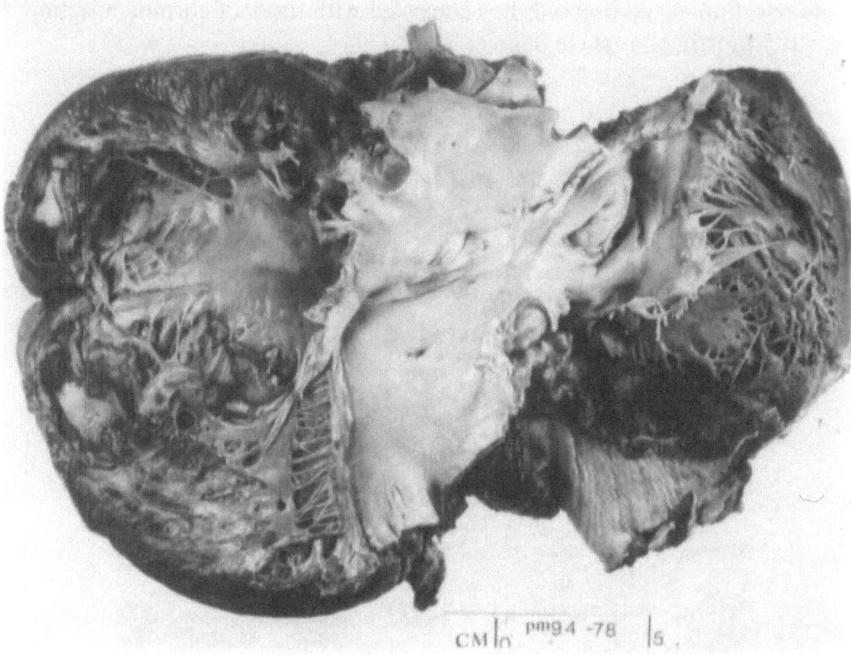

Figure 16.2 Heterotopic cardiac transplant performed for chronic rheumatic valvular disease. Postoperative survival 0.64 years. The recipient ventricle is on the left and the donor ventricle on the right. Both contain antemortem mural thrombus. The donor heart showed acute on chronic vascular rejection

MICROSCOPIC APPEARANCES

The microscopic changes of chronic rejection were usually detectable 30 days postoperatively, but in one of our cases the intimal thickening of early chronic vascular rejection was observed as early as 20 days after transplantation[6]. A gradual progression of the changes characterizing acute rejection to those of chronic rejection was observed, depending upon the survival time of the patient and whether death was primarily due to infection, late acute rejection or chronic rejection. However, even in cases who survived periods from 1 to 12 years, a proportion of the hearts at autopsy showed evidence of persisting acute rejection. These changes, similar to those already described, took the form of focal infiltrates of lymphoid cells in the interstitium and subendo-cardial connective tissue (Figure 16.3). Many of these cells had acquired abundant RNA-rich pyroninophilic cytoplasm. Active myofibre damage mani-festing as fibre swelling and myocytolysis (Figure 16.4) was occasionally seen, while acute vascular rejection, presenting as fibrinoid necrosis of the media of large and medium-sized coronary artery radicles associated with an infiltrate of lymphoid cells, infrequently persisted (Figure 16.5). Where the signs of acute rejection were observed they coexisted with those of chronic rejection, the latter mostly of a severe degree.

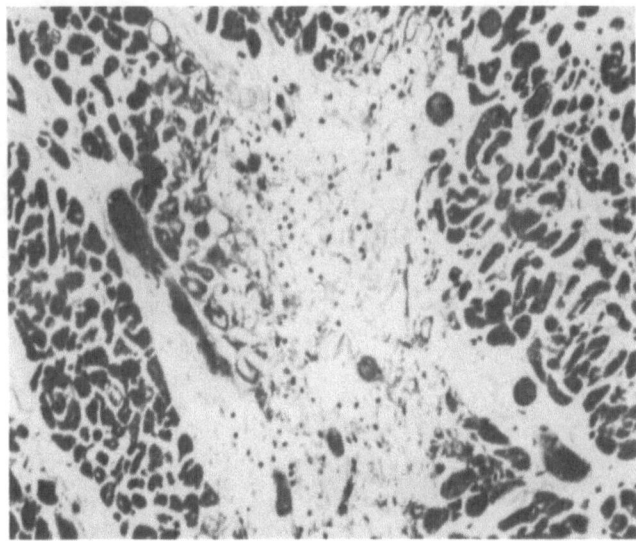

Figure 16.3 Persisting acute rejection. Focal myocytolysis of fibres, interstitial oedema and a mild interstitial lymphocytic infiltrate. Patient survived 2.7 years. Donor age 15 years. H & E × 150

The most striking and significant component of chronic rejection was the process of chronic vascular rejection which, due to continued proliferation of intimal lining cells, mainly myofibroblasts, led to progressive obliteration of the lumina of the epicardial branches of the main coronary arteries and its penetrating medium-sized branches (Figures 16.6, 16.7). The cellular thick-ened intima also showed lipid deposition of varying degrees and an increase of intercellular collagen, which further contributed to the luminal occlusion.

Initially, the lipid was observed in myofibroblasts and macrophages. With progressive accumulation, these cells disintegrated and released free-lying lipid. There was a variable lymphoid cellular infiltrate of the walls of the affected vessels in a few cases. The internal elastic lamina was either intact or fragmented. These lesions of chronic rejection in the large coronary artery branches, particularly when associated with abundant lipid deposition in the

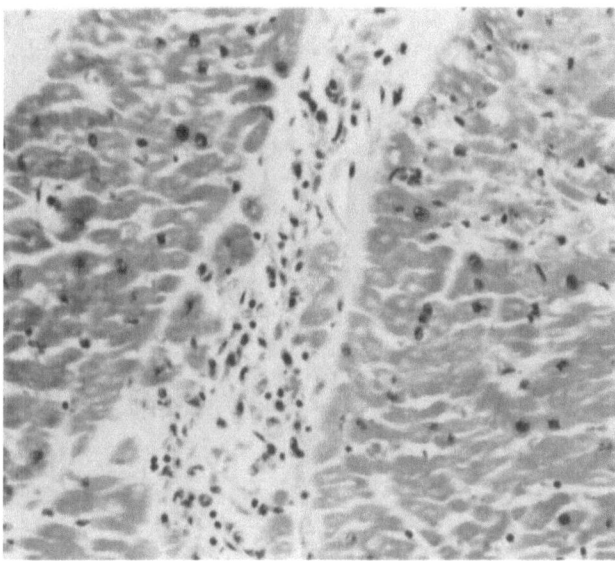

Figure 16.4 Persisting acute rejection. Focal interstitial infiltrate of lymphoid cells, some of which have acquired pyroninophilic cytoplasm. Patient survival 1.6 years. Donor age 25 years. H & E × 180

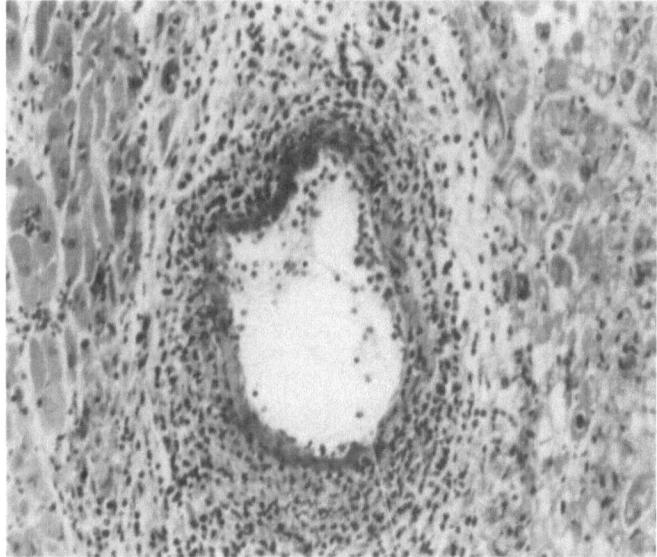

Figure 16.5 Persisting acute rejection. Fibrinoid necrosis of the wall of a small coronary artery radicle accompanied by an intense infiltrate of lymphoid cells in the vessel wall and perivascular connective tissue. Graft survival 80 days. H & E × 150

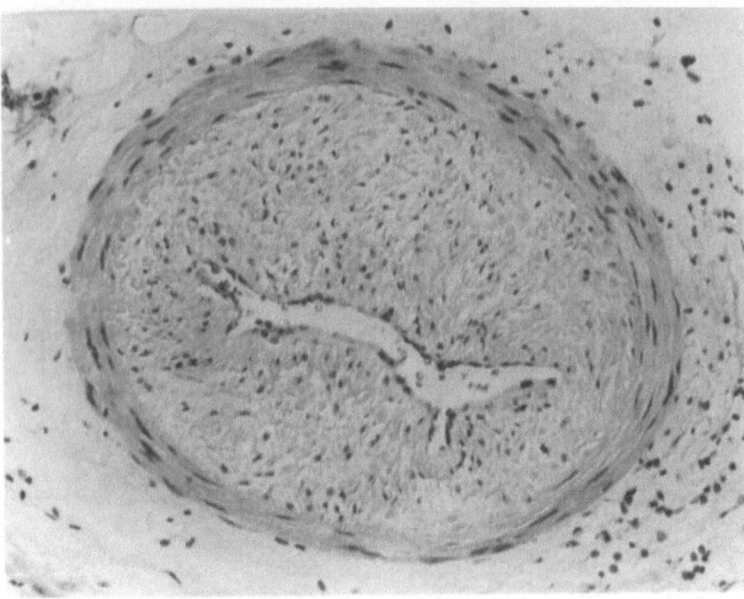

Figure 16.6 Chronic vascular rejection. Proliferation of intimal myofibroblasts has reduced the lumen of this small penetrating branch of the coronary artery to a mere slit. This is unassociated with lipid deposition and a lymphocytic infiltrate in this instance. Graft survival 1.6 years. Donor age 25 years. H & E × 175

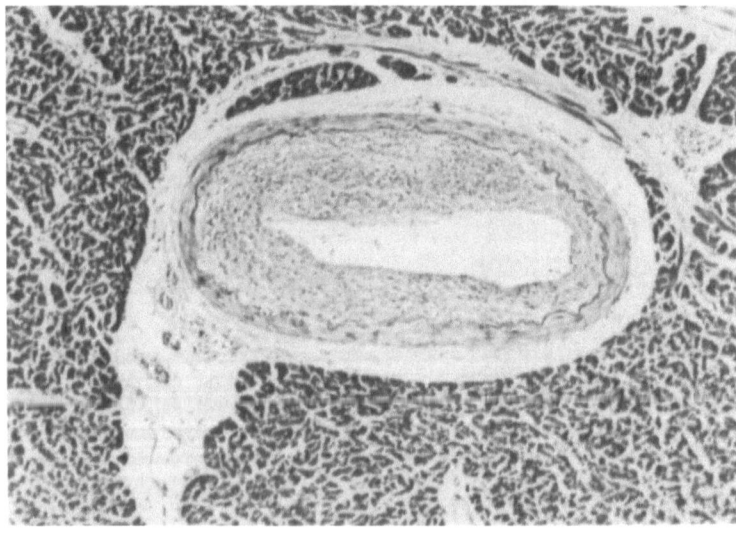

Figure 16.7 Chronic vascular rejection. Small coronary artery with severe intimal thickening due to myointimal cellular proliferation. Some fibrous replacement of media. Moderate lumen encroachment. Patient survival 12.5 years. Donor age 33 years. H & E × 70

thickened intima, bore a close resemblance to advanced atherosclerosis (Figures 16.8–16.10). The smaller coronary artery branches more often showed reparative fibrosis of previous medial necrosis, giving the lesion the appearance of a healed arteritis. These changes, in the more severely affected large arteries, predisposed to superadded thrombosis, which appeared as fresh thrombus in a few cases (Figure 16.11), but in the majority as old occlusive thrombus, which had undergone fibrous replacement and recanalization (Figure 16.12). It is of interest that veins were very seldom affected by this process.

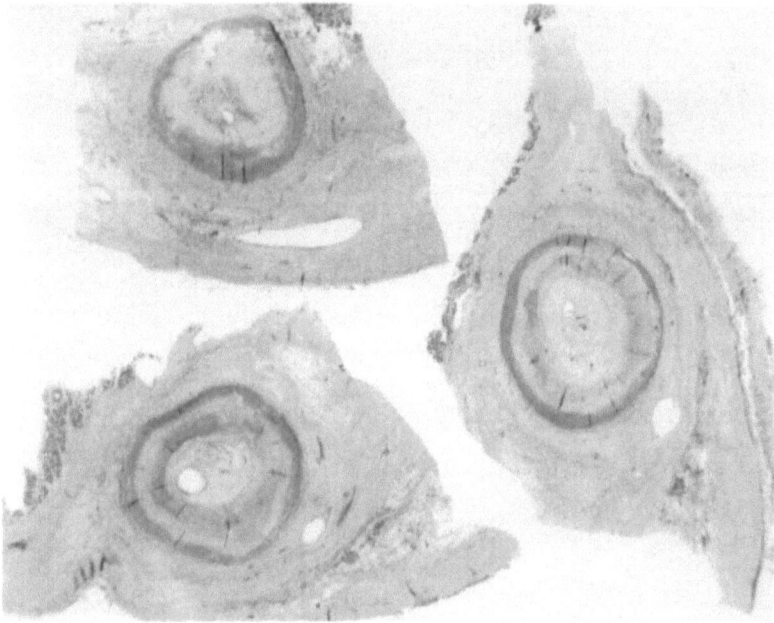

Figure 16.8 Chronic vascular rejection. The epicardial branches of the main coronary arteries are virtually obliterated by markedly thickened intima in which there is lipid deposition. Patient survival 12.5 years. Donor age 33 years. H & E × 5

In addition to the vascular changes, scanty interstitial and subendocardial lymphoid infiltrates still persisted. However, the lymphoid cells had acquired more cytoplasm and had the appearances of activated lymphocytes. Plasma cells were noted and became progressively more numerous. Frequent scars were noted in the myocardium. In some the remnants of degenerate myocardial fibres, occurring in collapsed stroma in the presence of a lymphoid infiltrate, suggested an origin in previous foci of myocytolysis (Figures 16.13, 16.14). In others the appearance of large acellular scars were indicative of fibrous replacement of ischaemic infarcts (Figure 16.15). Extensive acute infarction was observed in heterotopic transplants which had severe chronic rejection of the coronary arteries with added fresh thrombus formation.

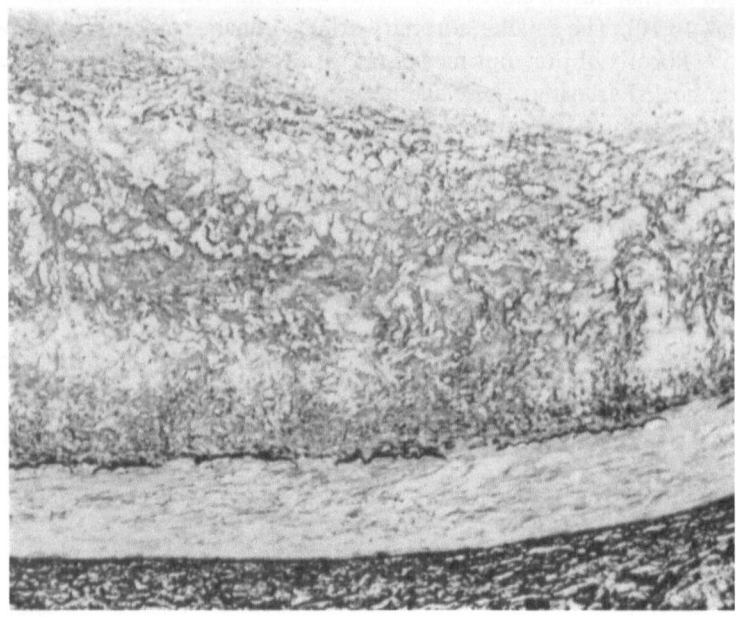

Figure 16.9 Chronic vascular rejection. A large coronary artery radicle shows intimal thickening with pronounced lipid deposition. There is loss of smooth muscle from the media and the internal elastic lamina is fragmented. Survival time 2.2 years. Donor age 30 years. H & E × 60

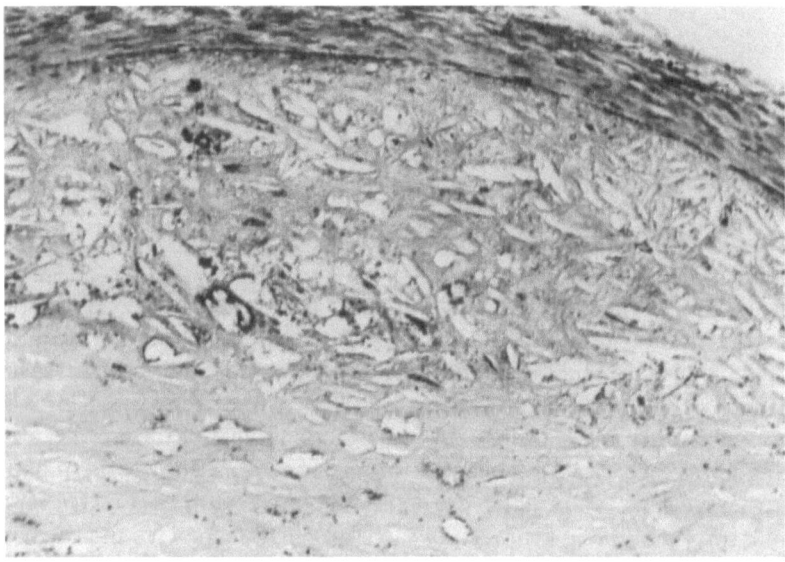

Figure 16.10 Chronic vascular rejection. Atherosclerotic-like appearance of advanced rejection. Patient survival 4.2 years. Donor age 35 years. H & E × 155

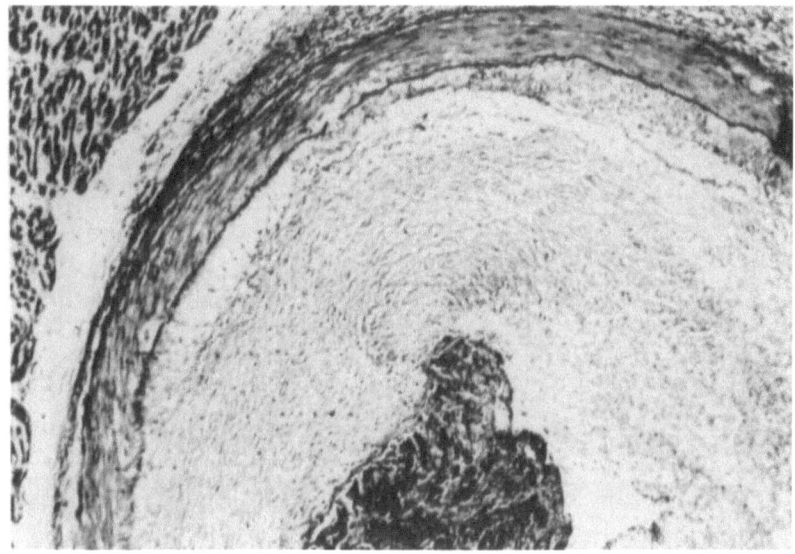

Figure 16.11 Advanced chronic vascular rejection. Pronounced lumen encroachment with superadded recent occlusive thrombus. Patient survival 2.7 years. Donor age 15 years. H & E × 60

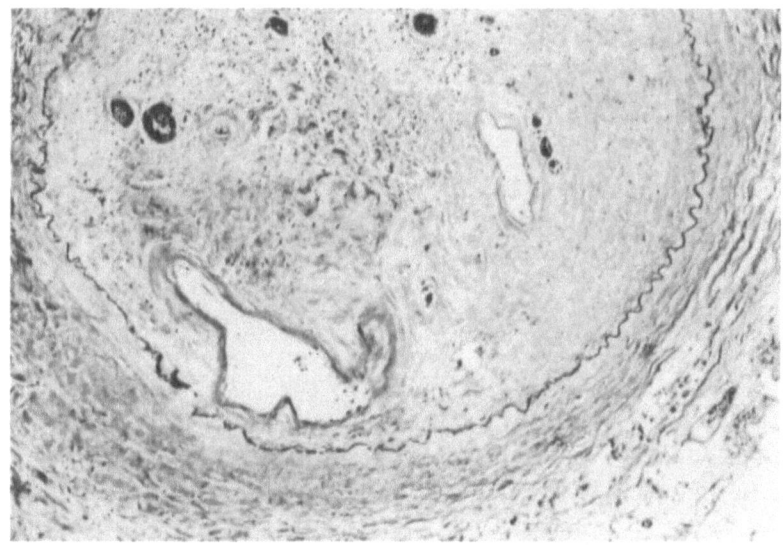

Figure 16.12 Advanced chronic vascular rejection. Lumen of altered artery obliterated by old organized and recanalized thrombus. Patient survival 2.2 years. Donor age 30 years. H & E × 60

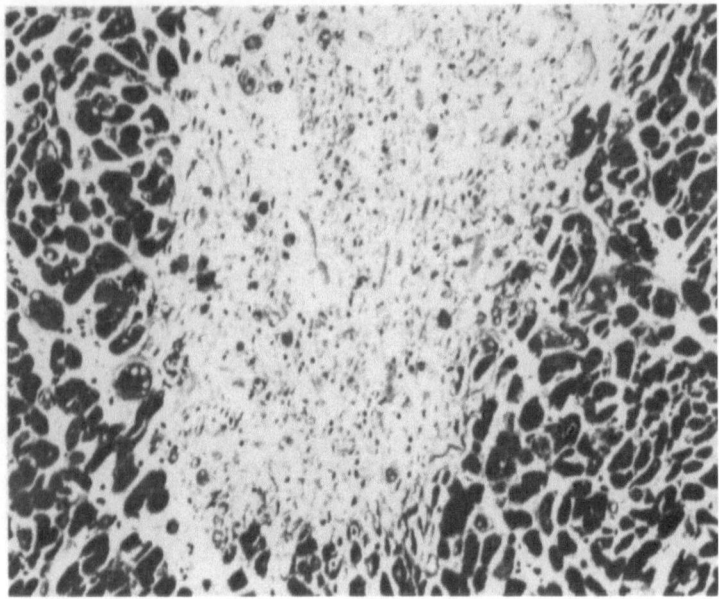

Figure 16.13 Scar showing remnants of degenerate myocardial fibres and persisting lymphoid infiltrate which suggest a previous focus of myocytolysis. Patient survival 2.7 years. Donor age 15 years. H & E × 150

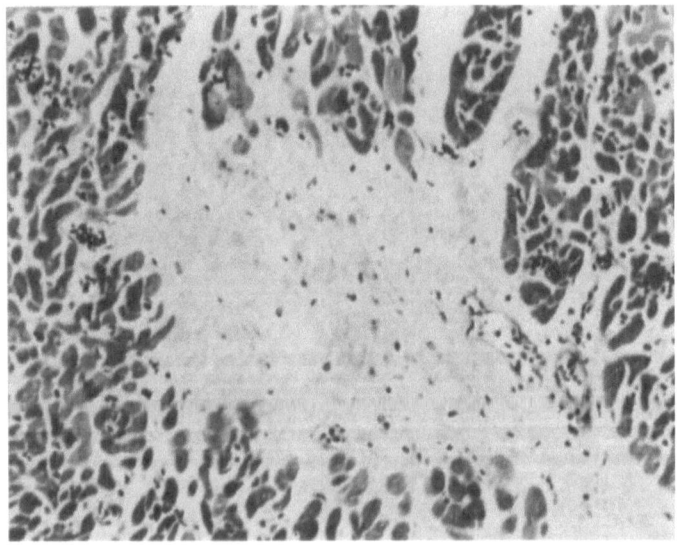

Figure 16.14 Small dense acellular scar probably due to previous myocytolysis with collapse fibrosis. No persistent cellular response. Patient survival 1.6 years. Donor age 25 years. H & E × 175

Other cardiac structures were surprisingly little affected. Some loss of medial smooth muscle architecture was observed in the aorta and pulmonary arteries with little accompanying cellular infiltrate. Only in the presence of severe rejection were the valves affected by a focal lymphoid infiltrate. Some valves thus affected showed incipient platelet deposition along contact lines.

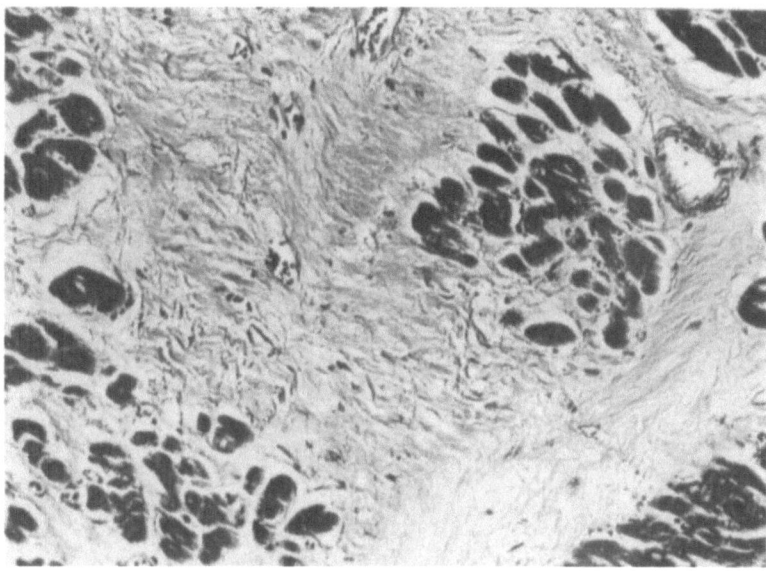

Figure 16.15   Large acellular fibrous scar of healed myocardial infarct. Patient survival 12.5 years. Donor age 33 years. H & E × 175

INCIDENCE OF CHRONIC REJECTION

The frequency with which chronic rejection changes occur in long-surviving cardiac transplants is illustrated in a study of 12 patients with 14 cardiac transplants, which had survival times longer than 1 year[19]. These consisted of three orthotopic and nine heterotopic transplants examined at autopsy, and two surgical specimens from patients who underwent heterotopic retransplantation. The grafts survived 1.1–12.5 years with a mean of 2.7 years. Microscopically, 28.5% of hearts showed evidence of persisting acute rejection and 92.9% showed signs of significant chronic rejection. In the response of chronic vascular rejection, severe myointimal proliferation was present in most cases (85.7%), while a cellular infiltrate of the vessel wall was generally absent (71.4%). The degree of lipid deposition bore no relation to the degree of rejection. Severe luminal encroachment of between 51% and 100% resulting from these changes were frequently present (78.6%), while superadded thrombosis of the affected arteries was present in 71.4% of cases. Myocardial scars were present in 92.9% of hearts, while extensive acute infarction was present in 42.9% of heterotopic transplants. In only one case, with a survival time of 1.7 years, was there an almost complete absence of rejection, and the arteries were virtually normal (Figure 16.16). Further, it is striking that in those 14 cases there was an almost complete absence of infective lesions, while a significant degree of rejection was responsible for the patient's death or graft failure in 78.6%.

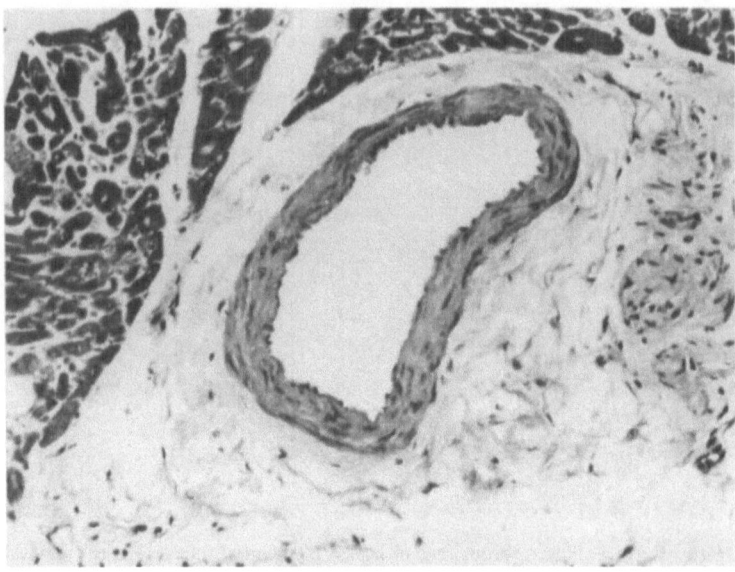

Figure 16.16 Normal looking coronary artery in the only transplant which showed no chronic rejection changes. Patient survival 1.7 years. Donor age 35 years. H & E × 175

COMMENT

The appearances of the vascular lesions described above are those of a reparative process following immune-mediated intimal and medial damage to the artery. These probably represent the cumulative effect of multiple acute rejection episodes, whether these be overt or clinically silent. In severity these lesions bear no constant relationship to the survival time of the graft or patient, and took from 1.1 to 12.5 years to evolve ultimately. The determining factor for graft survival, in the presence of chronic rejection, was myocardial ischaemia manifesting as extensive recent or old infarction. The fact that the donor hearts were generally procured from young people (mean age 28.3 years) further underlined the significance of this event. This is an ironical situation as ischaemic heart disease is a frequent indication for cardiac transplantation.

While the endomyocardial biopsy is an effective means of monitoring acute rejection episodes, it is less so in chronic rejection. Experience has shown that extensive myocardial fibrosis may exist which is not detected in the rather superficial endomyocardial biopsy, in which the subendocardial myofibres remain viable. Neither does the biopsy include medium-sized or large coronary arteries which are the vessels affected by the process of chronic rejection.

Another feature in our series of cases, with predominating numbers of heterotopic transplants, which deserves highlighting, is the advanced nature of the chronic rejection reaction in the donor hearts, and of the ischaemic lesions in the recipient hearts. These patients enjoy the benefit of two hearts, which jointly are able to maintain vital function in the presence of severely incapacitating lesions far beyond a stage possible in a single heart. Consequently, the donor hearts generally show more advanced chronic rejection than orthotopic transplants, and the recipient hearts reveal a degree of atherosclerosis with accompanying ischaemic manifestations more severe than would be possible in the natural state. Both lesions predispose to extensive mural thrombus formation (present in 50% of donor hearts with chronic rejection), which in turn results in increased potential for peripheral embolization.

References

1. Barnard, C. N. (1967). The operation. A human cardiac transplant: an interim report of a successful operation performed at Groote Schuur Hospital, Cape Town. *S. Afr. Med. J.*, **41**, 1271

2. Jamieson, S. W., Oyer, P. E., Reitz, B. A., Baumgartner, W. A., Bieber, C. P., Stinson, E. B. and Shumway, N. E. (1981). Cardiac transplantation at Stanford. *Heart Transplant.*, **1**, 86

3. Baumgartner, W. A., Reitz, B. A., Oyer, P. E., Stinson, E. B. and Shumway, N. E. (1979). Cardiac homotransplantation. *Curr. Probl. Surg.*, **16**, 3

4. Cooper, D. K. C., Lanza, R. P., Oliver, S., Forder, A. A., Rose, A. G., Uys, C. J., Novitzky, D. and Barnard, C. N. (1983). Infectious complications of heterotopic heart transplantation. *Thorax*, **38**, 822

5. Uys, C. J., Rose, A. G. and Barnard, C. N. (1979). The pathology of human heart transplantation. An assessment after 11 years' experience at Groote Schuur Hospital. *S. Afr. Med. J.*, **56**, 887

6. Uys, C. J. and Rose, A. G. (1983). Cardiac transplantation. Aspects of the pathology. In Sommers, S. C. and Rosen, P. P. (eds.) *Pathology Annual*. Vol. 17, pp. 147–178. (New York: Appleton-Century-Crofts)

7. Lower, R. R., Stofer, R. C. and Shumway, N. E. (1961). Homovital transplantation of the heart. *J. Thorac. Cardiovasc. Surg.*, **41**, 196

8. Lower, R. R., Dong, E. and Shumway, N. E. (1965). Long-term survival of cardiac homografts. *Surgery*, **58**, 110

9. Lower, R. R., Kontos, H. A., Kosek, J. C., Sewell, D. H. and Graham, W. H. (1968). Experiences in heart transplantation. *Am. J. Cardiol.*, **22**, 766

10. Thomson, J. G. (1969). Production of severe atheroma in a transplanted heart. *Lancet*, **2**, 1088

11. Bieber, C. P., Stinson, E. B., Shumway, N. E., Payne, R. and Kosek, J. (1970). Cardiac transplantation in man. VII. Cardiac allograft pathology. *Circulation*, **41**, 753

12. Milam, J. P., Shipkey, F. H., Lind, C. J., Nora, J. J., Leachman, D., Rochelle, D. G., Bloodwell, R. D., Hallman, G. L. and Cooley, D. A. (1970). Morphologic findings in human allografts. *Circulation*, **41**, 519
13. Kosek, J. C., Bieber, C. P. and Lower, R. R. (1974). Heart graft arteriosclerosis. *Transplant. Proc.*, **3**, 512
14. Sinclair, R. A., Andres, G. A. and Hsu, K. C. (1974). Immunofluorescent studies of the arterial lesion in rat cardiac allografts. *Arch. Pathol.*, **94**, 331
15. Laden, A. M. K. (1972). Experimental atherosclerosis in rat and rabbit cardiac allografts. *Arch. Pathol.*, **93**, 240
16. Laden, A. M. K., Sinclair, R. A. and Ruskiewicz, M. (1973). Vascular changes in experimental allografts. *Transplant. Proc.*, **5**, 737
17. Alonso, D. R., Storek, P. K. and Minick, C. R. (1977). Studies in the pathogenesis of atherosclerosis induced in rabbit cardiac allografts by the synergy of graft rejection in hypercholesterolaemia. *Am. J. Pathol.*, **87**, 415
18. Rose, A. G., Uys, C. J., Cooper, D. K. C. and Barnard, C. N. (1982). Donor heart morphology twelve and a half years after orthotopic transplantation. *Heart Transplant.*, **1**, 329
19. Uys, C. J. and Rose, A. G. (1984). The pathology of long-term cardiac transplants. *Arch. Pathol. Lab. Med.*, **108**, 112

17
The Management of Chronic Rejection: Retransplantation

INTRODUCTION

When allograft failure or severe dysfunction occurs following acute or chronic rejection of an orthotopically or heterotopically transplanted heart, replacement of the heart, or the addition of a further heart, can substantially extend patient survival. There are very few reported data on the indications for retransplantation, or on the complications and results of these procedures[1-4].

INDICATIONS FOR RETRANSPLANTATION

Retransplantation should be considered in any patient in whom the cardiac allograft undergoes failure or severe dysfunction from acute and/or chronic rejection. Retransplantation has also been performed on occasion for intractable arrhythmias of the donor heart, and for acute donor right ventricular failure due to an excessive pulmonary vascular resistance following orthotopic transplantation[1]. Refinements of criteria for selection of both recipients and donors have made these indications for retransplantation rare.

Intractable acute rejection of an orthotopic graft is clearly an urgent indication for retransplantation; when occurring in a heterotopic graft, the urgency is less acute, but nevertheless a second donor should be found as quickly as possible.

The decision to retransplant a patient undergoing chronic rejection (graft arteriosclerosis) and, in particular, the timing of the procedure, may be difficult, as the patient's general condition may remain good, despite evidence of increasing coronary arteriosclerotic changes. Both surgeon and patient may be reluctant to undertake retransplantation whilst the patient remains asymptomatic; delay, however, may result in sudden death from major myocardial infarction. Alternatively, the patient's general condition may have deteriorated from chronic infection or other complications of long-term immunosuppression, creating doubt as to his suitability for retransplantation.

SELECTION OF PATIENTS FOR RETRANSPLANTATION

All of the criteria for transplantation should be reassessed before retransplantation is performed[5], since significant changes may have occurred since the patient was assessed initially. In particular, the increased immunosuppression that is necessary during acute rejection episodes, or the prolonged immunosuppression in patients who have survived long enough to develop graft arteriosclerosis, may have resulted in foci of infection. These infections must be eradicated or suppressed before retransplantation is undertaken. The patient should also be carefully reassessed from a psychological standpoint to ascertain whether he or she can cope with the stresses and strains of a further transplant procedure. Particular attention should be paid to the patient's compliance with medical guidance and his or her adherence to therapy during the course of the first transplant. Retransplantation may be inadvisable if non-compliance had contributed towards failure of the initial allograft.

Meticulous testing of the recipient for the presence of lymphocytotoxic antibodies must be carried out, and antibodies against any new potential donor excluded. Antibody formation has occurred to a greater or lesser degree in many of the patients who have received cardiac allografts at our institution and, although it has not prohibited retransplantation in any one case, it would appear to have been a major factor in the lack of success of retransplantation in one patient (Table 17.1, case 2); this patient has been discussed fully elsewhere[6].

TIMING OF RETRANSPLANTATION IN INTRACTABLE ACUTE REJECTION

Intractable acute rejection occurring in a patient with an orthotopic transplant is, of course, a surgical emergency. A second donor must be found within a day or two, or death of the patient will occur. Heterotopic heart transplantation, however, may allow patient survival even when the donor heart has ceased functioning entirely[7]. This is particularly likely in patients who undergo acute rejection of the graft within the first few weeks or months following retransplantation, at which stage the patient's own heart is likely to remain sufficiently functional to allow patient survival until a second transplant procedure is performed.

At our own institution, excision of the irreversibly acutely rejected heart in such patients has been delayed, whenever possible, until the time of retransplantation. The patient has been maintained on methylprednisolone 20 mg/kg

Table 17.1 Clinical data and results of retransplantation in seven patients at Groote Schuur Hospital

	Date of first transplant	Age	Underlying primary cardiac pathology	Immuno-suppressive therapy	Survival of first heterotopic graft	Cause of failure/dysfunction	Period of support by recipient heart	Date and type of second transplant	Immuno-suppressive therapy	Survival of second graft	Cause of graft failure/patient death	Overall patient survival (months)
1.	7/7/78	44	IHD	A+M	13 months	Acute-on-chronic	5 months	27/1/80 Heterotopic	A+M	24 days	Pneumonia/septicaemia	20
2.	16/2/79	25	CM	A+M	35 days	Acute	31 months	4/10/81 Heterotopic	A+M	5 days	Acute rejection*	48
3.	11/11/79	34	IHD	A+M	14 months	Acute-on-chronic	4 months	26/5/81 Heterotopic	A+M	33 months	Alive and well	51
4.	24/10/80	45	IHD	A+M	35 days	Acute	1 day	29/11/80 Heterotopic	A+M	3 months	Pneumonia	4
5.	31/7/81	14	CM	A+M	24 months	Graft arterio-sclerosis	—	2/8/83 Orthotopic	CYA+M	6 months	Alive and well	30
6.	30/12/82	36	IHD	A+M	45 days?	Acute	21 days	15/2/83 Heterotopic	A+M	12 months	Alive and well	13
7.	5/1/80	14	CM	A+M	48 months	Graft arterio-sclerosis	—	29/12/83 Orthotopic	CYA+M	2 months	Alive and well	50

*Patient survived on own heart for a further 17 months before dying from his underlying cardiomyopathy
Dates are day/month/year
IHD = ischaemic heart disease; CM = cardiomyopathy; A + M = azathioprine + methylprednisolone; CYA + M = cyclosporin A + methylprednisolone

per day orally in an effort to prevent symptoms from the toxic effects of tissue necrosis. This has been successful in all cases except one, when the patient developed a high fever and was clearly unwell, necessitating immediate excision of the rejected donor organ (Table 17.1, case 2); the patient survived over 2 years after the donor heart was excised, at which time retransplantation was undertaken[6].

This particular patient also illustrates the difficulty of accurately assessing the long-term prognosis for a patient with cardiomyopathy. Following acute rejection of the second donor heart within 5 days, he again survived for a period of 17 months, before dying of his underlying disease. He therefore survived, albeit in New York Heart Association functional class 4, for more than 4 years from the time of his first heart transplant. A potential advantage of heterotopic heart transplantation is demonstrated here, since the patient would almost certainly have died from acute rejection if he had originally undergone orthotopic transplantation, particularly in a geographic area such as ours where potential donors are few.

DIAGNOSIS OF CHRONIC REJECTION

Clinical

Graft arteriosclerosis is, of course, not accompanied by angina, as the donor heart remains denervated. In our experience, a steady deterioration in the patient's exercise tolerance has proved to be the main symptom related to progressive chronic rejection, though some patients remain surprisingly symptom-free even in the presence of advanced disease. Other symptoms and signs related to a low cardiac output may also occur, and we have observed significant weight loss in some patients.

Electrocardiography and exercise stress testing

Myocardial ischaemia or infarction may be demonstrated on the electrocardiogram at rest, and, particularly, on exercise.

Echocardiography

A progressive reduction in ejection fraction on sequential echocardiograms may be observed. Abnormalities of regional wall motion may be associated with the development of ischaemic or infarcted areas.

Radionuclide angiography

In some patients a progressive reduction in left ventricular ejection fraction on multigated equilibrium blood pool scanning (MUGA) using technetium-99[m] labelled red cells in the absence of features of acute rejection (Chapter 11) has proved a clear indicator that myocardial function is deteriorating (Figure 17.1). (The left ventricular ejection fraction of the donor heart rises significantly after either orthotopic or heterotopic transplantation in both the human and the baboon, increasing some 10%. Studies in our laboratory have shown that this increase in ejection fraction follows total denervation of the heart. In baboons with autografted hearts, ejection fraction falls at a time when significant re-innervation is believed to have occurred (Novitzky *et al.*, unpublished data). In the patient with chronic rejection, therefore, the ejection fraction may remain relatively high when measured by this technique, despite a significant reduction in exercise tolerance.)

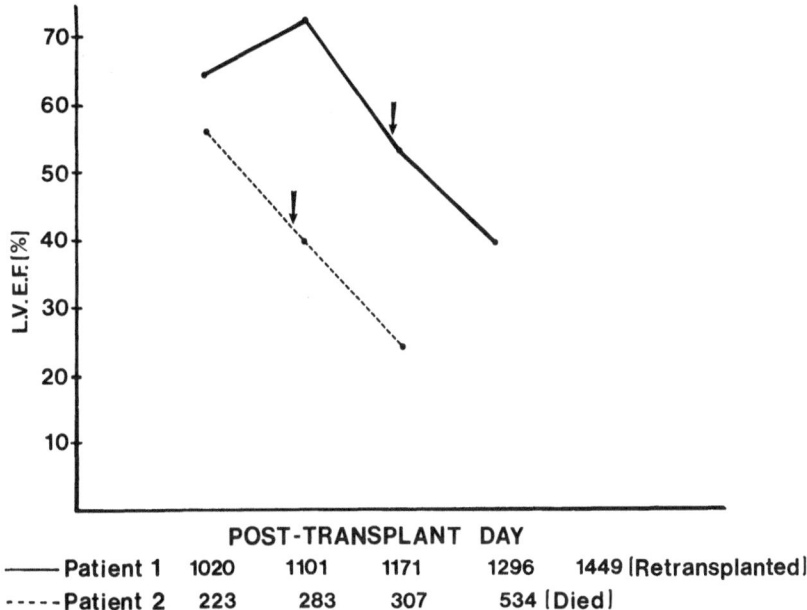

Figure 17.1 Sequential left ventricular ejection fractions (L.V.E.F. (%)) estimated by multigated equilibrium blood pool scanning using technetium-99^{m} labelled red cells in two patients (1 and 2) undergoing chronic rejection of heterotopic heart transplants. (The normal left ventricular ejection fraction of the transplanted heart using this technique is 70–80%.) (↓ marks the onset of symptoms of cardiac failure)

Thallium scanning

Further non-invasive investigation in the form of radionuclide scanning of the myocardium using thallium-201 may prove helpful in assessing the extent of myocardial ischaemia and infarction, and in estimating prognosis. Sequential scans may indicate the rate of deterioration.

Coronary arteriography and left ventriculography

These invasive procedures may carry a risk of cardiac arrest in patients with advanced graft arteriosclerosis, but will confirm the state of left ventricular function and the degree of occlusion of the coronary arterial tree (Figure 17.2). Coronary arteriography shows features indistinguishable from those seen in non-transplanted patients with coronary atheroma, though graft arteriosclerosis tends to be widespread and there is frequently a conspicuous absence of small peripheral vessels. Occasionally, there is an absence of large vessel disease; in such cases, coronary arteriography will not reflect the true state of the disease process, though ventricular wall motion and ejection fraction on ventriculography may be grossly abnormal.

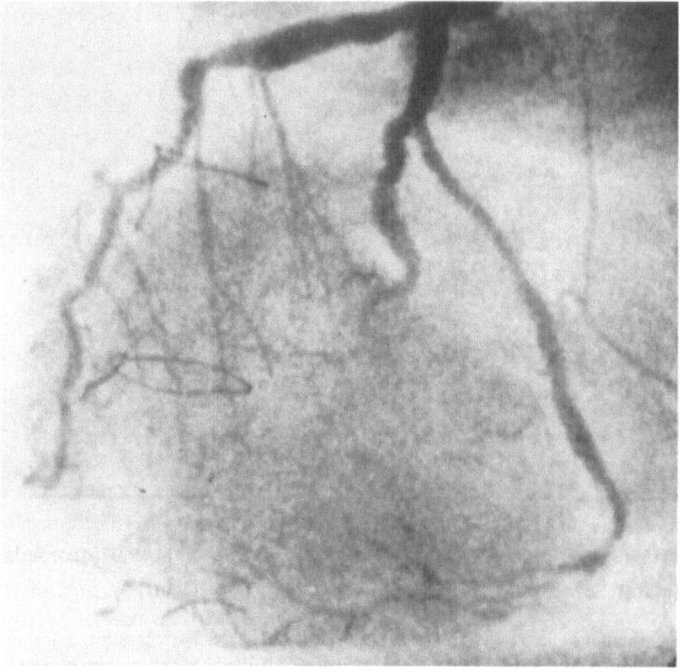

Figure 17.2 Coronary arteriogram of the left coronary artery in a patient 11 years after orthotopic heart transplantation. (The right coronary artery was totally occluded at its origin.) A 60% stenosis of the left anterior descending coronary artery and diffuse disease of the circumflex arteries can be noted. Left ventriculography demonstrated infero-apical dyskinesia

Endomyocardial biopsy

Chronic rejection can rarely be diagnosed with accuracy from endomyocardial biopsy. The myocardium may show areas of fibrosis, though these may have resulted from previous acute rejection episodes. Only if the biopsy includes an artery of appreciable size, which is relatively unusual, and that artery seen to be significantly affected by graft arteriosclerosis, can the diagnosis be confirmed by this technique. Even then, the extent of the process and the involvement of the major arteries remains uncertain.

MANAGEMENT OF CHRONIC REJECTION

In 1970 the Stanford group took several measures to counteract the series of events considered responsible for accelerated graft arteriosclerosis. A regimen was introduced involving anticoagulation with warfarin sodium, the administration of an antiplatelet agent (dipyridamole), limitation of the dietary intake of lipids, and of calories to maintain a normal body weight, and encouragement to follow a programme of daily exercise. These measures resulted in a significant delay in the incidence of graft arteriosclerosis[8]. The incidence of this complication, documented by yearly coronary arteriographic examinations, was reduced from 58% to 5% at 1 year, 88% to 17% at 2 years, and 100% to 20% at 3 years[1]. By 5 years, however, graft arteriosclerosis was seen in 42% of patients.

Most groups involved in the care of patients with heart transplants continue to prescribe a diet low in lipids (irrespective of the underlying primary cardiac pathology), attempt by strict calorie control to prevent the patient from becoming overweight, prohibit smoking, which frequently proves exceedingly difficult, continue antiplatelet agents indefinitely, and encourage regular moderate exercise, in the hope that these measures will reduce the progress of the condition. Long-term anticoagulation is generally now not thought to be helpful; the frequency of this complication in patients with heterotopic heart transplants, who receive long-term anticoagulation, is no lower than in those with orthotopic transplants, who generally do not. A cholesterol-reducing agent, such as cholestyramine, is probably indicated in patients with persistent hypercholesterolaemia, but the value of such medication in preventing graft arteriosclerosis remains uncertain and would appear unlikely.

It is too early to know whether immunosuppression with cyclosporin A will reduce the high incidence or rate of progession of graft arteriosclerosis in patients with cardiac transplants.

In view of the generalized nature of the disease process and the involvement of small peripheral arteries, myocardial revascularization procedures such as aorto-coronary artery bypass grafting using, for example, saphenous vein, are not indicated in these patients. Supportive medical measures in the form of anti-failure therapy (digoxin, diuretics, etc.) may improve the patient symptomatically for a while, but retransplantation provides the only potentially curative answer.

THE TIMING OF RETRANSPLANTATION IN ADVANCED CHRONIC REJECTION

As with acute rejection, complete failure of an orthotopic allograft from chronic rejection results in the death of the patient; it is usually clear, however, that chronic rejection is occurring, and time is available to plan the retransplant procedure.

Our experience with patients with heterotopic allografts has been that recipient heart function steadily deteriorates during the months following transplantation, irrespective of the underlying cardiac pathology. By the time graft arteriosclerosis has occurred, recipient heart function has frequently ceased altogether or has become inadequate to sustain life. As with orthotopic transplants, complete graft failure, therefore, is frequently followed by the death of the patient.

The timing of retransplantation may prove difficult, therefore, in patients with either heterotopic or orthotopic grafts in whom chronic rejection is occurring. The decision to retransplant must not be delayed until graft function becomes totally inadequate, yet, on the other hand, retransplantation should not be undertaken until absolutely essential. The exact timing is influenced by many factors, notably the ease or difficulty with which a suitable donor will be obtained; for example, if the patient has a high level of circulating lymphocytotoxic antibodies, some delay may occur in obtaining a suitable donor, and the search should begin earlier rather than later.

The policy of the Stanford group has been to offer retransplantation to patients with evidence on coronary arteriography of life-threatening occlusive lesions in the major coronary arteries, irrespective of the patients' exercise tolerance[2]. This policy evolved following the sudden death of three long-term survivors with such lesions. At our own centre, we have not seen sudden death in an otherwise asymptomatic patient, and have therefore been possibly rather less aggressive in offering retransplantation. We have generally waited until exercise tolerance has significantly deteriorated, and coronary arteriography and thallium scanning have confirmed advanced disease.

The rate of development and progression of graft arteriosclerosis is extremely variable. We have seen advanced disease as early as 3 months, yet no disease as late as 13 years after transplantation. In our experience, the development of even moderately advanced disease may be compatible with an acceptable quality of life for several further months or even years. In one of our patients, a 50% stenosis of the right coronary artery was demonstrated 6 years before death; this progressed to complete occlusion of this vessel at its origin and widespread disease of the left coronary system over the next 4 years (Figure 17.2). Some 2 years later the patient finally succumbed to the disease, retransplantation having been contraindicated on other grounds[9, 10].

RETRANSPLANTATION—OPERATIVE CONSIDERATIONS

In patients with orthotopic allografts

The operation of retransplantation in a patient with an existing orthotopic allograft presents the same technical problems and risks of reoperation as in any patient who has previously undergone cardiac surgery. Adhesions have invariably developed between pericardium and heart, frequently making the initial dissection time-consuming. As myocardial function in these patients is poor, particular care must be taken not to handle or disturb the heart more than is absolutely essential before pump oxygenator support has been initiated; for this reason, occasionally it may be necessary to resort to use of the femoral artery to commence cardiopulmonary bypass.

In patients with heterotopic allografts

After the operation of heterotopic transplantation, the pericardium cannot be closed. Unless a sheet of prosthetic material has been inserted between heart and anterior chest wall, adhesions are likely to develop between the right ventricle of the recipient's own heart and the posterior aspect of the sternum; the donor heart, lying in the right chest, adheres to the right lung and anterior chest wall. Retransplantation may, therefore, be a technically difficult procedure. Great care is required in opening the sternum and in dissecting out the structures in the chest. In one of our patients (Table 17.1, case 5), the recipient right ventricle was inadvertently opened during sternotomy, necessitating emergency femoro–femoral cardiopulmonary bypass to maintain the circulation whilst the situation was controlled[11].

If the first donor heart is to be removed, this is carried out once cardiopulmonary bypass has been initiated. Air leaks may result following dissection in the region of the right lung, though in no case have these caused significant postoperative problems in the patients under our care. The heart is removed, and the second donor heart inserted using the standard surgical technique of heterotopic heart transplantation.

Orthotopic transplantation in patients with a previous heterotopic allograft

Two patients in our series now survive with two donor hearts within their chests (Table 17.1, cases 5 and 7), the first (heterotopic) donor heart having been left *in situ*, and the patient's own heart having been replaced[11]. One of the advantages of heterotopic transplantation is that the recipient's own heart may assist the circulation during periods of severe acute rejection of the donor heart; such episodes have been well documented[7]. By the same principle, the first donor heart, though severely affected by graft arteriosclerosis, may lend support to the second donor organ should it be compromised by a severe acute rejection episode. For this reason, we felt it advisable to leave the first donor heart *in situ* in both of these cases.

In addition, in one of these two patients (Table 17.1, case 5) the donor heart that was available was taken from a 14-year-old girl weighing only 22 kg. Since the recipient weighed 56 kg it was felt that the small size of the donor heart might be insufficient to support the entire circulation alone during the initial few weeks or months, and the first donor heart might lend some support throughout this period, during which time the second donor heart would gradually hypertrophy. Heterotopic heart transplantation has occasionally been performed for a similar reason at other centres[12].

In such cases where the first donor heart is to be left *in situ* and the patient's own heart to be replaced, less dissection is required. Following excision of the recipient's heart, the standard operation of orthotopic transplantation is performed (Figure 17.3)[11].

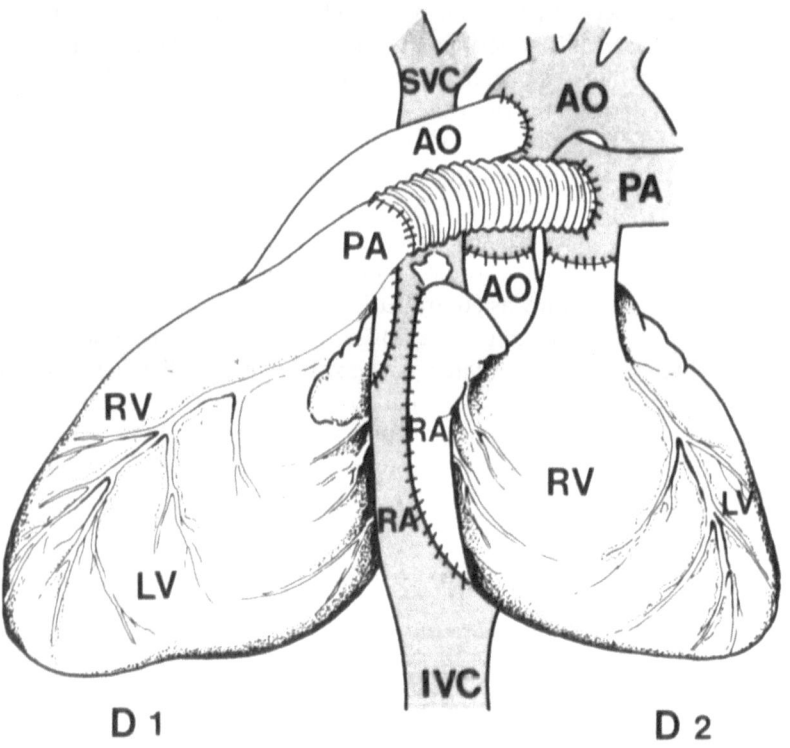

Figure 17.3 The completed operation of orthotopic geart transplantation in a patient with a previous heterotopic transplant. The shaded structures are the patient's original tissues. D 1 = first (heterotopic) donor heart; D 2 = second (orthotopic) donor heart, SVC = superior vena cava; IVC = inferior vena cava; RA = right atrium; RV = right ventricle; PA = pulmonary artery; LV = left ventricle; AO = aorta

In both of these cases, excision of the first donor heart would have been technically difficult in view of tight adhesions between this heart and the surrounding tissues, notably the lung. By leaving this heart *in situ* the operating time was reduced and potential postoperative complications avoided.

The first donor heart, affected as it is by severe graft arteriosclerosis, will eventually cease to function altogether. The retention of a chronically rejected, non-functioning heart has not caused problems in other patients, even when such hearts have remained *in situ* for several months before the death of the patient has occurred from his underlying recipient heart failure whilst awaiting retransplantation.

With conventional immunosuppression using azathioprine and methylprednisolone, episodes of life-threatening, severe acute rejection were relatively common, and the support given by the recipient heart at such times valuable. The diminished incidence of severe acute rejection episodes associated with cyclosporin A therapy have reduced this advantage, and, in future cases, the retention of a first heterotopic donor heart may not prove necessary, unless the pulmonary vascular resistance remains high. In such cases, both hearts would then be excised, and the second donor heart transplanted orthotopically.

Though the operative procedure of retransplantation is rather more difficult due to the presence of adhesions, we have experienced few significant technical complications. Apart from the case mentioned above in which the recipient right ventricle was inadvertently opened during sternotomy, one other patient developed adult respiratory distress syndrome (shock lung) in the early postoperative period, possibly resulting from a difficulty in venting the recipient left ventricle during operation (Table 17.1, case 1).

Excision of an acutely rejected heterotopic allograft in a patient with a functioning recipient heart

In patients with an irreversibly acutely rejected heterotopic allograft (and a functioning recipient heart), when the donor heart requires excision as a semi-emergency following the development of toxic symptoms from tissue necrosis, and when retransplantation cannot yet be performed due to the absence of a suitable donor or other contraindication, excision has been achieved without the need for cardiopulmonary bypass. The operation is performed through a median sternotomy. Vascular clamps are applied across the four sites of anastomosis (i.e. aorta, pulmonary artery, right atrium and left atrium), the donor tissue divided and excised, and the residual cuffs of tissue oversewn. There have been no complications associated with leaving cuffs of donor aorta or atria in the chest. If a second heterotopic heart transplant is anticipated, the vacated cavity in the right chest has been maintained by filling it with a suitable foreign body, such as a silastic breast prosthesis. If this is not done, the space will fill with blood and other fluid and dense adhesions will form, making subsequent heterotopic transplantation exceedingly difficult, if not impossible.

POSTOPERATIVE CARE AND IMMUNOSUPPRESSION

The immediate postoperative care of patients who have undergone retransplantation does not differ significantly from that following the initial procedure. Apart from the patient with adult respiratory distress syndrome, the seven patients in our own series recovered from the retransplant operation as quickly and as uneventfully as from the first operation.

If retransplantation is performed during or immediately following an irreversible acute rejection episode, care must be taken not to over-immunosuppress the patient, as he will almost certainly already have received a considerable amount of immunosuppressive therapy; preoperative 'loading' doses of the various drugs are probably unnecessary.

RESULTS OF RETRANSPLANTATION

Between January 1980 and January 1984 seven patients, all with heterotopic cardiac grafts, underwent second cardiac transplant procedures at our institution[4]. The retransplant operation was performed between 47 days and 4 years after the primary operation. Details of these patients are shown in Table 17.1. The operation was for acute rejection in two cases, acute-on-chronic rejection in two, and graft arteriosclerosis in three. In five patients the first heterotopic donor heart was excised and replaced. In two, the first heterotopic donor heart was left in situ and the patient's own heart (now non-functioning) was excised and replaced by the second donor heart. These two patients, therefore, underwent orthotopic transplantation and now have two functioning donor hearts. Both of these operations were performed in patients with chronic rejection.

There was no operative mortality in our small series. One patient developed adult respiratory distress syndrome (case 1) and required tracheostomy on the 5th postoperative day; he developed a pneumonia and died of septicaemia on the 24th post-transplant day. A second patient (case 4) also died from infection, developing pneumonia 3 months after transplantation, having otherwise made good progress. A third patient (case 2), discussed earlier, rejected the second graft within 5 days and eventually died of his underlying disease[6].

The four other patients remain alive and well 2, 7, 13 and 33 months after retransplantation.

At Stanford University Medical Center, cardiac retransplantation of orthotopic allografts was performed on more than 20 occasions between 1968 and 1983[3]. In a review of the first seven of these patients[1], three recipients died 12,

15 and 91 days after retransplantation from infectious complications (systemic candidiasis, multiple infections, and aspergillus mediastinitis respectively). A fourth patient died after 21 days from a cerebrovascular accident, and a fifth after 18 months from arrhythmia. At the time of the review, two patients were alive 22 and 44 months after retransplantation.

The results of our experience would suggest that cardiac retransplantation can be undertaken with little extra operative risk, and can substantially prolong the life of patients when primary allograft failure occurs following acute or chronic rejection. It is likely that the procedure will be undertaken increasingly during the next few years as transplant patients who had been immunosuppressed with conventional therapy present with chronic rejection. It remains to be seen whether cyclosporin A or a derivative of this drug will be effective in preventing this complication; if this proves not to be the case, retransplantation may become a common procedure if the supply of donor organs proves sufficient.

References

1. Copeland, J. G., Griepp, R. B., Bieber, C. P., Billingham, M., Schroeder, J. S., Hunt, S., Mason, J., Stinson, E. B. and Shumway, N. E. (1977). Successful retransplantation of the human heart. *J. Thorac. Cardiovasc. Surg.*, **73**, 242
2. Baumgartner, W. A., Reitz, B. A., Oyer, P. E., Stinson, E. B. and Shumway, N. E. (1979). Cardiac homotransplantation. *Curr. Probl. Surg.*, **16**, 1
3. Copeland, J. G. and Stinson, E. B. (1979). Human heart transplantation. *Curr. Probl. Cardiol.*, **4**, 4
4. Novitzky, D., Cooper, D. K. C., Lanza, R. P. and Barnard, C. N. (1984). Further cardiac transplant procedures in patients with heterotopic heart transplants. *Am. Thorac. Surg.* (In press)
5. Cooper, D. K. C., Charles, R. P., Beck, W. and Barnard, C. N. (1982). The assessment and selection of patients for heterotopic heart transplantation. *S. Afr. Med. J.*, **61**, 575
6. Lanza, R. P., Campbell, E., Cooper, D. K. C., Du Toit, E. and Barnard, C. N. (1983). The problem of the presensitized heart transplant recipient. *Heart Transplant.*, **2**, 151
7. Novitzky, D., Cooper, D. K. C., Rose, A. G. and Barnard, C. N. (1984). The value of recipient heart assistance during severe acute rejection following heterotopic cardiac transplantation. *J. Cardiovasc. Surg.* (In press)
8. Griepp, R. B., Stinson, E. B., Bieber, C. P., Reitz, B. A., Copeland, J. G., Oyer, P. E. and Shumway, N. E. (1977). Control of graft arteriosclerosis in human heart transplant recipients. *Surgery*, **81**, 262
9. Cooper, D. K. C., Charles, R. P., Fraser, R. C., Beck, W. and Barnard, C. N. (1980). Long-term survival after orthotopic and heterotopic cardiac transplantation. *Br. Med. J.*, **281**, 1093
10. Rose, A. G., Uys, C. J., Cooper, D. K. C. and Barnard, C. N. (1982). Donor heart morphology 12½ years after orthotopic transplantation. *Heart Transplant.*, **1**, 329
11. Novitzky, D., Cooper, D. K. C. and Barnard, C. N. (1984). Orthotopic heart transplantation in a patient with a heart heterotopic transplant. *Heart Transplant.*, **3**, 257
12. Melvin, K. R., Pollick, C., Hunt, S. A., McDougall, R., Goris, M. L., Oyer, P. E., Popp, R. L. and Stinson, E. B. (1982). Cardiovascular physiology in a case of heterotopic cardiac transplantation. *Am. J. Cardiol.*, **49**, 1301

18
Other Complications of Transplantation and Immunosuppression

INTRODUCTION

The major problem associated with cardiac transplantation is undoubtedly rejection, both acute and chronic. The prevention or treatment of rejection by immunosuppressive drugs leads to complications, notably infection and, to a lesser extent, malignant tumour formation. There are many other potential complications, however, that are related to the transplantation operation or, particularly, to the immunocompromised status of the patient. These complications will be outlined and discussed below in the light of our own experience.

COMPLICATIONS OF THE OPERATION OF CARDIAC TRANSPLANTATION

Any of the complications of open heart surgery can, of course, occur following orthotopic or heterotopic transplantation. Technical complications are fortunately rare, and none of our orthotopic or heterotopic patients has required reoperation for such problems.

Haemorrhage

Haemorrhage is a potential early complication that may occur following the operation of either orthotopic or heterotopic transplantation. In both procedures there are long suture lines involving both low pressure venous systems and high pressure arterial systems. With care, however, postoperative bleeding should not be a major problem, though it would appear to be more difficult to prevent following transplantation of the heart and both lungs (Chapter 21).

Technical complications

In the preparation of the donor heart for both orthotopic and heterotopic transplantation, care must be taken to avoid the region of the sinoatrial node. In heterotopic heart transplantation, the recipient sinoatrial node must also be avoided.

Inadequate surgical technique may lead to narrowing at anastomotic suture lines, particularly following the rather more difficult operation of heterotopic heart transplantation. In three patients in our series, difficulty was met in manipulating the endomyocardial biopsy catheter and bioptome into the donor right atrium through the superior vena cava–right atrial anastomosis, which was narrowed as a result of inadequate operative surgical technique or sub-sequent contraction from fibrosis. The avoidance of this problem is discussed in Chapter 8. In two of these patients the biopsy forceps could be passed through this anastomosis without difficulty when access to the venous system was by the femoral vein, but not when access was via the jugular vein.

Neither route could be used successfully in the third patient; left ventricular endomyocardial biopsy had to be performed by the transarterial route. The patient died after 2 years from an unrelated problem; postmortem exam-ination confirmed contraction of the right atrial anastomosis to 2 mm in diameter. This had resulted in haemodynamic derangement of the normal heterotopic heart transplant circulatory system. Blood returning from the systemic circulation was directed almost entirely through the recipient right heart; after passage through the lungs, the blood passed predominantly through the more compliant donor left heart. Though the circulation was unusual, the patient remained asymptomatic until she died from a cerebral embolus after failing to take her anticoagulants regularly.

Wound infection

Wound infection is fortunately relatively rare after major cardiac surgery, including transplantation, but can, of course, be potentially disastrous in the immunosuppressed patient.

Two patients in our series have developed severe postoperative sternal wound infections that were extremely difficult to eradicate. The original infecting organism in one was *Staphylococcus aureus*, though seven further organisms were subsequently grown from discharging sinuses in this region. Over the course of a 2-year period the patient unsuccessfully underwent nine operative procedures to try to eradicate the sternal and retrosternal infection. Chronic discharging sinuses remained for approximately 36 months but then spontaneously healed. The patient died from chronic rejection in his fifth postoperative year. In the second patient the original infecting organism remains uncertain, though *Enterobacter sp.* and *Staphylococcus epidermidis* were the first organisms cultured from the pus exuding from the wound. Eight further organisms, including *Aspergillus sp.* and *Clostridium perfringens* were subsequently cultured. The patient, who underwent three surgical drainage procedures before the infection was eradicated permanently, remains alive and well 8 years later.

Systemic and pulmonary emboli

One of our original orthotopically transplanted patients experienced multiple pulmonary emboli from deep vein thrombosis that resulted in his death 61 days after transplantation. The orthotopic patients, however, were not routinely anticoagulated as are the heterotopic patients. Pulmonary emboli have also been reported arising from a residual recipient right atrial appendage following orthotopic transplantation[1]; this appendage should be excised at operation.

During the first heterotopic heart transplant operation performed at Groote Schuur Hospital, particles of atheromatous tissue that arose from a severely diseased aorta embolized mainly to the brain[2]; similar complications have been documented following other surgical manipulations[3,4]. Though the patient recovered from the cardiac operation, he remained bedridden, which may have been a contributing factor to the development of bilateral femoral vein thrombosis, which in turn resulted in recurring pulmonary embolism and infarction. He died after 111 days; infarcts of different ages were found in both lungs at necropsy.

The need to anticoagulate all patients with heterotopic heart transplants has been discussed in Chapter 9, and this disadvantage of the operation considered in Chapter 20. Relatively few of our patients, however, have been seriously troubled by emboli. Non-compliance of the patient with regard to meticulous attention to anticoagulant therapy has been a major contributing factor in all cases.

Three heterotopic patients suffered from one or more major systemic emboli (arising in the poorly contracting recipient left ventricle) when anticoagulation was poorly controlled, one of which proved fatal. A further patient experienced multiple small emboli arising from a thrombosed aortic prosthetic valve in the recipient heart, which was also affected by bacterial endocarditis (Chapter 20). The patient recovered fully following excision of the prosthesis. The presence of a prosthetic valve is now considered an absolute contraindication to heterotopic heart transplantation.

COMPLICATIONS OF ENDOMYOCARDIAL BIOPSY

Endomyocardial biopsy is associated with an approximate 4% incidence of complication at our institution[5], though these have generally been minor complications such as pneumothorax and transient recurrent laryngeal nerve or brachial plexus paresis induced by local anaesthesia.

A rare but potentially serious complication is perforation of the right ventricular myocardium at the time of taking the biopsy. This has occurred on at least one occasion at our institution. In this particular case, chest radiography of the hypotensive patient revealed a right haemothorax, which was drained by intercostal tube insertion; the patient recovered uneventfully. On one other occasion the histopathologist reported seeing normal lung tissue in the biopsy specimen, but this patient remained asymptomatic.

Pulmonary embolism (or systemic embolism in the case of left ventricular biopsy) from dislodgement of mural thrombus, which may result from decreased myocardial contractions due to rejection, is a potential hazard of endomyocardial biopsy following orthotopic or heterotopic transplantation. Ventricular ectopic activity induced by the catheter or bioptome may occur but has not been a problem in our experience.

The risk of introducing infection at the time of biopsy remains a potential hazard. Our policy of antibiotic prophylaxis for 24 hours at the time of biopsy, however, would appear to have averted this complication in our own series.

COMPLICATIONS FROM IMMUNOSUPPRESSIVE DRUG THERAPY

The major potential complications of the various drugs presently used to immunosuppress patients with cardiac allografts are listed in Table 18.1. Drug-related complications form the majority of complications occurring after heart transplantation, though hopefully the reduced dosages of steroid now possible with the introduction of cyclosporin will reduce this incidence.

Corticosteroids

Impotence

There are few data available on the incidence of impotence in other cardiac transplant groups. In renal transplant series, however, impotence has been reported in 22–43% of male recipients[6].

Secondary impotence was a complaint in five of our heterotopic male patients (an overall incidence of 11%, and an incidence of 20% of those who lived longer than 1 year). Whether this is related solely to steroid therapy or influenced by psychological factors, such as living under the long-term stress of the fear of rejection and infection, etc., is uncertain. Most patients are reluctant to talk about this complication, and so it is possible that the incidence is even higher than we report. All the patients were men who had previously had children, and all psychologically desired to have sexual relations with their wives. One suffered from the Leriche syndrome.

Table 18.1 Major potential complications from immunosuppressive drug therapy

Corticosteroids
  Fluid and electrolyte disturbances
  Musculoskeletal disorders (including osteoporosis, vertebral compression fractures, pathological bone fractures, aseptic necrosis, muscle weakness, steroid myopathy, and loss of muscle mass)
  Gastrointestinal disorders (including peptic ulcers, pancreatitis, abdominal distension, and ulcerative oesophagitis)
  Dermatological disorders
  Neurological disorders (including psychiatric complications and convulsions)
  Endocrine disorders (including development of Cushingoid state, suppression of growth in children, menstrual irregularities, decreased carbohydrate tolerance, and manifestations of latent diabetes mellitus, impotence)
  Ophthalmic disorders (including cataracts, increased intraocular pressure, glaucoma, and exophthalmos)
  Metabolic disorders (including negative nitrogen balance)

Azathioprine
  Haematopoietic disorders (including leukopenia, thrombocytopenia, and chronic anaemia)
  Gastrointestinal disorders (including nausea and vomiting, and hepatitis with biliary stasis)
  Others (including skin rashes, alopecia, fever, arthralgias, diarrhoea, steatorrhoea, and negative nitrogen balance)

Cyclophosphamide
  Haematopoietic disorders (including leukopenia, thrombocytopenia, and anaemia)
  Gastrointestinal disorders (including anorexia, nausea and vomiting)
  Genito-urinary disorders (including sterile haemorrhagic cystitis)
  Gonadal suppression
  Pulmonary disorders (including interstitial pulmonary fibrosis)

Antithymocyte globulin
  Anaphylactic shock
  Others (including musculoskeletal pains, rash, fever, chills, and bronchospasm)

Cyclosporin
  Nephrotoxicity
  Lymphoma (greater incidence than with other immunosuppressive agents)
  Others (including hypertrichosis, gingival hyperplasia, tremor, hyperaesthesia, hypertension, hepatic dysfunction, and gastrointestinal intolerance)

Four of the patients were treated with testosterone. One experienced severe nausea, vomiting, and malaise early in the treatment and did not receive further therapy. Within 1 month the other three patients reported satisfactory sexual relations with their wives. It remains uncertain, however, whether this was a direct physiological result of the drug therapy or a placebo effect.

Diabetes mellitus

True steroid diabetes is usually mild and may reflect exacerbation of a pre-diabetic state or the discovery of a previously latent or unrecognized diabetes.

Frequently it can be controlled by diet and a reduction in the daily steroid dosage alone. The need for insulin is rare, though oral hypoglycaemic agents are occasionally necessary.

At our own centre, diabetes mellitus has occurred as a transient phenomenon, lasting a few days or weeks at most, in four patients (6%), and has always occurred early in the post-transplant period in patients receiving large doses of methylprednisolone for acute rejection. We have not seen it, to date, in patients receiving cyclosporin and low-dose methylprednisolone therapy.

A similar incidence of steroid diabetes has been reported from other cardiac transplant centres using conventional immunosuppression. The University of Arizona and the Medical College of Virginia have reported incidences of 10% and 8% respectively[7,8]. In renal transplant patients there is a similar incidence[9].

Because of the well-known effect of steroids on gluconeogenesis and on insulin activity we have been careful in our selection of potential recipients to exclude those with insulin-requiring diabetes mellitus. It may prove possible to offer such patients heart transplantation using cyclosporin and low-dose methylprednisolone, though the risk of infection in such patients will probably remain higher than in those with no tendency towards diabetes.

Osteoporosis and aseptic necrosis of bone

There are two mechanisms by which corticosteroids may produce aseptic necrosis of bone. There is considerable evidence from both experimental animals and man that steroids induce hyperlipidaemia, fatty infiltration of the liver, and systemic fat embolization that leads to ischaemic necrosis of bone[10,11]. An alternative hypothesis is that bone resorption results from persistent hyperparathyroidism induced by steroids, leading to trabecular collapse and subsequent bone necrosis[12,13].

In our own series these complications of steroids have taken the form of vertebral compression in two patients and aseptic necrosis of the head of the humerus in one, though both patients with vertebral collapse were asymptomatic.

Aseptic osteonecrosis is a relatively common problem at many renal and cardiac transplantation centres, with an incidence varying from 4 to 41%[12-16]. The hip is the joint most commonly involved, followed by the knee, shoulder, and elbow. Both surgical and non-surgical means of treatment can be used, usually depending on the severity of the symptoms. Limitation of weight-bearing for several months by the joint concerned often suffices. Obviously a reduction in steroid dosage to the lowest possible levels reduces the risk of extension of the damage. Hip joint replacement, however, may be necessary, though when knee joints are affected, joint replacement is less successful. At Stanford, approximately 2% of cardiac transplant patients have developed aseptic necrosis of the head of the femur and have required hip replacement[14,17].

High levels or prolonged use of steroids can also lead to vertebral collapse or facilitate bone injury. At the Medical College of Virginia 4% of cardiac transplant patients developed vertebral collapse[8], and at La Pitié Hospital in Paris 9% suffered from complications of osteoporosis[18].

Growth retardation and delayed onset of puberty

Both of these complications have occurred in our two youngest recipients, boys 14 years old at the time of transplantation, despite efforts to reduce the steroid dosage to the minimum. Neither boy showed signs of pubertal changes during the first 2 post-transplant years. This caused one of the boys embarrassment at school—the other received private tuition at home—and he was therefore given a course of testosterone. Such therapy, however, can minimize further growth by causing permanent closure of the epiphyses. Its timing is therefore important, and expert guidance from an endocrinologist is clearly necessary.

Because of the complication of growth impairment, many renal, liver and cardiac transplantation units are reluctant to accept children as potential recipients. It has been our own view that, though inhibition of growth in a teenager may result in short stature, this may be acceptable and not create insurmountable psychological problems. Growth retardation in children under the age of 12 or 13, however, may lead to such gross dwarfism that severe psychological problems may ensue. The proportion of children who demonstrate normal growth following organ transplantation varies considerably from 13% to over 60% from one series to another[19]. Decisions of this nature are clearly difficult, but hopefully will become easier as immunosuppression with cyclosporin permits lower dosages of steroid to be used, thus inhibiting growth less. It may prove possible to withdraw steroid therapy altogether in some patients with cardiac transplants. A compensatory growth spurt ensues when steroid dosages are reduced to below growth-suppressing levels ($< 45\,mg$ cortisone/m^2 per day) or when the drug is discontinued[20].

There is some evidence that the growth retardation effect is minimized by administering a double dosage of steroids on alternate days with no therapy on intervening days[21,22]. Although alternate-day therapy was considered in our two 14-year-old patients, we chose to retain the daily dose as both boys continued to experience episodes of moderately severe acute rejection throughout the first year.

Gastrointestinal tract haemorrhage

Gastrointestinal tract bleeding is a well-known complication of steroid therapy, but has been relatively uncommon in our own patients, occurring on only three occasions. Its risk is increased by the addition of both anticoagulant and antiplatelet therapy, which patients with heterotopic heart transplants receive.

The routine administration of cimetidine and antacids appears to have success-fully minimized its incidence.

We have, however, been at pains to investigate and treat any patients with clinical symptoms or history of peptic ulcer before we undertake transplan-tation. One patient with a strong history of ulcer was submitted to partial gastrectomy before being accepted for transplantation; he suffered no further gastrointestinal problems and remains well 8 years later.

Gastrointestinal complications, including peptic ulcer, perforation and gastrointestinal haemorrhage, with or without detectable gastric or duodenal ulcer, have been reported by a number of renal and cardiac transplant centres[7,9,23,24]. In one early renal series such complications were responsible for more than 6% of patient deaths[23]. With the introduction of routine prophylactic therapy with atropine-like drugs, alkaline powders or gels, and cimetidine, these complications have been greatly reduced[25]. Rejection episodes have been reported after the use of cimetidine in transplant recipients[26], though most groups, including our own, have been successfully using this drug to pre-vent gastrointestinal ulceration and bleeding without any such complication.

Gastrointestinal complications arising in transplant patients are managed by the standard surgical and medical methods of investigation and treatment.

Lenticular cataracts

Cataracts can be induced by prolonged steroid therapy, and have occurred in two of our own patients 3 years after transplantation. Other centres have reported a high incidence of cataract after organ transplantation. At the Cleveland Clinic and Peter Bent Brigham Hospital cataracts accounted for no less than 52% and 24%, respectively of late complications following renal transplantation[9,24]. In cardiac transplant patients at the Medical College of Virginia, cataracts occurred in only 6% of patients[8].

Low-dose corticosteroids never provoke the development of cataracts, even with prolonged use[27]. The high dose administered during rejection episodes, however, produce subcortical crystalline opacities which invariably affect only the posterior pole of the lens. These cataracts usually do not progress and cause little impairment of visual acuity. Surgical excision, therefore, is rarely required.

Psychiatric complications

The incidence of psychiatric complications in patients receiving steroid therapy has been reported to be between 4% and 36%[28,29]. Symptoms vary in severity from insomnia, nervousness and slight mood changes, to manic-depressive or schizophrenic psychoses and suicide attempts. At the University of Arizona, 12% of the cardiac transplant patients have developed psychiatric compli-cations (one psychosis and three depressions)[7]. Although a number of other cardiac transplant centres have sporadically reported psychiatric complications, details and overall incidences are not available.

At our own centre, one patient committed suicide by jumping out of a hospital window 21 days after transplantation following the onset of a severe acute depressive illness. A second patient developed a psychosis, and others have shown varying degrees of depression and personality change. It is, however, difficult to determine whether such disorders are drug-related or occur as a result of the isolation and stress of the post-transplant period.

Pancreatitis

The cause of post-transplant pancreatitis remains uncertain. Several aetiologies have been implicated; these include drugs (corticosteroids, azathioprine, frusemide, adrenaline and alcohol)[30-34], infections (cytomegalovirus, viral hepatitis, mumps, coxsackie and enteroviruses)[35-38], autoimmune disorders[39, 40], ischaemia[41], and biliary tract or peptic ulcer disease[42].

The University of Arizona has reported a 6% incidence in cardiac transplant patients within the first 3 months[7]. Incidences of up to 7%, with a mortality rate of more than 50%, have been reported from several renal transplant centres[42]. Though clinically severe acute pancreatitis occurred in only one of our own patients, accounting for his death some 3 weeks after transplantation, a low-grade, asymptomatic pancreatitis has been noted in 49% of patients coming to necropsy[43]. Similarly, at Stanford, pancreatitis was found at necropsy in 70% of cardiac transplant patients[42].

Azathioprine

We have found azathioprine an easy and safe drug to use, and to be relatively free from serious complication, though its role in the occurrence of pancreatitis (see above) and hepatitis remains uncertain. Though hepatitis has not been reported as a significant complication at most cardiac transplant centres, it has been an important cause of morbidity and mortality in the renal transplant patient[44-46]. The incidence of transient or permanent liver function abnormality in renal patients varies from 7 to 67%, with chronic liver disease developing in some 6 to 16%[47-50]. Possible causes include hepatotoxic drugs, especially azathioprine, and viruses.

Bone marrow suppression, involving both red and white cell precursors, has rarely proved a problem, as it occurs relatively slowly and recovers relatively quickly in the cardiac patient. Adjustment of dosage prevents severe suppression from occurring. Long-term therapy with azathioprine, however, may result in chronic anaemia, requiring iron therapy and even periodic blood transfusion. We have switched one patient to cyclosporin A for this reason, even though he remained well immunosuppressed with azathioprine and methylprednisolone for over 2 years following transplantation.

Cyclophosphamide

We have occasionally added small doses of cyclophosphamide to the 'conventional' immunosuppressive regimen in patients with unresponsive severe acute rejection, when the total white blood count (WBC) remained high, despite large doses of azathioprine and actinomycin D. If successful in reducing the white blood count and reversing the rejection episode, then we have on occasion discontinued the azathioprine and continued cyclophosphamide and methylprednisolone as maintenance therapy. One such patient continued well controlled (with regard to acute rejection) for 4 years with no cyclophosphamide-associated complication, though he has recently undergone retransplantation for chronic rejection. A low dose (1–2 mg/kg per day) of this drug was sufficient to maintain a total white blood count within the range 3–5000/mm³, but has not been effective in preventing the development of chronic rejection changes. A second patient maintained on cyclophosphamide developed a severe haemorrhagic aseptic cystitis, which resolved when the drug was replaced with azathioprine.

Though cyclophosphamide has undoubtedly been valuable on occasions, we have found it a difficult drug to use. Unlike azathioprine, a fall in white blood count may be precipitous and result in a severe leukopenia (WBC < 1000/mm³), which may persist for several days before recovery occurs. In our experience, cyclophosphamide-induced leukopenia has been life-threatening on at least three occasions. As a result of these experiences, we have avoided the use of cyclophosphamide whenever possible.

Antithymocyte globulin

There is a small risk of anaphylactic shock following the administration of antithymocyte globulin (ATG). This complication has occurred in two of our patients receiving intravenous rabbit antithymocyte globulin (RATG). At Stanford, approximately 2% of patients have exhibited frank anaphylaxis with the intramuscular use of ATG[17]. The risk of anaphylaxis may be reduced by administering a test done subcutaneously and observing for a severe histamine skin reaction, and by administering steroids and an antihistamine before the ATG.

Patients who experience anaphylactic shock may require urgent steroid and adrenaline therapy, vasopressor support, and mechanically assisted respiration. They may, however, cautiously receive further ATG on subsequent occasions; in our experience, this reaction may be related to the batch of ATG used rather than to the ATG *per se*. Should the complication occur again, ATG produced in a second species of animal (e.g. horse or goat rather than rabbit) may be found not to provoke the reaction, and may be used safely.

We have no experience with the intramuscular administration of RATG. The Stanford group, however, reports that pain at the site of injection is invariable and can become intense once an immune response has developed to the heterologous antisera[17]. This pain can be greatly reduced by mixing ATG with a local anaesthetic; the patient is encouraged to exercise his legs for several hours after injection, thus increasing the lymphatic uptake of the ATG.

Approximately 10% of the patients receiving RATG at both Stanford and our own centre develop a combination of symptoms, which include rash, fever, chills, back and joint pain and, less frequently, bronchospasm. During acute rejection episodes the chills and fever can be prevented by giving intravenous steroid therapy prior to the intravenous administration of RATG. Bronchospasm is treated as for anaphylaxis. Aspirin and antihistamines are useful in the treatment of joint pain and fever, and rash, respectively.

The clinical syndrome of serum sickness (fever, hepatomegaly, splenomegaly and lymphadenopathy, associated with upper abdominal discomfort and pain) was seen during intravenous RATG administration in two patients in our own series, which resolved after discontinuation of therapy. Although three additional patients have complained of severe generalized muscular pains some hours after intravenous ATG administration, treatment with analgesics and antihistamines has been successful on each occasion.

Blood chemistry features of a low-grade hepatitis, associated with upper abdominal discomfort, were noted for a few weeks in one patient. Although ATG was considered as a possible aetiological factor, this was never confirmed; the aetiology of minor liver dysfunction frequently remains unclear in transplant patients[51].

Cyclosporin A

To date, using the regimen outlined in Chapter 9, we have seen relatively few complications from cyclosporin therapy. Like many fungal antibiotics, cyclosporin is nephrotoxic and has been reported to cause primary and secondary anuria in some patients receiving renal allografts[52, 53]. Primary anuria may be avoided if patients are deliberately hydrated and given mannitol or frusemide[53]. Impairment of renal function in cardiac transplant recipients responds to reduced levels of cyclosporin and, when severe, to complete discontinuation of the drug for 1–2 days[54]. Frusemide is also helpful in reversing the accompanying oliguria. Cyclosporin-induced renal toxicity appears to be relatively well tolerated, though short-term haemodialysis may be required on occasion. Close attention must be paid to monitoring both renal function and cyclosporin levels in the blood if the risk of renal failure is to be minimized.

Cyclosporin has also been reported to cause liver dysfunction, though it is doubtful whether this is a serious problem[55]. Liver dysfunction is usually dose-dependent and returns to normal levels when the dosage is reduced.

Persistent hypertension has been noted as a side-effect of cyclosporin administration in some recipients. A large number of other side-effects has been described (Table 18.1). The effects of truly long-term administration of this drug remain as yet uncertain.

Benign skin lesions

Patients on long-term immunosuppression not infrequently develop multiple benign skin lesions, which may require no treatment. Warts and kerato-acanthomas are not uncommon. Several renal transplant groups have reported a greater than 40% incidence of warts, which are thought to result from reactivation of latent viruses rather than from primary infection[56, 57]. It is important, however, to differentiate benign lesions from malignant tumours, such as squamous and basal cell carcinomata, which are the most common malignancies in immunocompromised patients (Chapter 14). All suspicious lesions should be biopsied or excised.

Long-term immunosuppressive therapy is clearly associated with a large number of side-effects and complications. Some of these can be avoided or minimized by careful selection of the patient or by pretransplant prophylactic treatment (e.g. for peptic ulcer), and others by post-transplant prophylactic medication. Avoidance of all such complications, however, cannot be ensured, and the potential risks must be considered when the potential recipient is initially assessed for cardiac transplantation.

COMPLICATIONS OF THE ORIGINAL DISEASE PROCESS

A few of our heterotopic heart transplant patients with underlying ischaemic heart disease have continued to show features of progressive atheroma of either the coronary arteries or the peripheral arterial system. One patient suffered a massive myocardial infarction of the recipient heart 3 months after transplantation. He experienced diaphoresis and severe typical ischaemic chest pain radiating to the arms; an electrocardiogram confirmed the sudden onset of ventricular fibrillation. Throughout this episode, however, the donor heart maintained a steady rhythm and a systemic blood pressure of 110/70 mmHg. He did not demonstrate any other clinical features of shock. Analgesia was all that was necessary in the form of therapy.

Other patients with ischaemic heart disease have subsequently lost co-ordinated electrical function of the recipient heart, but have suffered no adverse effects. Several of our patients with underlying cardiomyopathy have also lost function of the recipient heart. This has not led to problems, though we have been careful to continue anticoagulation. In one long-surviving patient ventricular fibrillation was demonstrated on one occasion, and co-ordinated contractions on subsequent occasions some months later, though it is unlikely that ventricular function was sufficient to open the aortic valve.

Patients with widespread atheroma are, of course, at risk from progression of this disease in vessels other than the coronaries. One of our patients who remains well over 4 years after his original transplant operation, and almost 3 years after retransplantation for acute-on-chronic rejection, has recently undergone below-knee amputation for painful ischaemic ulceration of the right lower leg and foot, associated with a progressive peripheral arteriopathy; all of the major arteries of both legs from groin to feet show calcification on radiography.

References

1. Ross, D. (1968). Report of a heart transplant operation. *Am. J. Cardiol.*, **22**, 838
2. Uys, C. J., Rose, A. G. and Barnard, C. N. (1975). The autopsy findings in a case of hetero-topic ardiac transplantation with left ventricular bypass for ischemic heart failure. *S. Afr. Med. J.*, **49**, 2029
3. Harrington, J. T., Sommers, S. C. and Kassiver, J. P. (1968). Atheromatous emboli with progressive renal failure. *Ann. Intern. Med.*, **68**, 152
4. Schinella, R. A. and Porensky, R. (1974). Atheromatous emboli associated with external cardiac massage. *Arch. Pathol.*, **97**, 319
5. Cooper, D. K. C., Fraser, R. C., Rose, A. G., Ayzenberg, T., Oldfield, G., Hassoulas, J., Novitzky, D., Uys, C. J. and Barnard, C. N. (1982). Technique, complications and clinical value of endomyocardial biopsy in patients with heterotopic heart transplants. *Thorax*, **37**, 727
6. Penn, I. and Makowski, E. L. (1981). Parenthood in kidney and liver transplant recipients. *Transplant. Proc.*, **13**, 36
7. Copeland, J., Fuller, J., Sailor, M. J. and McAleer, M. J. (1983). Heart transplantation at the Health Sciences Center of the University of Arizona. *Heart Transplant.*, **2**, 246
8. Hess, M. L., Hastillo, A., Goldman, M., Rider, S., Mohanakumar, T., Ducey, K., Wolfgang, T., Szentpetery, S. and Lower, R. R. (1983). Cardiac transplantation at the Medical College of Virginia. *Heart Transplant.*, **2**, 246
9. Kirkman, R. L., Strom, T. B., Weir, M. R. and Tilney, N. L. (1982). Late mortality and morbidity in recipients of long-term renal allografts. *Transplantation*, **34**, 347
10. Fisher, D. E. and Bickel, W. H. (1971). Corticosteroid-induced avascular necrosis—a clinical study of seventy-seven patients. *J. Bone J. Surg.*, **53A**, 859
11. Fisher, D. E., Bickel, W. H., Holley, K. E. and Ellefson, R. D. (1972). Corticosteroid-induced necrosis. II. Experimental study. *Clin. Orthop.*, **84**, 200
12. Briggs, W. A., Hampers, C. L., Merrill, J. P., Hager, E. B., Wilson, R. E., Birtch, A. G. and Murray, J. E. (1972). Aseptic necrosis in the femur after renal transplantation. *Ann. Surg.*, **175**, 282
13. Solomon, L. (1973). Drug-induced arthropathy and necrosis of the femoral head. *J. Bone J. Surg.*, **55B**, 246
14. Burton, D. S., Mochizuki, R. M. and Helpern, A. A. (1978). Total hip arthroplasty in the cardiac transplant patient. *Clin. Orthop.*, **130**, 186
15. Morris, P. J., Oliver, D. O., Bishop, M., Cullen, P., Fellows, G., French, M., Ledingham, J. G., Smith, J. C., Ting, A. and Williams, K. (1978). Results from a new renal transplantation unit. *Lancet*, **2**, 1353
16. Merrill, J. P. (1978). Dialysis versus transplantation in the treatment of end-stage renal disease. *Annu. Rev. Med.*, **29**, 243
17. Jamieson, S. W., Bieber, C. P. and Oyer, P. E. (1981). Suppression of immunity for cardiac transplantation. In Salaman, J. R. (ed.) *Immunosuppressive Therapy*. pp. 177–9. (Lancaster: MTP Press)

18. Cabrol, C., Gandjbakhch, I., Pavie, A., Cabrol, A., Mattei, M. F., Lienhart, A., Gluckman, J. C. and Rottembourg, J. (1983). Cardiac transplantation at La Pitié Hospital. *Heart Transplant.*, **2**, 244

19. Crosnier, J. and Broyer, M. (1979). Treatment of chronic renal failure in children. In Hamburger, J., Crosnier, J. and Grunfield, J. P. (eds.) *Nephrology.* p. 1361. (New York: Wiley).

20. Blodgett, F. M., Burgin, L., Iezzoni, D., Ciribetz, D. and Talbot, N. B. (1956). Effects of prolonged cortisone therapy on the statural growth, skeletal maturation and metabolic status of children. *N. Engl. J. Med.*, **254**, 636

21. Soyka, L. F. and Saxena, K. M. (1965). Alternate-day steroid therapy for nephrotic children. *J. Am. Med. Assoc.*, **192**, 225

22. Potter, D. E., Holliday, M. A., Wilson, C. J., Salvatierra, O. and Belzer, F. O. (1975). Alternate-day steroids in children after renal transplantation. *Transplant. Proc.*, **7**, 79

23. Crosnier, J., Leski, M., Kreis, H. and Descamps, D. (1969). Non-renal complications of kidney allotransplantations. In Alwall, N. *et al.* (eds.) *Proceedings of the Fourth International Congress of Nephrology, Stockholm.* Vol. 3, p. 270. (Basel and New York: Karger)

24. Abele, R., Novick, A. C., Braun, W. E., Steinmuller, D., Buszta, C., Greenstreet, R. and Hinton, J. (1982). Long-term results of renal transplantation in recipients with a functioning graft for two years. *Transplantation*, **34**, 264

25. Jones, R. H., Rudge, C. J. Bewick, M., Parsons, V. and Weston, M. J. (1978). Cimetidine: prophylaxis against gastrointestinal haemorrhage after renal transplantation. *Br. Med. J.*, **1**, 398

26. Primack, W. A. (1978). Cimetidine and renal allograft rejection. *Lancet*, **1**, 824

27. Crosnier, J. (1981). Extrarenal complications. In Hamburger, J., Crosnier, J., Bach, J. F. and Kreis, H. (eds.) *Renal Transplantation.* p. 232. (Baltimore/London: Williams & Wilkins)

28. Quarton, G. C., Clark, L. D., Cobb, S. and Bauer, W. (1955). Mental disturbance associated with ACTH and cortisone: a review of explanatory hypotheses. *Medicine*, **34**, 13

29. Ritchie, E. A. (1956). Toxic psychosis under cortisone and corticotropin. *J. Ment. Sci.*, **102**, 830

30. Bourne, M. S. and Dawson, H. (1958). Acute pancreatitis complicating prednisolone therapy. *Lancet*, **2**, 1209

31. Mallory, A. and Kern, F. (1980). Drug-induced pancreatitis: a critical review. *Gastroenterology*, **78**, 813

32. Nakashima, Y. and Howard, J. M. (1977). Drug-induced acute pancreatitis. *Surg. Gynecol. Obstet.*, **145**, 105

33. Kawanishi, H., Rudolph, E. and Bull, F. E. (1973). Azathioprine-induced acute pancreatitis. *N. Engl. J. Med.*, **289**, 357

34. Jones, P. E. and Oelbaum, M. H. (1975). Furosemide-induced pancreatitis. *Br. Med. J.*, **1**, 133

35. Tilney, N. L., Collins, J. J. and Wilson, R. E. (1966). Hemorrhagic pancreatitis: a fatal complication of renal transplantation. *N. Engl. J. Med.*, **275**, 1051

36. Hume, D. M. (1968). Kidney transplantation. In Rapaport, F. T. and Dausset, J. (eds.) *Human Transplantation.* p.110. (New York: Grune & Stratton)

37. Werbitt, W. and Mohsenifar, Z. (1980). Mononucleosis pancreatitis. *South. Med. J.*, **73**, 1094

38. Imrie, C. W., Ferguson, J. C. and Sommerville, R. G. (1977). Coxsackie and mumps virus infection in a prospective study of acute pancreatitis. *Gut*, **18**, 53

39. Fujii, G. and Nelson, R. A. (1963). The cross-reactivity and transfer of antibody in transplantation immunity. *J. Exp. Med.*, **118**, 1037

40. Amos, D. B. and Stickel, D. L. (1968). Human transplantation antigens. *Adv. Intern. Med.*, **14**, 15

41. Feiner, H. (1976). Pancreatitis after cardiac surgery. *Am. J. Surg.*, **131**, 684

42. Karrer, F. M., Mammana, R. B. and Copeland, J. G. (1982). Survival following pancreatitis and surgical drainage of a pancreatic pseudocyst in a heart transplant recipient. *Heart Transplant.*, **1**, 325

43. Uys, C. J., Rose, A. G. and Barnard, C. N. (1979). The pathology of human cardiac transplantation. *S. Afr. Med. J.*, **56**, 887

44. Rubin, R. H. (1981). Infection in the renal transplant patient. In Rubin, R. H. and Young, L. S. (eds.) *Clinical Approach to Infection in the Compromised Host.* (New York: Plenum Press)

45. Rubin, R. H., Wolfson, J. S., Cosimi, A. B. and Tolkoff-Rubin, N. E. (1981). Infection in renal transplant recipients. *Am. J. Med.*, **70**, 405

46. Ware, A. S., Luby, J. P., Hollinger, B., Eigenbrodt, E. H., Cuthbert, J. A., Atkins, C. R., Shorey, J., Hull, A. R. and Combes, B. (1979). Etiology of liver disease in renal transplant recipients. *Ann. Intern. Med.*, **91**, 368

47. Moore, T. C. and Hume, D. M. (1969). The period and nature of hazard in clinical renal transplantation: the hazard to patient survival. *Ann. Surg.*, **170**, 1

48. Ware, A. J., Luby, J. P., Eigenbrodt, E. H., Long, D. L. and Hull, A. R. (1975). Spectrum of liver disease in renal transplant recipients. *Gastroenterology*, **68**, 755

49. La Quaglia, M. P., Tolkoff-Rubin, N. E., Dienstag, J. L., Cosimi, A. B., Herrin, J. T., Kelly, M. and Rubin, R. H. (1981). Impact of hepatitis on renal transplantation. *Transplantation*, **32**, 504

50. Anuras, S., Piros, J., Bonney, W. W., Forker, E. L., Colville, D. S. and Corry, R. J. (1977). Liver disease in renal transplant recipients. *Arch. Intern. Med.*, **137**, 42

51. Sopko, J. and Anuras, S. (1978). Liver disease in renal transplant recipients. *Am. J. Med.*, **64**, 139

52. Calne, R. Y., White, D. J., Thiru, S., Evans, D. B., McMaster, P., Dunn, D. C., Craddock, G. N., Pentlow, B. D. and Rolles, K. (1978). Cyclosporin A in patients receiving renal allografts from cadaver donors. *Lancet*, **2**, 1323

53. Calne, R. Y., Rolles, K., White, D. J. G., Thiru, S., Evans, D. B., McMaster, P., Dunn, D. C., Craddock, G. N., Henderson, R. G., Aziz, S. and Lewis, P. (1979). Cyclosporin A initially as the only immunosuppressant in 34 recipients of cadaveric organs: 32 kidneys, 2 pancreases and 2 livers. *Lancet*, **2**, 1033

54. Griffith, B. P., Hardesty, R. L., Thompson, M. E., Dummer, J. S. and Bahnson, H. T. (1983). Cardiac transplantation with cyclosporine: the Pittsburgh experience. *Heart Transplant.*, **2**, 251

55. Green, C. F. (1981). Cyclosporin A. In Salaman, J. R. (ed.) *Immunosuppressive Therapy.* p. 75. (Lancaster: MTP Press)

56. Koranda, F. C., Dehmel, E. M., Kahn, G. and Penn, I. (1974). Cutaneous complications in immunosuppressed renal homograft recipients. *J. Am. Med. Assoc.*, **229**, 419

57. Spencer, E. S. and Anderson, H. K. (1970). Clinically evident, non-terminal infections with herpes viruses and the wart virus in immunosuppressed renal allograft recipients. *Br. Med. J.*, **3**, 251

19
Results of Cardiac Transplantation and Factors Influencing Survival

INTRODUCTION

Only three cardiac transplant centres have had continuing programmes for more than 10 years—our own, Stanford Medical Center in California, and the La Pitié Hospital in Paris. More recently, 20 or so new centres have initiated programmes. Sixty-eight cardiac transplant operations were performed at the University of Cape Town on 61 patients between December 1967 and February 1984. Twelve of these transplants were orthotopic and 56 heterotopic; seven procedures were retransplants and two involved the use of xenografts. At Stanford University Medical Center, where approximately one-third of all heart transplants have been performed, 286 orthotopic and one heterotopic transplant operations were carried out between January 1968 and April 1983[1]. At La Pitié Hospital in Paris, 67 orthotopic and one heterotopic transplants were performed between December 1972 and December 1982[2].

Other major centres with clinically active programmes in cardiac transplantation that have reported their results from time to time include: in the USA, the Medical College of Virginia[3], Columbia-Presbyterian Medical Center[4], the University of Arizona[5], and the University of Pittsburgh[6]; in the UK, Papworth Hospital in Cambridge[7]; and in France, the Cardiologic Hospital of Lyon[8].

RESULTS OF CARDIAC TRANSPLANTATION

The results of cardiac transplantation in Cape Town are shown in Figure 19.1.

Actuarial patient survival rates for the early orthotopic, heterotopic using conventional immunosuppression (excluding the two xenografts), and

287

heterotopic using cyclosporin A groups have been 40%, 77%, 80% at 3 months, and 40%, 58% and 80% (projected) at 1 year after transplantation, respectively. Survival rates for the early orthotopic and conventional heterotopic groups at 2, 3, 4 and 7 years were 20% and 43%, 20% and 34%, 20% and 28%, and 20% and 17%, respectively. Two of the 10 (20%) patients in the orthotopic group survive or survived more than 12 years. Three of the first five conventional heterotopic patients remain alive 8 or more years later. The improvement in early survival between the three groups is almost certainly due to improvements in patient selection, management and immunosuppression, rather than in the surgical techniques employed.

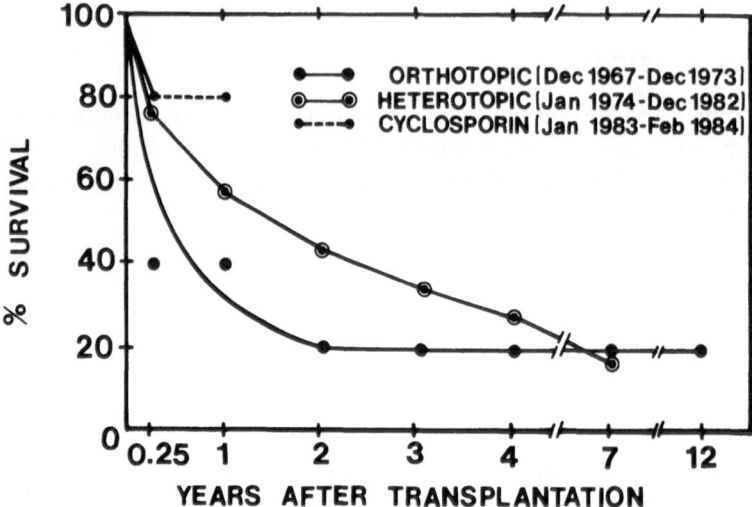

Figure 19.1   Actuarial survival of patients undergoing cardiac transplantation at Groote Schuur Hospital, Cape Town: 1967–83

Patient survival rates at Cape Town, Stanford and Paris at 3 months and 1 year are compared in Figure 19.2. Approximately 69–74% of the patients survived the initial 3-month period and 42–57% survived 1 year or more after transplantation.

Actuarial survival curves of patients at these three centres using conventional immunosuppression are shown in Figure 19.3. All of the patients in Cape Town received heterotopic transplants, whereas the patients at Stanford and Paris underwent orthotopic transplantation. Survival rates ranged from 42 to 63%, 35 to 55%, 33 to 51%, and 28 to 44% at 1, 2, 3 and 4 years after transplantation, respectively.

More recently, since cyclosporin replaced azathioprine as the primary immunosuppressant at several centres, higher survival rates have been obtained (Figure 19.4). One- and 2-year survival rates of approximately 65–80% have been reported. Results vary considerably from centre to centre, though a

number of new centres have reported very good results with a small group of
patients.

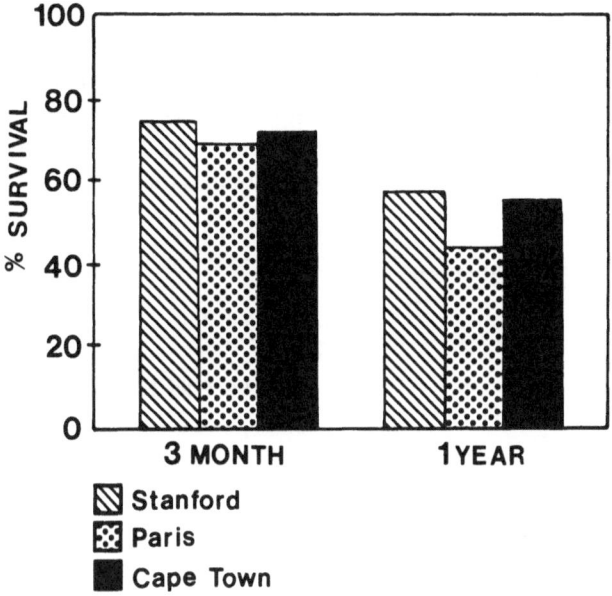

Figure 19.2   Three-month and 1-year overall survival rates at Stanford Medical Center, La Pitié
Hospital (Paris) and Groote Schuur Hospital (Cape Town)

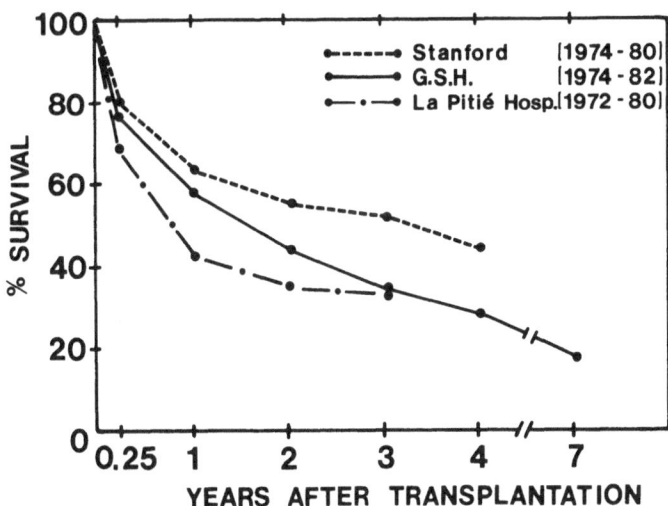

Figure 19.3   Actuarial survival of patients undergoing cardiac transplantation using conventional immunosuppression at Stanford Medical Center, La Pitié Hospital (Paris) and Groote
Schuur Hospital (Cape Town)

In patients with heterotopic heart transplants, graft failure from rejection may occur and yet the patient may survive and be retransplanted. If a second suitable donor does not become available, death may occur at some considerable interval of time after graft failure. At Cape Town, the overall mean heterotopic allograft survival with conventional immunosuppression was only 1.6 years. Similarly, the patient with an orthotopic transplant may survive failure of the allograft if retransplantation can be carried out in time. At Stanford, 24 retransplant procedures have been carried out. Allograft survival at both centres, therefore, is somewhat less than patient survival.

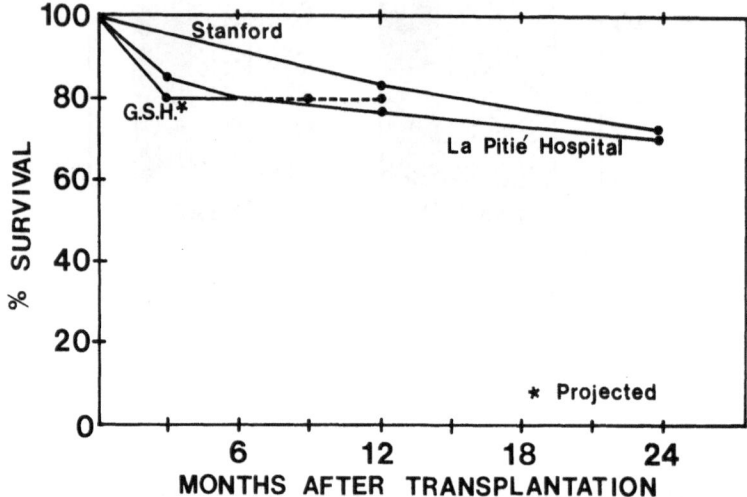

Figure 19.4 Actuarial survival of patients undergoing cardiac transplantation using cyclosporin A immunosuppression at Stanford Medical Center, La Pitié Hospital (Paris) and Groote Schuur Hospital (Cape Town)

MORTALITY AND GRAFT FAILURE

Of the 66 allotransplants in 59 patients performed in Cape Town during the past 16 years, death of the patient and/or graft failure (with survival of the patient with a heterotopic transplant) has occurred in 50 cases. Maximum survival has been 12.5 years. The causes and timing of death and/or graft failure are shown diagrammatically in Figure 19.5.

Infection accounted for 10 deaths within the first 3 months and a further five within the first year; two deaths occurred from infection after the first year. Though the risk of infection is possibly greatest in patients who have required heavy immunosuppression for severe and repeated episodes of acute rejection, life-threatening infection can also occur in patients who have not required increased therapy. Acute rejection accounted for seven graft failures within

3 months (five of these patients with heterotopic transplants survived longer for varying periods, including two who were retransplanted). Three further patients died from repeated episodes of acute or acute-on-chronic rejection within the first and second years. Chronic rejection (graft arteriosclerosis), confirmed by postmortem examination, accounted for 12 deaths, of which two-thirds occurred after the first year. Eleven other causes of death are listed in Table 19.1.

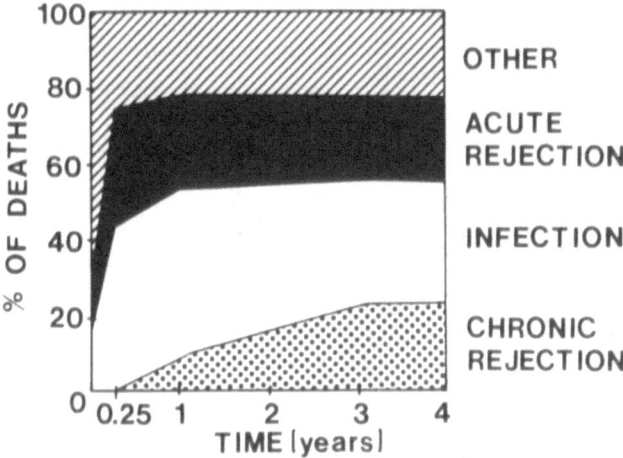

Figure 19.5 Cumulative causes of death and/or allograft failure following cardiac transplantation at Groote Schuur Hospital, Cape Town

A diagrammatic representation of the causes of death at Stanford Medical Center is shown in Figure 19.6.

Infection

Thirty-three per cent of deaths in Cape Town were from infection (Figure 19.5), which was the major cause of death in our patients. At Stanford, infection was also the most common cause of death, accounting for 58% of all deaths. Mortality from infection is greatest in the first few months when immunosuppression is heaviest[9, 10]. The greater percentage of deaths from infection at Stanford is possibly related to a rather heavier immunosuppressive regimen (resulting in a lower incidence of graft failure from acute rejection); a greater emphasis has been placed on antithymocyte globulin (RATG) administration at Stanford than at Cape Town[11,12]. The aetiologic agents responsible for these infections at the two centres were very similar[10]; bacterial organisms predominated, followed by viral and fungal.

At the transplant centres in Paris, Virginia and Arizona, infection was the second most common cause of mortality, accounting for approximately one-quarter (27%, 24% and 25%, respectively) of all deaths. The lower proportion of deaths due to infection at these three centres may be due to a less aggressive immunosuppressive policy; this is also suggested by the high proportion of patients (approximately 50%) who died from acute rejection in these three series.

Table 19.1 Causes and timing of deaths other than from infection and acute or chronic rejection at Groote Schuur Hospital, Cape Town

(1) Donor heart failure—day 1 (orthotopic transplant)
(2) Intravenous potassium cardiac arrest of both hearts—day 1 (heterotopic transplant)
(3) Unclear—failure of both hearts—day 7 (heterotopic transplant)
(4) Multiple organ failure—day 7
(5) Unclear—failure of both hearts—day 7 (heterotopic transplant)
(6) Suicide—acute depressive disorder—day 21
(7) Acute haemorrhagic pancreatitis—4 weeks
(8) Pulmonary emboli—16 weeks
(9) Kaposi's sarcoma—14 months
(10) Carcinoma of stomach—21 months
(11) Cerebral emboli—24 months

Acute rejection

Although acute rejection was only the third most common cause of death and/or graft failure in Cape Town, it was the primary cause of death at several centres and emerged as the second most common cause of death at Stanford. At both Cape Town and Stanford acute rejection accounted for approximately

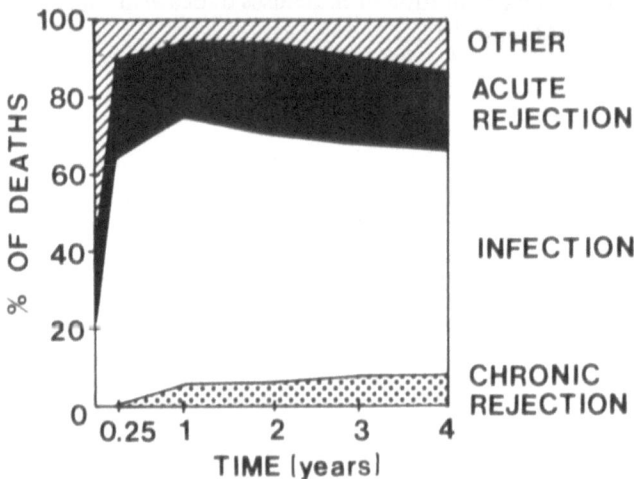

Figure 19.6 Cumulative causes of death following cardiac transplantation at Stanford Medical Center

20% of deaths, and, as would be expected, was seen primarily during the first postoperative year and was rare subsequently.

At Paris, Virginia and Arizona, acute rejection was by far the most common cause of mortality, accounting for approximately one-half (50%, 53% and 50%, respectively) of all deaths.

Clearly, those groups who are more aggressive and successful in the management of acute rejection pay a price by exposing their patients to greater risk of infection.

Chronic rejection (graft arteriosclerosis)

There are relatively few data on the incidence of this complication. This is possibly partly due to the fact that few centres have undertaken heart transplantation for a long enough period to have gained much experience of graft arteriosclerosis, which occurs generally late in the course of the patient's progress.

Chronic rejection was the second leading cause of death and/or graft failure at Cape Town (26% of deaths and/or graft failure) and the third most common cause of death at Stanford (11% of deaths). The incidence of chronic rejection at Stanford, however, may be somewhat higher, since at least 11 patients who have undergone retransplantation for this condition are not included in this figure.

At La Pitié Hospital in Paris, chronic rejection accounted for approximately 10% of deaths and/or graft failures. Although graft arteriosclerosis is thought to be the result of immunological damage followed by reparative myointimal proliferation[13-16], Thomson[17] and others[18,19] attribute the lipid deposition in the thickened intima to a combination of immune-related damage and co-existent hypercholesterolaemia. This latter conclusion is consistent with the finding of a significantly higher incidence of hyperlipidaemia in those of our patients who died or underwent graft failure from chronic rejection when compared with the other patients in our series[20]. The Stanford group has also reported finding a significantly increased incidence of graft arteriosclerosis in patients with high triglyceride levels[9].

Although a slightly greater percentage of patients undergoing heart transplantation in Cape Town had underlying ischaemic heart disease (57%) when compared with those operated on at Stanford (48%), this difference does not adequately account for the difference in incidence of graft arteriosclerosis seen between the two groups (Cape Town 26%; Stanford 11%). Heavier immunosuppression of the patients at Stanford may explain their lower incidence of chronic rejection (and higher incidence of infection). Other factors may also play a part. For example, the less rigorous psychiatric screening of potential recipients at Cape Town, with possibly a higher incidence of non-compliance with regard to drug therapy, may contribute to the higher incidence of chronic rejection.

FACTORS INFLUENCING SURVIVAL AFTER CARDIAC TRANSPLANTATION

We recently analysed the first 50 heart transplants (ten orthotopic and 40 heterotopic) performed in Cape Town in an effort to distinguish any factors which might have influenced survival[21]. Thirty-eight of these 50 patients had subsequently died or undergone graft failure (but survived until undergoing retransplantation). Duration of graft survival was from 1 day to 12.5 years. Various factors which might have influenced graft survival in these patients were investigated. These included: (1) recipient and (2) donor age, sex and race, (3) aetiology of the recipient's underlying primary cardiac disease, (4) recipient ABO blood group, (5) influence of pretransplantation blood transfusion in the recipient and (6) HLA compatibility between recipient and donor.

All of the patients received conventional immunosuppression; cyclosporin A may prove efficient enough to overcome some hitherto adverse factors.

Our findings are summarized below, together with relevant data from other centres. There are, however, few such reports from other groups, except Stanford.

1. Recipient age, sex and race

There was statistically significant longer survival in patients under 40 years when compared with those of a greater age ($p < 0.05$) (Figure 19.7). The increased mortality of the older age group was most marked within the first year. No recipient 50 years or older at the time of transplantation survived beyond the second year.

The Stanford group has reported a significant difference in survival rate between patients 45 years of age or older and younger patients. Survival for 3 years was approximately four times more likely for those under the age of 40 at transplantation than for those over 50[11,22]. The Arizona group, however, has observed no increased survival in younger patients[23].

The younger patients at Stanford and Cape Town probably did better due to a greater tolerance to the debilitating effects of immunosuppression and a greater resistance to infection; there was a statistically increased mortality at Cape Town from infection in patients over the age of 35 ($p < 0.05$)[10].

Survival has not been found to be influenced by the sex or race of the recipient at Cape Town or at any other centre.

2. Donor age, sex and race

There was no relationship between donor age or sex and allograft survival in our own series. At Stanford, however, patients who received grafts from donors under the age of 35 had a lower incidence of graft arteriosclerosis than those who received grafts from donors over the age of 35[24].

At our own centre the 15 recipients of allografts from white donors survived for a mean period of 9.2 months, while the 35 receiving allografts from non-white donors survived for an average of 27.6 months ($p < 0.05$) (Figure 19.8). There were only five black donors in this series, as in this ethnic group there are certain religious and social factors which make them reluctant to donate. Nevertheless, when the non-white group was subdivided into black and mixed race (Cape Coloured) donors, survival of the recipients averaged 41.2 and 25.3 months respectively. Although the 4.5-fold difference in survival between black and white donor groups was statistically significant ($p < 0.005$), the difference between the white and Coloured groups reached significance only at the 3-year survival point ($p < 0.05$). The difference between the black and Coloured groups did not reach statistical significance. Three (60%) of the five patients receiving hearts from black donors were alive at least 4 years after transplantation, whereas only four (9%) of the remaining 45 patients survived 4 years or more ($p < 0.001$).

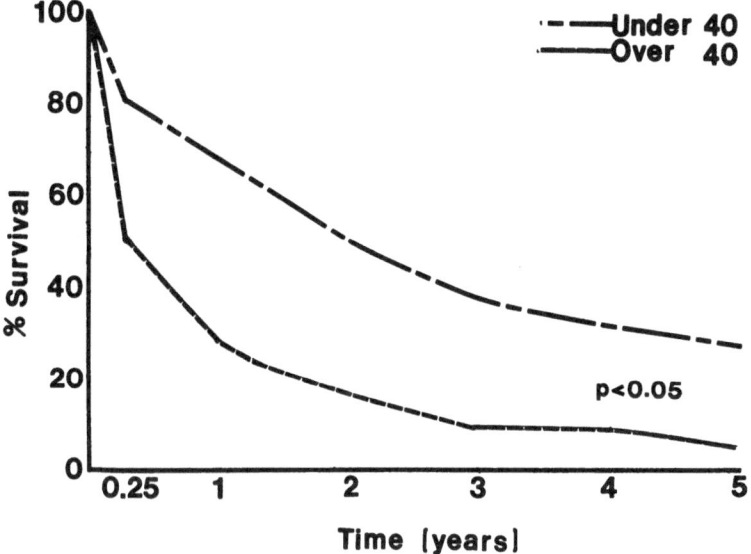

Figure 19.7   Patient survival related to recipient age (Groote Schuur Hospital, Cape Town)

We were unable to detect any differences in donor or recipient characteristics which might explain the improved survival of patients receiving hearts from non-white donors. It seems likely that this observed difference in graft survival is associated with the HLA differences that are known to exist between different racial groups[25], though we have been unable to identify any 'beneficial' HLA antigens or the lack of any 'detrimental' antigens. There appear to have been no reports on the effect of donor race on survival of patients undergoing cardiac transplantation elsewhere.

Although a number of transplant centres have reported poor survival of kidney grafts transplanted into black recipients when compared with white[26–28], the influence of the race of the donor of kidney grafts remains uncertain. In our own centre, survival of recipients of kidneys is not influenced by the race of the donor[29], though Opelz and his colleagues have shown that in the USA recipients of black donor kidneys survived for a significantly shorter period[26,27]. There may, however, be considerable HLA differences between the black population in the USA, which almost certainly contains a large number of patients of mixed racial background, and the black population of Southern Africa.

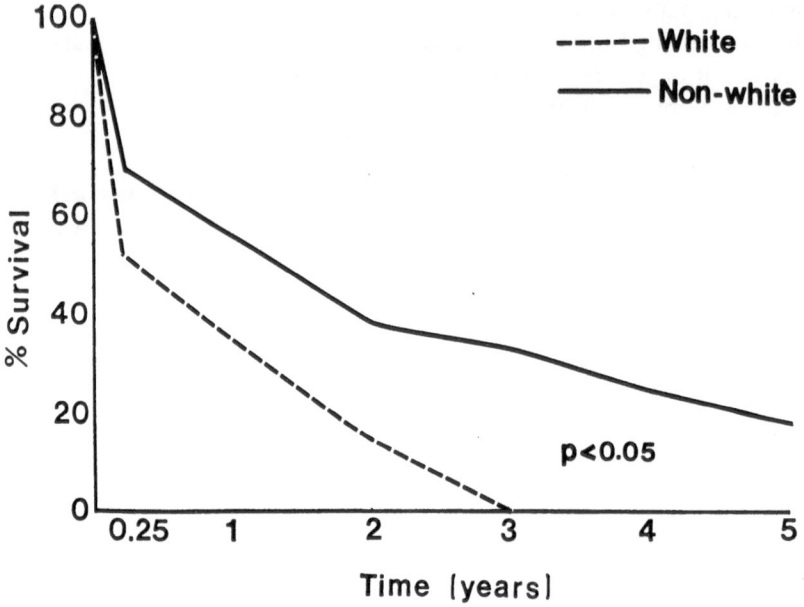

Figure 19.8 Patient survival related to donor race—white vs. non-white (Groote Schuur Hospital, Cape Town)

3. Aetiology of the underlying primary cardiac disease

The underlying condition necessitating transplantation at Cape Town was ischaemic heart disease (IHD) in 29 of the recipients, cardiomyopathy (CM) in 13, rheumatic heart disease (RHD) in four, endomyocardial fibrosis in two and mixed pathology (RHD and IHD) in two. Patients in the IHD group were significantly older (mean of 42 years) when compared to those with CM (mean of 30 years) ($p < 0.01$). Patients with RHD had an average age of 39 years.

The patients with RHD survived over three times as long as the patients from the IHD and CM groups ($p < 0.01$); the cumulative period of survival of the four RHD patients exceeded that of all 13 CM patients ($p < 0.05$)

(Table 19.2). Although there was a trend for IHD patients to survive longer than CM patients this did not reach statistical significance.

Table 19.2 Relationship of survival of cardiac transplant recipients to under-lying primary cardiac pathology (Groote Schuur Hospital, Cape Town)

Underlying heart disease	Number of recipients	Cumulative survival (months)	Mean survival/ recipient (months)
Ischaemic (IHD)	29	614.8	21.2
Cardiomyopathy (CM)	13	225.9	17.4
Rheumatic (RHD)	4	247.2	61.8

The increased survival of patients with RHD may be related to an immuno-logical effect of RHD, as it does not appear (after an analysis of covariance) to be related to a better combination of other factors which might influence survival[20]. One of the patients was, at 12.5 years, the longest surviving orthotopic cardiac transplant recipient in the series. Another, at over 7 years, was the longest surviving heterotopic recipient.

When correction was made for other factors influencing survival, the difference in survival between IHD and CM patients was nearly always twofold, the IHD group surviving longer, though statistical significance was not achieved. This is of particular interest considering the patients with CM were on average over a decade younger, and on this basis, might have been expected to have survived longer.

The Stanford group has reported no significant differences in survival between transplanted patients with underlying CM and IHD[30]. Furthermore, 1-year survival in CM patients was not affected by age, identical survival rates being observed for patients 40 years or older and for those under 40.

4. Recipient ABO blood group

Twenty-six recipients at Cape Town were of blood group A, 17 of group O, five of B, and two of AB. When each ABO blood group was considered separately, there was no significant relationship between the recipient's blood group and survival, though there was an obvious trend for prolonged survival in recipients with blood groups A or O, that is, those without B antigen (Table 19.3).

When survival of patients with B antigen on their red blood cells was compared with those without B antigen, mean survival of the latter group was almost four times as long as the former; this difference still did not quite reach statistical significance. When those patients who died from technical or other early complications were excluded, and only those surviving at least 2 months considered, then there was a statistically significant difference between the B and non-B groups, the non-B group surviving for a mean period (33.6 months), almost five times as long as the B group (6.7 months) ($p < 0.005$)[31].

Table 19.3   Relationship of survival of cardiac transplant recipients to ABO blood group antigens (Groote Schuur Hospital, Cape Town)

Blood group antigens	Number of recipients	Cumulative survival (months)	Mean survival/ recipient (months)
B antigen	7	47.0	6.7
Non-B antigen:	43	1008.1	23.4
Blood group A	26	579.0	22.3
Blood group O	17	429.1	25.2

The reason for this difference in survival is unknown, although it might result from a greater immune response of group B individuals. No other cardiac transplantation centres, however, have reported any differences in survival between patients with different ABO blood groups.

5. Pretransplant blood transfusions

Statistically significant improved survival related to previous blood transfusion has been well documented in patients undergoing renal transplantation, but has not been reported in patients undergoing cardiac transplantation, though a beneficial effect was reported by the Stanford group as long as a decade ago[32].

We also observed a beneficial effect from transfusion, though it did not reach overall statistical significance. At the 3-year interval, however, there were significantly more survivors from the former group than the latter ($p < 0.05$). This topic has been discussed more fully in Chapter 6.

6. HLA compatibility

In our own series, there was no relationship between overall survival and HLA-A and B matching. There was, however, an improved survival at 1 year when one or two HLA identical antigens were present in both donor and recipient ($p < 0.05$).

No significant difference in survival has been observed at Stanford on the basis of HLA-A and B matching of donors and recipients[11, 33], although incompatibility at the HLA-A2 and A3 loci has been found to be associated with a higher incidence of graft arteriosclerosis[24]. This topic has also been discussed further in Chapter 6.

Other factors which influence patient survival

Selection of patients

At this relatively early stage in the development of clinical heart transplantation, the results at any one centre can be greatly influenced by the centre's policy of selecting recipients. Obviously, if the selection policy is rigorous and only 'ideal' patients chosen to undergo this procedure (that is, patients under the age of 40, who are not yet terminal and therefore do not require inotropic support, who are well motivated personally, and who are well supported by family and friends) then the results are likely to be relatively good at that centre. The selection policy of any one centre is to a certain extent dictated by the number of potential recipients referred to that centre. Clearly, if the centre is referred a very large number of patients, then the selection of recipients can and, in fact, needs to be rigorous; any patient with a condition which might be considered even a mild contraindication may be excluded. If the centre is referred a small number of patients, then it is likely that their selection policy will become less rigorous, and this may result in relatively poorer results following transplantation.

At our own institution, we are referred a small number of patients for consideration for transplantation each year. Our own policy has, therefore, been relatively liberal, and we have on occasions accepted patients for transplantation even when there have been mild doubts as to their suitability on physical or psychological grounds. Many of our patients have not been 'ideal' candidates. In the early period of our transplant experience, many patients were accepted for transplantation who, by today's standards, were clearly too old or had other major adverse physical conditions[34]. More recently, our selection process has not been as rigorous as it should have been in the psychological assessment of these patients, and several have been transplanted who have subsequently been non-compliant[35]; this topic is discussed further below.

From our experience we have concluded that, since heart transplantation is a time-consuming and expensive form of therapy, which places great demands on the resources of any hospital, it should only be offered to patients with a very high chance of benefiting from the procedure. When carried out as a 'last-resort' procedure in terminally ill patients, it is followed by a high early mortality. As the number of donor hearts available to any one centre rarely equates with the number of potential recipients awaiting transplantation, it would seem only logical to offer such hearts to patients who are most likely to survive the many potential complications of this form of surgical therapy.

Physicians continue to refer patients late in the course of their illness. Approximately one-third of the patients referred to us have been bed-ridden and have required continuous inotropic support. Although we have transplanted several such patients, experience has shown that they are too advanced in the course of their illness, and few have the physical reserves to survive the early months after transplantation. As the results of transplantation steadily improve, patients will be referred rather earlier in the course of their illness and in a generally better physical condition, and are therefore likely to do well after transplantation. The overall results will improve further.

Patient non-compliance

Recently, we reviewed our series of heterotopic cardiac transplant patients and assessed the influence of non-compliance on long-term survival[35]. Failure of patients to conform to the advice and recommendations of their physician, resulting in less than optimal therapy, was a major factor in morbidity and mortality in these patients. The possible reasons for this are many and are discussed more fully in Chapter 15. Clearly, the initial selection of the patient may be a major factor, but a number of other factors are involved, such as the effects of drug therapy and the psychological stress of the early postoperative period.

Twenty-three per cent of the patients had suffered a major complication related to non-compliance. Of the 39 patients in this study, non-adherence was a direct cause or major contribution to irreversible graft failure or death in eight, and to reversible graft failure in one.

Though the number of patients in this study was small, non-compliance was found to be more common in certain groups (Table 19.4). A statistically significant increased incidence of non-compliance was found in (1) those under the age of 40 years ($p < 0.05$), (2) those less well educated ($p < 0.05$), (3) unskilled workers ($p < 0.025$) and (4) single or divorced patients ($p < 0.05$). Those with underlying cardiomyopathy, rather than ischaemic or rheumatic heart disease, also had a higher incidence of non-compliance, though this did not reach statistical significance. There were only two women in the study, but both showed features of non-compliance. The interest and influence of the surgical team at the heart transplant centre was demonstrated by the fact that there was a twofold increase in the incidence of non-compliance in patients not directly under our care at the time, though this did not reach statistical significance.

It would appear that the more mature, better educated patient with professional or executive employment and good family support, and with underlying ischaemic heart disease, would be the patient most likely to comply with the rigours of the post-transplant course.

Experience at Stanford has also shown that a history of non-compliance, psychosocial instability, or drug abuse correlates inversely with postoperative rehabilitation[36], and that a strong supportive social structure is important to help overcome the many postoperative stresses that all heart transplant patients face.

Table 19.4 Non-compliance in heterotopic heart transplant recipients (Groote Schuur Hospital, Cape Town)

	Compliant	Non-compliant	Total	Significance*
(1) Age				
>40	15	1 (6%)	16	
<40	15	8 (35%)	23	$p < 0.05$
	30	9 (23%)	39	
(2) Sex				
Male	30	7 (19%)	37	
Female	0	2 (100%)	2	NS
	30	9 (23%)	39	
(3) Ethnic group				
White	25	8 (24%)	33	
Black/mixed race	5	1 (17%)	6	NS
	30	9 (23%)	39	
(4) Marital status †				
Married	25	4 (14%)	29	
Single/divorced	3	5 (63%)	8	$p < 0.05$
	28	9 (24%)	37	
(5) Education ‡				
Tertiary	11	0 (0%)	11	
Secondary	16	9 (36%)	25	$p < 0.05$
	27	9 (25%)	36	
(6) Employment				
Senior executive/professional	7	0 (0%)	7	
Skilled manual	9	2 (18%)	11	
Clerical (unskilled)	8	5 (38%)	13	
Unskilled manual	0	3 (100%)	3	
Housewife	0	2 (100%)	2	
Scholar/student	3	0 (0%)	3	$p < 0.025$
	27	12 (31%)	39	
(7) Underlying cardiac pathology				
Ischaemic	17	4 (19%)	21	
Cardiomyopathic	9	5 (36%)	14	
Rheumatic	2	0 (0%)	2	
Other	2	0 (0%)	2	NS
	30	9 (23%)	39	

NS = Not statistically significant
*Fisher's Exact Test or extensions of Fisher's Exact Test
†Excludes two children
‡Excludes three patients still studying

References

1. Jamieson, S. W., Oyer, P. E., Bieber, C. P., Hunt, S. A., Billingham, M., Miller, J., Gamberg, P., Stinson, E. B. and Shumway, N. E. (1983). Cardiac transplantation at Stanford. *Heart Transplant.*, **2**, 243

2. Cabrol, C., Gandjbakch, I., Pavie, A., Cabrol, A., Mattei, M. F., Lienhart, A., Gluckman, J. C. and Rottembourg, J. (1983). Cardiac transplantation at La Pitié Hospital. *Heart Transplant.*, **2**, 244

3. Hess, M. L., Hastillo, A., Goldman, M., Rider, S., Mohanakumar, T., Ducey, K., Wolfgang, T., Szentpetery, S. and Lower, R. R. (1983). Cardiac transplantation at the Medical College of Virginia. *Heart Transplant.*, **2**, 246

4. Rose, E. A., Reemtsma, K., Drusin, R. E., Powers, E. R., Blood, D. K., Reison, D. S. and Lamb, J. I. (1983). Clinical cardiac transplantation at Columbia-Presbyterian Medical Center. *Heart Transplant.*, **2**, 248

5. Copeland, J., Fuller, J., Sailor, J. and McAleer, M. J. (1983). Heart transplantation at the Health Sciences Center of the University of Arizona. *Heart Transplant.*, **2**, 246

6. Griffith, B. P., Hardesty, R. L., Thompson, M. E., Dummer, J. S. and Bahnson, H. T. (1983). Cardiac transplantation with cyclosporine: the Pittsburgh experience. *Heart Transplant.*, **2**, 251

7. Wallwork, J., English, T. A. H. and Cory-Pearce, R. (1983). Cardiac transplantation at Cambridge. *Heart Transplant.*, **2**, 245

8. Dureau, G., Villard, J., Vial, P., Vacher, G., Hercule, C., George, M., Chuzel, M., Estanove, S., Marion, P. and Termet, H. (1983). Heart transplantation in Lyon. *Heart Transplant.*, **2**, 250

9. Pennock, J. L., Oyer, P. E., Reitz, B. A., Jamieson, S. W., Bieber, C. P., Wallwork, J., Stinson, E. B. and Shumway, N. E. (1982). Cardiac transplantation in perspective for the future: survival, complications, rehabilitation and cost. *J. Thorac. Cardiovasc. Surg.*, **83**, 168

10. Cooper, D. K. C., Lanza, R. P., Oliver, S., Forder, A. A., Rose, A. G., Uys, C. J., Novitzky, D. and Barnard, C. N. (1983). Infectious complications of heterotopic heart transplantation. *Thorax*, **38**, 822

11. Baumgartner, W. A., Reitz, B. A., Oyer, P. E., Stinson, E. B. and Shumway, N. E. (1979). Cardiac homotransplantation. *Curr. Probl. Surg.*, **16**, 3

12. Barnard, C. N., Barnard, M. S., Cooper, D. K. C., Curchio, C. N., Hassoulas, J., Novitsky, D. and Wolpowitz, A. (1981). The present status of heterotopic cardiac transplantation. *J. Thorac. Cardiovasc. Surg.*, **81**, 433

13. Bieber, C. P., Stinson, E. B., Shumway, N. E., Payne, R. and Kosek, J. (1970). Cardiac transplantation in man. VII. Cardiac allograft pathology. *Circulation*, **41**, 753

14. Milman, J. D., Shipkey, F. H., Lind, C. J., Nora, J. J., Leachman, R. D. and Rochelle, D. G. (1970). Morphologic findings in human cardiac allografts. *Circulation*, **41**, 519

15. Kosek, J. C., Bieber, C. P. and Lower, R. R. (1971). Heart graft arteriosclerosis. *Transplant. Proc.*, **3**, 512

16. Alsonson, D. R., Storek, P. K. and Minich, C. R. (1977). Studies on the pathogenesis of athero-arteriosclerosis induced in rabbit cardiac allografts by the synergy of graft rejection and hypercholesterolemia. *Am. J. Pathol.*, **87**, 415

17. Thomson, J. G. (1968). Heart transplantation in man—necropsy findings. *Br. Med. J.*, **2**, 511

18. Laden, A. M., Sinclair, R. A. and Ruskiewlez, M. (1973). Vascular changes in experimental cardiac allografts. *Transplant. Proc.*, **5**, 737

19. Laden, A. M. (1972). Experimental atherosclerosis in rats and rabbit cardiac allografts. *Arch. Pathol.*, **93**, 240

20. Lanza, R. P., Cooper, D. K. C., Boyd, S. T. and Barnard, C. N. (1984). A comparison of patients with ischemic, myopathic and rheumatic heart disease as cardiac transplant recipients. *Am. Heart J.*, **107**, 8

21. Cooper, D. K. C., Boyd, S. T., Lanza, R. P. and Barnard, C. N. (1984). Factors influencing survival following heart transplantation. *Heart Transplant.*, **3**, 86

22. Dong, E. and Shumway, N. E. (1977). Current results of human heart transplantation. *World J. Surg.*, **1**, 157

23. Fuller, J. F. and Copeland, J. G. (1983). The age criterion and recipient selection. (Presented at The International Society for Heart Transplantation, 3rd Annual Scientific Session, New Orleans.) *Heart Transplant.* (Suppl.), 30

24. Bieber, C. P., Hunt, S. A., Schwinn, D. A., Jamieson, S. A., Reitz, B. A., Oyer, P. E., Stinson, E. B. and Shumway, N. E. (1981). Complications in long-term survivors of cardiac transplantation. *Transplant. Proc.*, **13**, 207

25. Guttmann, R. D., Bach, F. B., Bach, M. K., Claman, H. N., David, J. R., Jeannet, M., Lindquist, R. R., McKhann, C. F., Papermaster, D. and Schwartz, R. S. (1981). *Immunology.* p. 102. (Kalamazoo: The Upjohn Company)

26. Opelz, G., Mickey, G. R. and Terasaki, P. I. (1977). Influence of race on kidney transplant survival. *Transplant. Proc.*, **9**, 137

27. Opelz, G. and Terasaki, P. I. (1980). International histocompatibility workshop study on renal transplantation. In Terasaki, P. I. (ed.) *Histocompatibility Testing.* p. 592. (Los Angeles: UCLA Tissue Typing Laboratory)

28. Jonasson, O. and Moses, V. (1981). Factors influencing first cadaver renal allograft survival. *Transplant. Proc.*, **13**, 44

29. Swanepoel, C. R., Campbell, E. and Cassidy, M. J. D. (1981). The influence of ethnic differences on the outcome of renal transplantation. Paper presented at the *8th Congress of the South African Transplantation Society*, 1981

30. Hassela, L. A., Fowles, R. E. and Stinson, E. B. (1981). Patients with congestive cardiomyopathy as cardiac transplant recipients. *Am. J. Cardiol.*, **47**, 1205

31. Lanza, R. P., Cooper, D. K. C. and Barnard, C. N. (1982). Effect of ABO blood group antigens on long-term survival after cardiac transplantation. *N. Engl. J. Med.*, **307**, 1275

32. Dong, E., Stinson, E. B., Griepp, R. B., Coulson, A. S. and Shumway, N. E. (1973). Cardiac transplantation following failure of previous cardiac surgery. *Surg. Forum*, **24**, 150

33. Stinson, E. B., Payne, R., Dong, E., Griepp, R. B. and Shumway, N. E. (1971). Correlation of histocompatibility matching with graft rejection and survival after cardiac transplantation in man. *Lancet*, **2**, 459

34. Losman, J. G., Levine, H., Campbell, C. D., Replogle, R. L., Hassoulas, J., Novitzky, D., Cooper, D. K. C. and Barnard, C. N. (1982). Changes in indications for heart transplantation: an additional argument for the preservation of the recipient's own heart. *J. Thorac. Cardiovasc. Surg.*, **84**, 716

35. Cooper, D. K. C., Lanza, R. P., Nash, E. S. and Barnard, C. N. (1984). Non-compliance in heart transplant recipients: the Cape Town experience. *Heart Transplant.*, **3**, 248

36. Christopherson, L. K. and Lunde, D. T. (1971). Selection of cardiac transplant recipients and their subsequent psychosocial adjustment. *Semin. Psychiatry*, **3**, 36

20
Advantages and Disadvantages of Heterotopic Transplantation

INTRODUCTION

Heterotopic heart transplantation has both advantages and disadvantages when compared with orthotopic heart transplantation (Table 20.1)[1]. In particular, the heterotopic procedure may allow recipient survival despite temporary or permanent loss of donor heart function following acute or chronic rejection; the circulation may be maintained by the recipient's own heart for at least

Table 20.1 Advantages and disadvantages of heterotopic over orthotopic heart transplantation

Advantages	Disadvantages

(1) Recipient heart acts as a built-in cardiac assist device and may maintain circulation:
(a) During reversible loss of donor heart function during:
  (i) period of recovery of donor heart from ischaemia sustained during transplantation
  (ii) severe acute rejection episodes
(b) Following irreversible loss of donor heart function from:
  (i) acute, or
  (ii) chronic rejection (whilst patient awaits retransplantation)
(c) During adaptation of a very small donor heart to the demands of the circulation
(2) Allows for possible recovery of recipient heart, e.g. after viral myocarditis
(3) Can be performed even in the presence of a high pulmonary vascular resistance as the hypertrophied recipient right ventricle continues to suppport the pulmonary circulation
	(1) Risk of systemic emboli from thrombus in poorly-contracting recipient left ventricle. Requires long-term anticoagulation
	(2) Continuing angina related to ischaemic recipient myocardium (rare)
	(3) Risk of infection and/or thrombus formation in relation to presence of valve prosthesis in recipient heart. This is a contraindication to heterotopic heart transplantation
	(4) Haemodynamically significant dysrhythmias of the recipient heart requiring high doses of antiarrhythmic agents

a period of time. This unique advantage of patient survival despite reversible or irreversible loss of donor heart function is documented below.

ADVANTAGES

1. Recipient heart acts as built-in cardiac assist device

Excision of the recipient's left ventricle in orthotopic transplantation can be criticized on the basis that, although diseased to the extent that the cardiac output is significantly reduced, it can still maintain a systemic circulation that is compatible with a restricted life. The recipient heart may lend valuable support both during the immediate postoperative period when the donor organ is recovering from the ischaemia sustained during transfer, and during periods when donor heart function is reduced from severe acute rejection. Recipient heart support in these situations has been well documented[2-5].

(a) *Reversible loss of donor heart function*

(i) *During recovery from the donor heart ischaemic period.* Recipient heart assistance during recovery of the donor heart from the initial ischaemic arrest period during transfer was highlighted in our clinical experience with hypothermic perfusion storage and is discussed and illustrated in Chapter 5 (Figure 20.1). Many other hearts, however, excised from haemodynamically unstable, brain-dead donors, who might have undergone periods of hypotension, hypoxia and even cardiac arrest, have taken several hours to recover optimum function. This observation has stimulated us to investigate the factors that bring about haemodynamic instability, and methods of correcting them, a study which is continuing (Chapter 3). There is no doubt that a number of our patients would have died at operation from inadequate donor heart function if orthotopic transplantation had been performed. We have had no operative mortality following heterotopic transplantation.

(ii) *During severe acute rejection episodes.* A recent review revealed that 25% (ten of 40) of our patients immunosuppressed with azathioprine and methylprednisolone had suffered acute rejection episodes severe enough to result in temporary or permanent loss of effective donor heart function, despite heavily increased immunosuppressive therapy[4].

Evidence for loss of effective donor heart function is based on arterial pulse wave (Figure 20.2) and electrocardiographic observations, such as ventricular fibrillation, in all patients, and on radionuclide scanning, intracardiac pressure monitoring and angiography at the time of endomyocardial biopsy in some patients. A non-existent donor heart arterial pulse trace or a pressure wave that falls to less than 25% of that of the recipient heart—all recipient hearts clearly had extremely poor function, with ejection fractions of between 7% and 27%—is considered evidence that donor heart function alone is inadequate

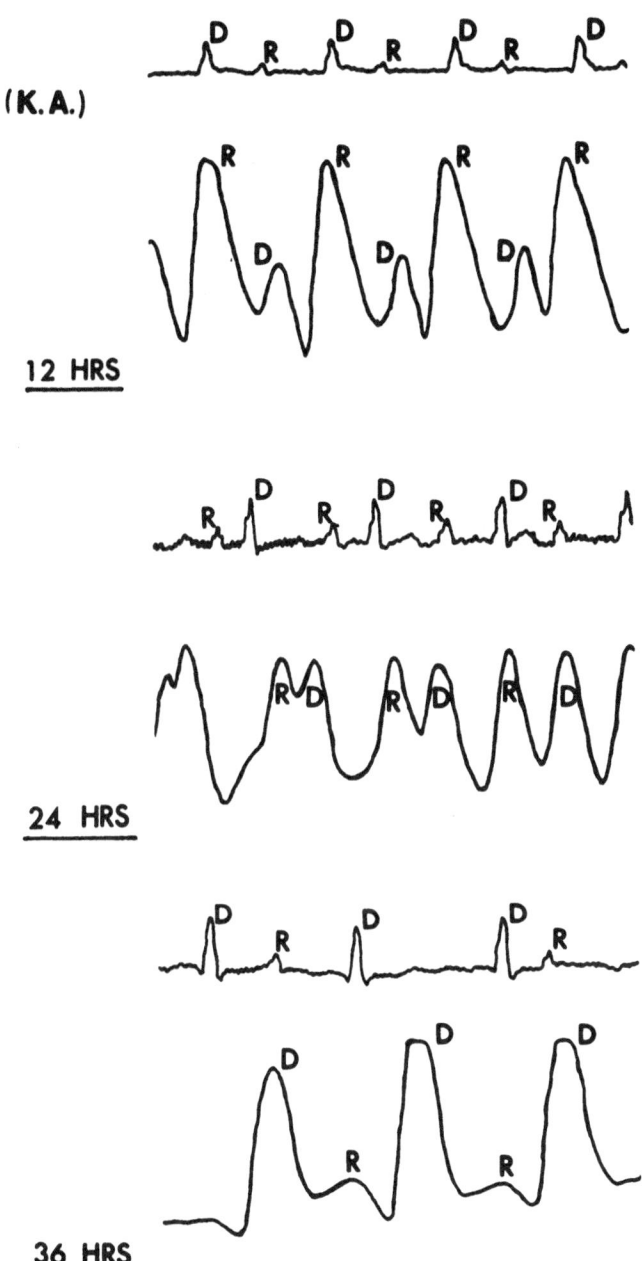

Figure 20.1 Diagram showing electrocardiogram (above) and femoral pulse trace (below) of donor (D) and recipient (R) hearts after heterotopic transplantation. Note the delayed recovery of the donor heart following transplantation after a 12-hour period of extracorporeal hypothermic perfusion storage

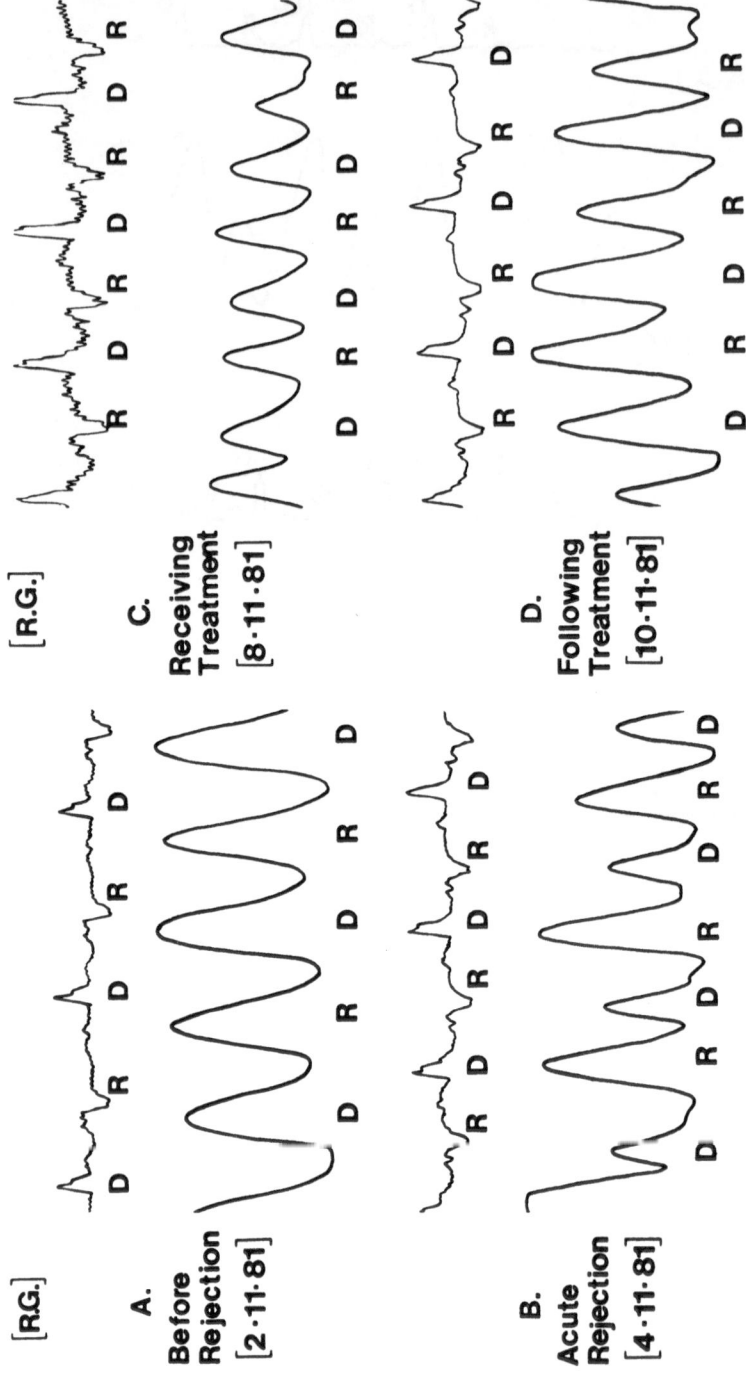

Figure 20.2 Diagram showing electrocardiogram (above) and femoral pulse trace (below) of donor (D) and recipient (R) hearts after heterotopic transplantation. Note the deterioration in the donor heart pulse in relation to the recipient heart pulse during an acute rejection episode, and the reversal of this trend following increased immunosuppressive therapy

to sustain a satisfactory circulation. It has been our experience that a good correlation exists between these observations of the arterial pulse trace and those of donor heart function made by radionuclide scanning and by direct haemodynamic studies at catheterization. When donor heart function deteriorates to this degree, these patients almost invariably require continuous inotropic support to sustain recipient heart output, which provides further evidence of the extreme deterioration in heart function.

Five of the ten patients who lost effective donor heart function during a severe acute rejection episode subsequently recovered full function (Table 20.2).

In one of these patients (case 1), who temporarily discontinued his medication, rejection progressed to the extent that the transplanted ventricles fibrillated[2]; electrical defibrillation and heavy immunosuppressive therapy were successful in restoring donor heart function. The patient remains alive and fully active 8 years later. Such a sequence of events could not have occurred, of course, if the patient had initially undergone orthotopic transplantation.

A second patient (case 5) developed acute rejection only 5 days after transplantation[5]. Despite heavy intravenous therapy with steroids and rabbit antithymocite globulin, severe rejection persisted. After 8 days of intensive therapy with no evidence of the return of donor heart function, cyclosporin A (CYA) (18 mg/kg per day) was added to the regimen. As all other therapy was continued for a further 7 days, we remain uncertain as to the exact role CYA played in the reversal of this rejection episode, though there was evidence of recovery of donor heart function within this period; after a further 14 days the donor heart was again the major support of the circulation. He has been maintained on a CYA and low-dose methylprednisolone regimen and has not suffered a further rejection episode during the 8 months that have elapsed.

(b) *Irreversible loss of donor heart function*

(i) *Following severe acute rejection.* Five patients suffered irreversible acute rejection that did not respond to intensive immunosuppression (Table 20.3). If there was no sign of significant reversal of the rejection episode after administration of a maximum of approximately 15 g of methylprednisolone, our policy has been to accept permanent loss of graft function rather than risk the increasing chance of infection. All immunosuppressive drugs were discontinued, except methylprednisolone 20 mg/day orally to prevent symptoms of toxicity from donor myocardial necrosis; retransplantation was then carried out if a suitable donor could be found.

Patients have survived for periods of up to approximately $2\frac{1}{2}$ years supported solely by their own hearts before undergoing retransplantation[6], though the quality of their lives has been extremely poor as they remained in New York Heart Association functional class 4. The continuous presence of the

Table 20.2　Details of five patients in whom donor heart function was reversibly lost during an acute rejection episode

Case	Age	Underlying cardiac pathology	Period after transplant of loss of donor heart function	Donor–recipient arterial pulse ratio (%)	Maximum endomyocardial biopsy score during rejection episode	Total intravenous methyl-prednisolone received	Number of days of loss of donor heart function	Clinical course and outcome
1	25	CM	10 months	0/100 (Donor heart in V.F.)	Inadequate specimen obtained	4 g	6	No further major episodes of acute rejection. Recovered excellent donor heart function. Alive and well at 7 years
2	36	CM	3 months	25/75	7.5	4 g	2	Recovered excellent donor heart function. Died from pneumonia at 8 months
3	32	CM	15 days	0/100	3.5 (after 4 g MP)	10 g	2	Suffered two further acute rejection episodes. Recovered excellent donor heart function until affected by early chronic rejection. Died from chronic rejection at 6 months
4	49	CM	31 days	25/75	4.5	8 g	3	Suffered a total of four acute rejection episodes. Recovered excellent donor heart function. Died at 10 months from tuberculous meningitis
5	47	CM	5 days	0/100	5.5 (after 8 g MP)	14 g (cyclosporin A added to regimen)	13	Recovered excellent donor heart function. No further rejection episodes. Alive and well at 8 months

CM = cardiomyopathy
VF = ventricular fibrillation
MP = methylprednisolone

Table 20.3 Details of five patients in whom donor heart function was irreversibly lost from acute rejection

Case	Age	Underlying cardiac pathology	Period after transplant of loss of donor heart function	Maximum endomyocardial biopsy score during rejection episode	Total intravenous methyl-prednisolone received	Clinical course and outcome
1	44	IHD	1 yr 5 d	5.0	2 g (Refused further therapy)	Recipient heart supported him for 5 months 16 days. Retransplanted. Died at 22 d from septicaemia
2	26	CM	(1) 36 d (2) 5 d	6.5	10 g	Recipient heart supported him for 2 years 7 months 14 days. Retransplanted. Suffered accelerated acute rejection. Recipient heart supported him for further 1 y 5 m 6 d. Strong circulating cytotoxic antibodies precluded a third transplant. Died from underlying disease (CM)
3	45	IHD	35 d	4.0 (Subsequent biopsy inadequate)	9 g	Retransplanted after 2 days' recipient heart support. Died at 3 months 3 days from pneumonia
4	31	IHD	36 d	7.0 (after 9 g MP)	9 g	Recipient heart supported him for 58 d. Died awaiting second donor
5	36	CM	25 d	6.0	16 g	Recipient heart supported him for 15 d. Retransplanted. Alive and well at 9 months

CM = cardiomyopathy
IHD = ischaemic heart disease
MP = methylprednisolone

patient's own heart has prolonged their lives and given them the opportunity to benefit from retransplantation, even though the ultimate outcome has not always been successful.

In our opinion the ten patients presented above would have died at the time of the severe acute rejection episode if they had undergone orthotopic rather than heterotopic heart transplantation. To date, none of the patients in our series has died at the time of an acute rejection episode, though one has died subsequently whilst awaiting a second donor following loss of donor heart function. Acute rejection has accounted for approximately half of the patients who have died at a number of centres[7-9]. We believe that the mortality from this complication would have been considerably reduced in these centres if heterotopic heart transplantation had been performed.

The ultimate results in this group of patients, however, are poor. Only two of the five patients who experienced reversible loss of donor heart function remain alive. Two of the remaining three died of infection, though at some considerable time interval after the acute rejection episode. It therefore seems unlikely that the occurrence of infection resulted directly from the increased immunosuppression necessary to overcome the rejection episode. It may be, however, that patients with heterotopic heart transplants receive greater total doses of immunosuppressive therapy (in an effort to reverse a rejection crisis) than those with orthotopic transplants, who might well have died before the crisis could have been brought under control. Theoretically, these patients may therefore be at a greater risk from infection in view of their heavily immunocompromised state. For the same reason, a greater incidence of malignant tumours might also be expected, though this has not proved to be the case (Chapter 14).

Of the five patients in this study who suffered irreversible loss of donor heart function, one died awaiting a second donor heart and four were retransplanted, though only one of the retransplanted patients remains alive today. The survival of one patient for 31 months between loss of donor heart function and retransplantation, and for a further 17 months following accelerated rejection of the second donor heart, draws attention to the difficulty of assessing prognosis with regard to longevity in patients with advanced myocardial disease. The presence of strong circulating cytotoxic antibodies precluded a third transplant in this patient[6].

Donor heart function may be lost when a severe acute rejection episode is not extreme, this has been exemplified in the present study by the findings of endomyocardial biopsy scores of as low as 4.5, even though the available evidence was that the donor heart was not contributing to the circulation. This observation has been further supported by studies in our experimental laboratories of orthotopic transplantation in baboons, where occasional histopathological scores of as low as 2.5 (moderate acute rejection) were obtained from hearts examined after death, for which no cause other than acute rejection could be found to account for the animal's demise[4]; it is hypothesized that cellular infiltration and oedema of the myocardium and, in particular, of the conducting system may lead to the onset of ventricular fibrillation.

(ii) *Following chronic or acute-on-chronic rejection.* We have also observed the survival of three patients for periods up to 5 months after permanent loss of donor heart function from chronic or acute-on-chronic rejection (Table 20.4). This phenomenon is less common, as the natural course of cardio-myopathy and ischaemic heart disease is for the heart to continue deteriorating further during the months following heterotopic heart transplantation; by the time donor heart function is lost from advanced chronic rejection, the recipient heart is no longer able to support the circulation.

Table 20.4 Details of three patients in whom donor heart function was irreversibly lost from chronic or acute-on-chronic rejection

Case	Age	Underlying cardiac pathology	Period after transplant of loss of donor heart function	Clinical course and outcome
1	42	IHD	2 years 9 months	Survived 1 month after donor heart failure. Died awaiting retransplantation
2	34	IHD	1 year 2 months	Survived 4 months after donor heart failure. Retransplanted. Alive and well 2 years 9 months later
3	52	IHD	9 months	Survived 5 months. Died awaiting retransplantation

IHD = ischaemic heart disease

One patient (Table 20.4, case 1), however, though requiring intermittent inotropic support, remained alive for 4 months until a second donor was obtained; he remains alive 2½ years after retransplantation and over 4 years since his original transplant operation. One other patient survived for 5 months following loss of donor heart function from chronic rejection but died before a suitable donor was found.

In heavily populated areas where a donor heart can be obtained within a few days, retransplantation for chronic rejection can be planned before donor heart function is lost. Any extra period of survival, whilst the patient is supported solely by his own heart, is therefore of less importance than when there is a relatively sudden loss of donor heart function associated with the onset of severe acute rejection. In areas where the acquisition of donor hearts is difficult and patients may have to wait several weeks or months for a suitable donor organ, however, the extra time provided by the presence of a functioning recipient heart may be life-saving.

(c) *When the donor heart is very small*

A further situation in which the recipient heart may give life-sustaining support is when the donor heart is particularly small, for example when obtained from a small child. The donor heart alone may be inadequate to sustain the necessary cardiac output, but, together with that of the recipient, the combined cardiac output may be satisfactory.

Though we have not met this exact situation, we have performed orthotopic transplantation in a patient with an existing heterotopic transplant for this reason[10]. The small second donor heart quickly supported the entire circulation, but the existing donor heart, though seriously diseased by graft arteriosclerosis, gave some support during the first 48 hours following operation.

The Stanford group has also performed heterotopic transplantation for this reason on one occasion[11], though again the small donor heart soon supported the full circulation. Heterotopic transplantation has also been performed elsewhere when the donor heart was particularly small (M. Yacoub, personal communication, 1983).

When there is doubt regarding the adequacy of cardiac output of a small donor heart, heterotopic transplantation would appear to be indicated, particularly in the presence of a high pulmonary vascular resistance. The recipient heart may lend valuable support for some weeks or months whilst hypertrophy of the donor myocardium is occurring.

2. Allows for possible recovering of the recipient heart

The possibility that certain myocardial diseases may spontaneously resolve, or at least improve significantly, if enough time is allowed for the disease to run its natural course, has been confirmed in one of our patients. At the time of heterotopic transplantation a 22-year-old patient was virtually moribund from what was presumed to be viral myocarditis, requiring heavy inotropic support to maintain a circulation. During the first 3 postoperative months the patient's own heart recovered substantially, so much so that, when a severe acute rejection episode (and marked changes of early chronic rejection) intervened, it was felt safe to excise the donor heart rather than risk infection from heavy immunosuppression. Investigations performed during the following 3-year period showed that his myocardial function remained subnormal, but was sufficiently improved to allow him to attend college and lead a basically normal life (in New York Heart Association class 2). There is no doubt that the support given by the heterotopic transplant averted death when he was critically ill. He died suddenly during the fourth year.

This patient remains unique in our experience. More commonly, the cardiomyopathic recipient heart tends to deteriorate slowly in function over the months following a successful heart transplant, until the circulation is supported entirely by the donor heart.

There is some evidence suggesting that even a short period of support by a satisfactorily functioning donor heart can lead to improved performance temporarily by the recipient heart. For example, one 36-year-old man with cardiomyopathy (Table 20.3, case 5) required complete bedrest and a continuous intravenous inotropic infusion to maintain a systolic arterial pressure of 80 mmHg before transplantation. He suffered early irreversible acute rejection, and 25 days after transplantation all immunosuppressive therapy (except 20 mg methylprednisolone daily) was discontinued. By this time, however, function of his own heart had improved to the state where he could be up and about in his hospital room all day. He required no inotropic support, maintaining a systolic pressure of approximately 100 mmHg and good peripheral perfusion. He remained in this stable condition for 15 days, at which time he underwent retransplantation; he remains alive and well 1 year later, supported almost entirely by the donor heart.

The phenomenon that a recipient heart dependent on inotropic drugs can, after as short a period as 3–4 weeks' support by a donor heart, support the circulation itself once again without inotropic therapy, warrants comment. It can probably be ascribed to a marked improvement in the fluid and electrolyte balance of the body brought about during the period of good cardiac output when the donor heart was functioning satisfactorily. This condition may be maintained for several weeks before the patient once again lapses into a state of gross failure, necessitating inotropic support, which may prove fatal should a second donor not be found quickly. In cardiomyopathic patients, the effect of immunosuppressive therapy on the original disease process cannot be excluded as a possible factor in the observed improvement in myocardial function.

3. Can be performed in the presence of a high pulmonary vascular resistance

The recipient's own right ventricle is often normal or only slightly diseased or, in some cases of longstanding left ventricular failure, hypertrophied in response to a raised pulmonary vascular resistance (PVR). It is unnecessary— indeed, unwise—to excise such a ventricle, as in orthotopic transplantation, since in the presence of an elevated PVR this may throw an acute burden on the donor right ventricle, which it may be unable to meet. It is generally accepted that a PVR of more than 30% of the systemic resistance, or of 8 Wood units, is an absolute contraindication to orthotopic transplantation. Observations have shown, however, that a high PVR in patients with advanced myocardial disease may be at least partly reversible, and that a significant fall in PVR may be observed after transplantation[12, 13]. The degree of reversibility can frequently be predicted before transplantation by recording the PVR both before and during the administration of 100% oxygen or of tolazoline or sodium nitroprusside[13], all of which may bring about a marked fall in PVR in patients with a large reactive component. If it has not already led to recipient right ventricular failure, residual pulmonary hypertension poses no danger to the heterotopically transplanted patient's life or to his speedy postoperative recovery; the patient's own hypertrophied right ventricle can accommodate these elevated pressures and continue to support the right-sided circulation, at least during the immediate postoperative period. If the recipient right ventricle is already showing signs of failure, however, it is unlikely that heterotopic transplantation will be successful.

This theoretical advantage has not been tested fully on many occasions, though we do have one patient alive and well 8 years after heterotopic transplantation who had a PVR of 8 units at the time of operation, and who was clearly unsuitable for orthotopic transplantation. The observations of the Columbia group[13], however, with regards to the reversibility of a high PVR in many cases, have reduced this indication for heterotopic transplantation.

DISADVANTAGES

1. Risk of emboli from thrombus formation in the poorly contracting recipient heart

The presence of a poorly contracting recipient left ventricle leads to a risk of systemic emboli from thrombus forming in the chamber. All patients, therefore, require long-term anticoagulation with warfarin sodium, together with antiplatelet agents, in an effort to avert this complication. In our experience, however, systemic emboli are relatively rare, and in nearly all cases occur in patients who are less than meticulous in attending for anticoagulation control and in taking warfarin sodium regularly. This complication led, however, to the death of one patient 2 years after transplantation, though the patient's non-compliance with regard to maintaining strict anticoagulation therapy was a significant factor.

Pulmonary emboli, possibly from similar clot formation in the right ventricle, have been documented in one patient, but it is possible that small emboli have gone undetected in other patients.

We have also seen both pulmonary and systemic emboli in patients with orthotopic transplants. Pulmonary emboli may arise from deep vein thrombosis in a patient with a poor circulation, and systemic emboli may arise from thrombus in a poorly contracting left ventricle that may be affected by either acute or chronic rejection.

2. Continuing angina from ischaemia of the recipient heart

Slight chest pains have recurred in two patients who underwent heterotopic transplantation for intractable angina. These pains, however, have been easily controlled by minimal medical treatment. Though the coronary atheroma remains in the recipient heart, the transfer of major responsibility for the circulation to the donor heart greatly diminishes the oxygen requirements of the recipient myocardium; continuing angina is therefore rarely a problem.

In four additional patients, coordinated contractions of the recipient heart have ceased altogether several months or years after heterotopic transplantation. One of the patients experienced a massive myocardial infarction of the recipient heart, which was associated with ventricular fibrillation, approximately 3 months after transplantation. During this episode the donor organ maintained a stable pressure, even though the patient experienced most of the symptoms of an infarction, including pain and diaphoresis. The patient led a normal life for a further year until he died of pneumonia. We have not noticed any prolonged morbidity or permanent disability resulting from the patient's own heart being left *in situ*, even when the heart is no longer functioning.

3. Risk of infection and/or thrombus formation when a valve prosthesis is present in the recipient heart (Absolute contraindication to heterotopic transplantation)

As a result of our experience with a patient who underwent left ventricular (rather than biventricular) bypass, we now believe that the presence of a prosthetic valve in the recipient heart, which might act as a source of systemic emboli or as a site for bacterial endocarditis, is an absolute contraindication to heterotopic transplantation[14].

This heterotopically transplanted patient developed a *Staphylococcus aureus* endocarditis on an aortic valve prosthesis in his own heart. Cardiac

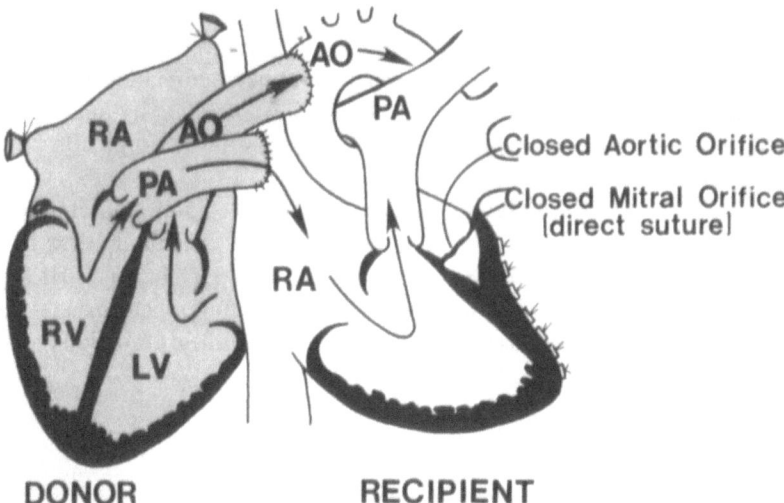

Figure 20.3 Diagram of circulation of a patient who underwent left ventricular bypass and subsequent recipient left ventriculectomy

catheterization showed that the prosthesis was not opening, probably because of thrombus. In an effort to remove the source of infection and potential systemic emboli, as well as to excise the focus of the recurrent episodes of ventricular tachycardia that he was also experiencing, the prosthesis was excised, the aortic root closed with the anterior leaflet of the mitral valve, the mitral valve orifice closed by direct suture, and left ventriculectomy performed (Figure 20.3)[14]. This operative therapy was successful and the patient remains alive and well over 8 years later.

The circulation is unusual in that the patient retains his own right ventricle, which supports his pulmonary circulation. The donor right ventricle returns only its own coronary venous return to the circulation. His systemic circulation is supported only by the donor left ventricle, since his own left ventricle was excised.

A prosthesis in the recipient heart may become immobile if the donor heart is functioning satisfactorily. The risk of thrombus formation with resulting systemic emboli is then extremely high. This complication has been reported to us from another centre (M. Yacoub, personal communication, 1983). A second patient in our own series has recently undergone orthotopic transplantation in view of the presence in his own heart of an aortic valve prosthesis.

4. Haemodynamically significant dysrhythmias of the recipient heart requiring high doses of antiarrhythmic agents

Several patients with advanced myocardial disease, regardless of the underlying primary pathology, exhibit troublesome dysrhythmias requiring antiarrhythmic agents. The majority of these dysrhythmias can be ignored as the heterotopically transplanted donor heart is unaffected and can support the circulation alone. In one patient, however, continuing paroxysmal dysrhythmias of the recipient heart caused significant haemodynamic instability, with hypotension. The administration of large doses of antiarrhythmic agents failed to control these dysrhythmias, and also further affected function of the donor heart.

It is not clear why dysrhythmias in this patient affected donor heart output. The hypotension led to renal failure, and the patient eventually died from multisystem failure. At necropsy, all anastomoses between the two hearts were widely patent, and there did not appear to be any anatomical reason why failure of the recipient heart should have affected donor heart function during a dysrhythmic episode.

CONCLUSIONS

Given the various advantages and disadvantages of both heterotopic and orthotopic transplantation, we have felt that, on balance, the advantages have outweighed the disadvantages under the circumstances that have existed at our own centre during the past 10 years. If cyclosporin A (or its descendants), however, continues to show its early promise in reducing the number and severity of acute rejection episodes, then one of the major advantages of heterotopic transplantation may be minimized. Orthotopic heart transplantation may then clearly be the operation of choice in the majority of patients.

References

1. Barnard, C. N. and Cooper, D. K. C. (1984). Heterotopic versus orthotopic heart transplantation. *Transplant Proc.* (In press)
2. Barnard, C. N., Losman, J. G., Curcio, C. A., Sanchez, H. E. and Wolpowitz, A. (1977). The advantage of heterotopic cardiac transplantation over orthotopic cardiac transplantation in the management of severe acute rejection. *J. Thorac. Cardiovasc. Surg.*, **74**, 918
3. Wicomb, W. N., Cooper, D. K. C., Novitzky, D. and Barnard, C. N. (1984). Cardiac transplantation following storage of the donor heart by a portable hypothermic perfusion system. *Ann. Thorac. Surg.*, **37**, 243
4. Novitzky, D., Cooper, D. K. C., Rose, A. G. and Barnard, C. N. (1984). The value of recipient heart assistance during severe acute rejection following heterotopic cardiac transplantation. *J. Cardiovasc. Surg.* (In press)
5. Novitzky, D., Cooper, D. K. C. and Barnard, C. N. (1984). Reversal of acute rejection by cyclosporin A in a heterotopic heart transplant. *Heart Transplant.*, **3**, 117
6. Lanza, R. P., Campbell, E. M., Cooper, D. K. C., Du Toit, E. D. and Barnard, C. N. (1983). The problem of the presensitized heart transplant recipient. *Heart Transplant.*, **2**, 151
7. Cabrol, C., Gandjbakch, I., Pavie, A., Cabrol, A., Mattei, M. F., Lienhart, A., Gluckman, J. C. and Rottembourg, J. (1983). Cardiac transplantation at La Pitié Hospital. *Heart Transplant.*, **2**, 244
8. Hess, M. L., Hastillo, A., Goldman, M., Rider, S., Mohanakumar, T., Ducey, K., Wolfgang, T., Szentpetery, S. and Lower, R. (1983). Cardiac transplantation at the Medical College of Virginia. *Heart Transplant.*, **2**, 246
9. Copeland, J., Fuller, J., Sailor, J. and McAleer, M. J. (1983). Heart transplantation at the Health Sciences Center of the University of Arizona. *Heart Transplant.*, **2**, 246
10. Novitzky, D., Cooper, D. K. C. and Barnard, C. N. (1984). Orthotopic heart transplantation in a patient with a heterotopic heart transplant. *Heart Transplant.*, **3**, 257
11. Melvin, K. R., Pollick, C., Hunt, S. A., McDougall, R., Goris, M. L., Oyer, P., Popp, R. L. and Stinson, E. B. (1982). Cardiovascular physiology in a case of heterotopic cardiac transplantation. *Am. J. Cardiol.*, **49**, 1301
12. Losman, J. G., Levine, H., Campbell, C. D., Replogle, R. L., Hassoulas, J., Novitzky, D., Cooper, D. K. C. and Barnard, C. N. (1982). Changes in indications for heart transplantation. *J. Thorac. Cardiovasc. Surg.*, **84**, 716
13. Pucillo, A. L., Reison, D. S., Rose, E. A., Drusin, R. E., Reemtsma, K. and Powers, E. R. (1983). Reversibility of elevated pulmonary vascular resistance after cardiac transplantation. (Abstract) *J. Am. Coll. Cardiol.*, **1**, 72
14. Losman, J. G., Curcio, C. A. and Barnard, C. N. (1978). Normal cardiac function with a hybrid heart. *Ann. Thorac. Surg.*, **26**, 177

21
Transplantation of the Heart and Both Lungs

INTRODUCTION

Transplantation of the heart and both lungs as a form of therapy is clearly still in its infancy. Most groups which have performed the operation have not yet overcome the considerable technical difficulties involved. For the foreseeable future, the number of patients submitted to this procedure will remain small, largely as a result of the strict selection requirements for potential donors. In recent years, however, an improved understanding of the blood supply of the trachea and bronchi has resulted in a better prospect of satisfactory healing at the site of the airway anastomosis. The introduction of cyclosporin A has allowed control of the acute rejection process without the need for corticosteroid therapy during the first 2–3 weeks. These recent advances, largely the work of the Stanford group, will almost certainly lead to an improved outlook for selected patients with pulmonary vascular disease, various advanced pulmonary diseases, and complex developmental abnormalities of the heart and lungs.

EXPERIMENTAL BACKGROUND

The early experimental work in this field has been reviewed fully elsewhere[1,2]. Although attempts to transplant the heart and lungs into the neck were made as early as 1907[3], and into the abdomen in 1951[4], it was Demikhov who made the first attempt to carry out orthotopic transplantation of these organs in the late 1940s and early 1950s[5]. Demikhov achieved survival for up to 6 days, death resulting mainly from thrombosis at the sites of blood vessel anastomosis, or from bronchopneumonia in the lower lobes.

With the advent of supportive techniques, such as hypothermia and cardiopulmonary bypass, further attempts were made in 1953 by Neptune et al.[6] and in 1957 by Webb and Howard[7], though in all cases the bronchi were the site of airway anastomosis. Lower et al. (1961)[8] and Longmore and his colleagues (1968)[9] introduced simplified techniques in which the trachea was the site of anastomosis, which have been the basis for the recent successful clinical attempts of transplantation of the heart and both lungs.

The results in the dog were poor, and there is evidence that this animal requires the presence of afferent pathways from the lungs to maintain spontaneous breathing[1, 9]. Primates, however, appear to tolerate total denervation of the lungs and do not require the Herring–Breuer reflex as the dog does[10]; spontaneous respiration, controlled by the midbrain, is preserved.

EARLY CLINICAL EXPERIENCE

Single lung transplantation

The results of transplantation of a single lung, with anastomoses of pulmonary artery, left atrial cuff, and bronchus, have been extremely disappointing[11]. Hardy was the first to carry out this operation clinically in 1963[12]. By 1980, 38 such transplants had been performed, with a mean survival of only 8.5 days; two patients survived for 6 and 10 months respectively[11]. Most of the deaths occurred from complications of the bronchial anastomosis, with necrosis of the bronchial stump and dehiscence of the suture line[13–15]. The second major complication was pneumonia. The differentiation between acute rejection, reimplantation response[16], and infection was, and remains, difficult, and may, on occasion, be impossible[14].

Strong evidence that a major limiting factor preventing the success of single lung transplantation is an inadequate blood supply to the bronchial stump was put forward by Haglin et al.[17]. Their patient underwent bilateral lung transplantation. A bronchial artery from the donor aorta was preserved for the left lung and reimplanted in the recipient's aorta. Due to technical difficulties, the right bronchus was not revascularized in this way. Eleven days later the patient died from septicaemia and pulmonary insufficiency. The postmortem findings showed the right bronchus to have necrotic changes, while the left bronchus was entirely normal. This problem of maintaining an adequate blood supply to the bronchus is minimized when the heart and both lungs are transplanted in a single unit as a block, preserving the carina and both bronchi intact. The blood supply to the airway from small branches of the coronary arteries in the region of the bare area of the heart is retained[18].

A second major advantage of this technique is that acute rejection of the lung and myocardium frequently occur together[19], and therefore pulmonary rejection can be strongly suspected by the findings of endomyocardial biopsy[20]. In all the earlier patients undergoing single lung transplantation conventional immunosuppression was used. The introduction of cyclosporin A and a concomitant reduction in the use of corticosteroids has improved the chances of bronchial healing[21]. In single lung transplantation, however, bronchial ischaemia remains a major factor in the failure of the operation.

Transplantation of the heart and both lungs

This operation was first performed clinically by Cooley on 31 August 1968[22]. The patient was a 2-month-old infant with a complete atrioventricular canal defect, pulmonary hypertension and pneumonia. The patient required re-opening for bleeding, and died 14 hours after the initial transplant operation. In December 1969, Lillehei performed the second such operation on a 43-year-old patient with emphysema and pulmonary hypertension[23]; the patient survived 8 days, dying from pneumonia.

The third operation was performed at our own institution in Cape Town in July 1971[24,25]. Details of this patient have been reported elsewhere, and only a brief summary will be presented here. The patient was a 49-year-old man with chronic respiratory failure from longstanding airways disease and bronchiectasis. By 1970 he had become bedridden, requiring oxygen therapy, and anti-failure therapy for cor pulmonale. The donor heart was intermittently perfused with blood from the recipient's cardiopulmonary bypass machine throughout the surgical procedure (Figure 21.1). Anastomoses were performed, in turn, between the donor and recipient bronchi, right atria, and aortae. The bronchi, rather than the trachea, were chosen as the site of anastomosis of the air passages, as it was believed at that time that this would preserve both the blood supply to the carina and the cough reflex at the carinal area more satisfactorily.

The patient recovered satisfactorily from the operation and was extubated within 20 hours. Immunosuppression was with azathioprine and corticosteroids. On the 8th postoperative day a right pneumothorax developed and, at right thoracotomy, a bronchopleural fistula on the posterior aspect of the bronchial anastomosis was repaired and covered with an intercostal flap; the air leak ceased. By the 18th day, however, the patient showed features of a right upper and middle lobe pneumonia, and the pneumothorax recurred. A second thoracotomy was performed, at which complete necrosis of the mucosa of the donor right bronchus was found, necessitating pneumonectomy. The patient tolerated this procedure moderately well, but developed a septicaemia and died on the 23rd day. Autopsy showed bronchopneumonia of the left lung, pericarditis, mediastinitis and meningitis, but no significant rejection of the transplanted organs. The cause of death was considered to be a klebsiella pneumonia and septicaemia.

It was not until another 10 years had elapsed that a fourth transplant of heart and lungs was performed, on this occasion at Stanford University[26]. The availability of an improved immunosuppressive regimen, including cyclosporin A[27], the better understanding of the reimplantation syndrome[28], the availability of endomyocardial biopsy to diagnose acute rejection[20, 28], and an improved understanding of the blood supply of the trachea and bronchi[28], resulted in the first long-term survival of such a patient.

INDICATIONS FOR HEART–LUNG TRANSPLANTATION

Though patients with a variety of pulmonary and cardiac disorders might be considered for heart and lung transplantation (Table 21.1), at the present time the operation is being restricted mainly to those with severe irreversible pulmonary vascular disease, either primary idiopathic or secondary to congenital heart disease (Eisenmenger's syndrome).

Table 21.1   Major indications for transplantation of the heart and both lungs

(1) *Cardiac*
    Cardiogenic pulmonary hypertension:
    (a) Congenital—Eisenmenger's syndrome
    (b) Acquired—high fixed pulmonary vascular resistance with right ventricular failure

(2) *Pulmonary*
    Primary (idiopathic) pulmonary hypertension
    End-stage chronic obstructive airways disease (emphysema)
    Interstitial pulmonary fibrosis (fibrosing alveolitis)
    Cystic fibrosis
    Toxic pneumonitis (e.g. Paraquat poisoning)

SELECTION OF THE RECIPIENT

The potential recipient must clearly have a severely restricted exercise tolerance and a life expectancy of less than 1 year[28]. He or she must otherwise fulfil the requirements for any patient being considered for cardiac transplantation, with the exception that a recent pulmonary infarction is not a contraindication for heart–lung transplantation. Patients requiring this operation are frequently within their third or fourth decades of life. They often have marked nutritional derangement, resulting from longstanding cardiac failure and hypoxaemia, and systemic hypoxaemia with an elevated haemoglobin and haematocrit. The onset of syncopal episodes or oxygen dependence indicate an extremely poor prognosis.

SELECTION OF THE DONOR

Selection criteria of the donor for heart and lung transplantation are much more strict than for heart transplantation alone. Probably only 25% of brain-dead donors can be used for donation of the heart and lungs[28], the remainder being excluded largely because of pulmonary problems. Potential donors have frequently undergone prolonged ventilation, and may have developed atelectasis or pulmonary infection. It is essential to exclude respiratory infection in such potential donors. The chest radiograph should be clear, with no evidence of pulmonary contusion or infection. Bronchial lavage is performed and microscopic examination carried out to exclude the presence of micro-organisms and pus cells; the presence of epithelial cells is considered normal.

The potential lungs should show good function. Simple tests, such as estimating the arterial blood gases with the donor ventilated temporarily on 100% oxygen, are carried out; the arterial PO_2 should rise above 350 mmHg under such conditions. Lung compliance should be shown to be normal for a normal tidal volume[28].

There must also be a close anatomical match between the sizes of the chest cavities of the potential recipient and donor. An excessively large lung placed

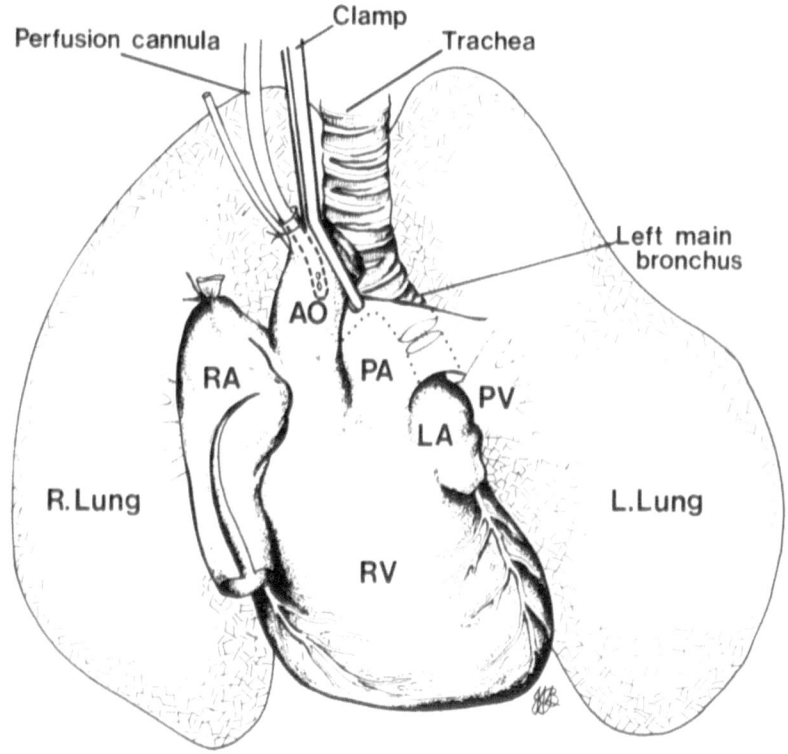

Figure 21.1   The donor organs as used in the Cape Town case (1971). Note transection of both bronchi. The donor aorta was perfused from the aortic line of the recipient cardiopulmonary bypass machine via a perfusion cannula inserted into the donor ascending aorta. RA = right atrium; RV = right ventricle; PA = pulmonary artery; PV = pulmonary vein; LA = left atrium; AO = aorta

in a small pleural cavity will be compressed, resulting in atelectasis and arteriovenous shunting[28]; there would be a high risk of infection in such atelectatic regions in an immunocompromised patient.

DONOR LUNG PRESERVATION

Methods of successfully preserving viable lung tissue during periods of ischaemia are still in their infancy. Experimental work has to date been disappointing. Flushing with a modified Collins' solution before storage by immersion in 4°C ice slush has not been shown to preserve lung integrity and function satisfactorily even after such a short period as 3 hours[29]. Maintaining lung inflation, flushing with and subsequently storing at 4°C in modified Sacks' solution has resulted in adequate short-term function of single canine lungs after periods of ischaemic storage ranging from 7 to 21 hours[30]. Flush cooling with cold blood followed by hypothermic storage has resulted in adequate storage for approximately 20 hours; these lungs showed minimal injury on light and electron microscopy, with normal ventilatory parameters and blood oxygenation during the first 24 hours after transplantation[31].

SURGICAL TECHNIQUE OF TRANSPLANTATION OF THE HEART AND BOTH LUNGS

As the preservation of lung tissue is unsatisfactory at the present time, the donor and recipient operations are performed simultaneously in adjacent theatres. Our own personal experience of this procedure is based on extensive experimental work in baboons (Novitzky et al., unpublished).

Anatomical considerations

The blood supply of the trachea is shared with that of the oesophagus and adjacent mediastinal tissues. It is derived from three major sources, between which there are poor collateral circulations. As a result, dissection of only 1–2 cm of trachea circumferentially may lead to ischaemic necrosis[32].

The upper portion of the trachea is supplied predominantly by branches of the inferior thyroid artery (Figure 21.2). The mid portion and carina derive blood directly from the bronchial arteries, which originate from the aorta. The bronchial collateral circulation around the hilum of the lung is fairly good, and permits segmental resection of the bronchus. The carina and both bronchi also receive small but important arteries which arise from the major coronary arteries, predominantly the left; small vessels penetrate the mediastinum in the region of the 'bare' area of the posterior aspect of the left atrium. (These arteries can be an important source of collateral blood supply to the

heart when both main coronary arteries are occluded at their origin[18, 33, 34].)
In their normal state the diameter of these vessels varies between 80 and
100 μm. Though in the normal subject they play but a small role in the blood
supply of the trachea, once the donor trachea has been transected for heart
and lung transplantation they become essential. They are crucial for adequate
healing at the tracheal suture line. The Stanford team has shown by angiography that after transplantation these arteries dilate and form a collateral
anastomotic network with branches from the descending bronchial arteries of
the recipient[28].

In patients with severe pulmonary hypertension, a further possible source
of blood supply to the bronchus is by retrograde flow from the pulmonary
artery, via a collateral circulation which develops with the bronchial arteries.
After transplantation, however, this pulmonary hypertension no longer exists
and any retrograde flow from the pulmonary artery will be negligible. The

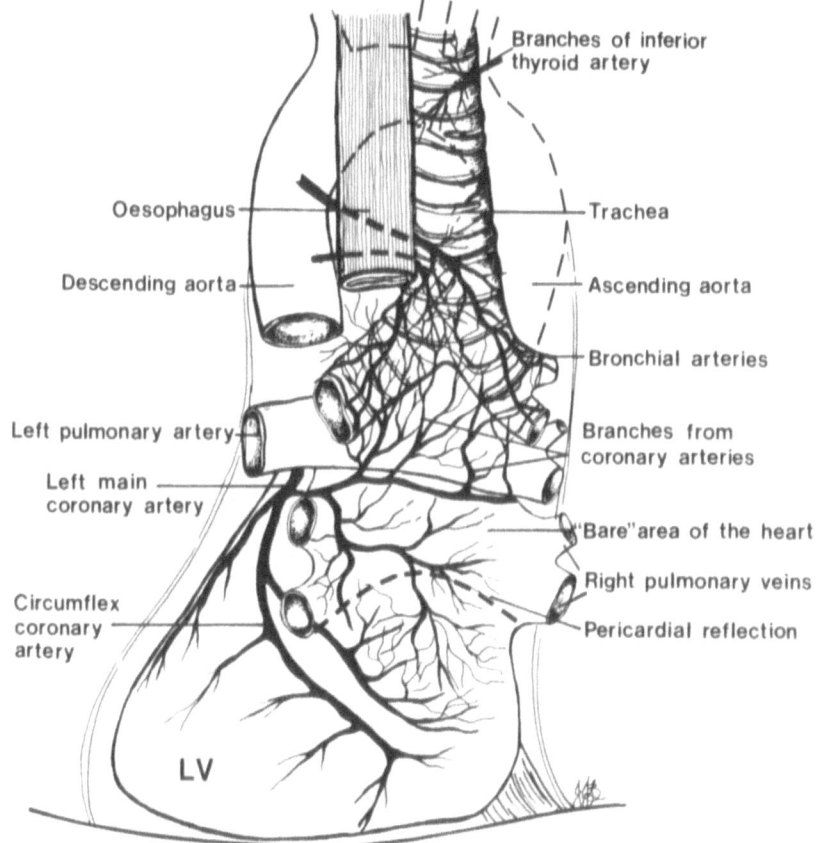

Figure 21.2 Posterior view of heart and trachea, showing blood supply to the trachea, carina
and bronchi. LV = left ventricle

absence of this retrograde supply may possibly contribute to a relative ischaemia and necrosis of the mucosa of the bronchus if the anastomosis is
performed at this level.

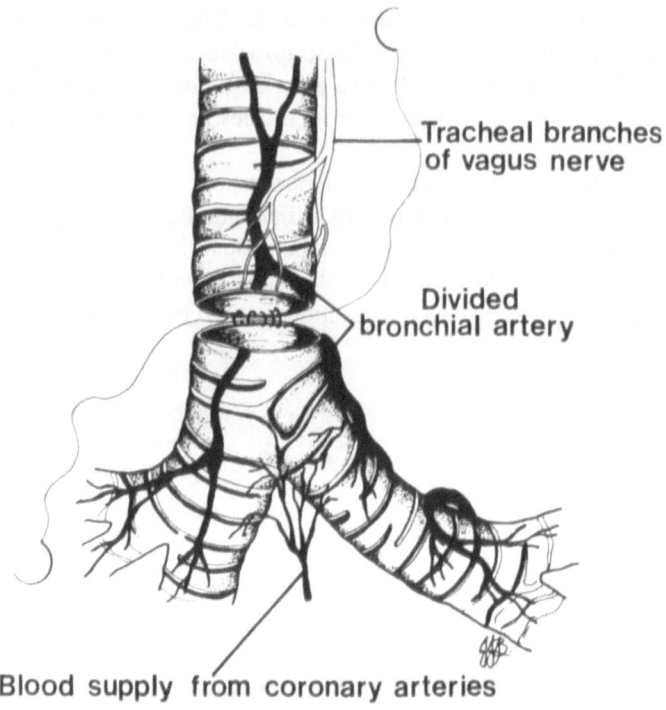

Tracheal branches
of vagus nerve

Divided
bronchial artery

Blood supply from coronary arteries

Figure 21.3   Donor trachea and bronchi, with transection above the carina, showing disruption
of the blood supply to the carina and bronchi from the bronchial arteries, and retention of the
blood supply from the coronary arteries

   To preserve the blood supply of the carina and bronchi from the coronary
arteries, it is essential to avoid dissection in the areolar fat tissue which is inter-
posed between the donor trachea and left atrium, through which these vessels
run. Retention of the carina in the donor heart–lung block would appear to be
advantageous as this blood supply from the coronary arteries is therefore
retained (Figure 21.3). The Stanford group has not reported significant air
leaks or dehiscence at the tracheal anastomosis in its series, suggesting that
there has been no significant ischaemia of the trachea following the transplant
operation. If the bronchi are used for the sites of anastomosis, as in our own
case in 1971 (Figure 21.4), the blood supply of the distal bronchus, derived
from both bronchial and coronary arteries, is divided, with a resulting high
risk of ischaemic necrosis at the suture line. The high incidence of this complication following single lung transplants is almost certainly for the same
reason.

Donor operation

Through a midline sternotomy the heart and ascending aorta are exposed. The superior vena cava is doubly ligated and divided proximal to the azygos vein, and the inferior vena cava clamped at the diaphragm and divided cephalad, thus decompressing the right side of the heart. The tip of the left atrial appendage is transected to decompress the left side of the heart. The aorta is then immediately cross-clamped at the level of the brachiocephalic artery, and cardioplegic solution infused into the root of the aorta. Cold saline is applied over the heart. Whilst the cardioplegic solution is still being infused, the pleuropericardium is incised on each side from the sternum to the hilum of the lung. The phrenic nerve is divided and the hilum dissected free. This dissection is extended posteriorly to mobilize the posterior aspect of the left atrium. The aorta is then transected at the level of the cross-clamp. The trachea is mobilized and transected superior to the carina. No attempt is made to mobilize the carina, thus preserving the blood supply from the coronary arteries. The donor heart and lungs can then be removed as a single block of tissue.

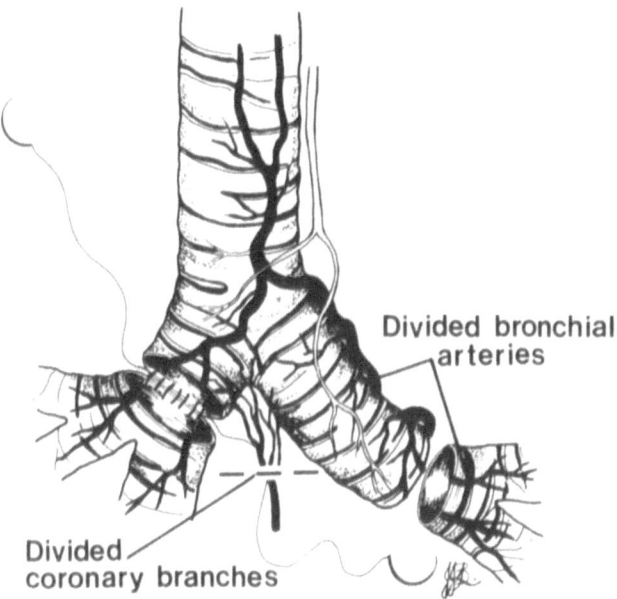

Divided bronchial arteries

Divided coronary branches

Figure 21.4 Donor trachea and bronchi, with transection at the level of the bronchi, showing disruption of both bronchial and coronary arterial supplies to the distal bronchi

These organs are placed in a bowl of cold saline, care being taken not to allow saline to run into the bronchial tree. An incision is made in the right atrium, beginning in the posterolateral aspect of the inferior vena caval orifice and extended up into the base of the right atrial appendage (as for orthotopic heart transplantation). The trachea is trimmed to within one or two cartilages of the carina. The heart and lungs are then transferred to the adjacent theatre for insertion into the recipient.

Recipient operation

Excision of the recipient organs

Through a midline sternotomy, cardiopulmonary bypass is initiated through an arterial cannula inserted into the aorta (at the origin of the brachiocephalic artery) and venous cannulae introduced through the lateral wall of the right atrium into both superior and inferior venae cavae. Snares are placed around both cavae, converting cardiopulmonary bypass to total bypass. Systemic cooling to reduce the body temperature to 20 °C is begun.

The aorta is cross-clamped proximal to the arterial cannula, and cardiectomy carried out as for orthotopic heart transplantation. Right and left pleural cavities are then entered through incisions in the pleuropericardium made parallel and posterior to the phrenic nerves, great care being taken to avoid any damage to these structures (Figure 21.5). Each lung can then be withdrawn through its corresponding pleuropericardial incision into the pericardial cavity. The right and left pulmonary arteries are divided, a cuff of pulmonary artery tissue being left *in situ* under the arch of the aorta to prevent

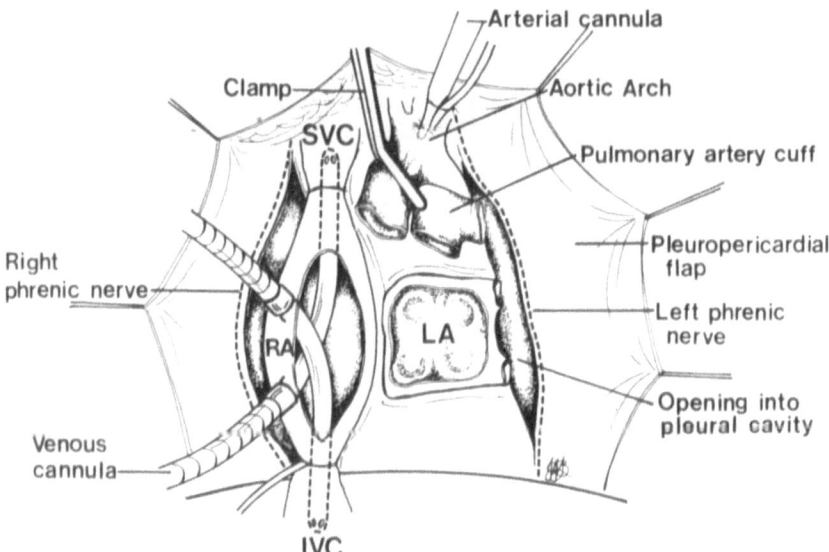

Figure 21.5 View of recipient pericardial cavity after resection of the recipient heart and lungs, showing the remnants of the right (RA) and left (LA) atria, aorta and pulmonary artery. The incisions in the pleuropericardium posterior to the right and left phrenic nerves are indicated

possible damage to the left recurrent laryngeal nerve. The pulmonary veins are transected close to the posterior wall of the left atrium. Great care is taken to obtain haemostasis in this region as it will be extremely difficult to examine at the end of the operation. The trachea is transected above the carina, a minimum of mobilization having been carried out (Figure 21.3). The two lungs can then be removed from the chest cavity. A further check is made to ensure that adequate haemostasis has been obtained.

The posterior pericardium is left intact where possible to avoid excessive dissection of the posterior mediastinum, and thus further reduce the risk of subsequent haemorrhage. In the dissection and division of the trachea, care must be exerted to prevent damage to the vagus nerve plexus which surrounds the oesophagus, or gastric dilatation and impaired pyloric function may result[35].

Implantation of the donor organs

The donor heart and lungs are then introduced into the pericardial cavity, each lung being passed through the respective opening in the pleuroperi-cardium, posterior to the phrenic nerve (Figure 21.6). The right lung is passed posterior to the remnant of the recipient right atrium. The recipient aorta and trachea are trimmed to the appropriate lengths. The recipient and donor tracheae are anastomosed using a continuous suture of 4/0 polypropylene. The lungs are gently inflated; cold saline is applied around the tracheal suture line to inspect for air leaks. If there is no leak, a few interrupted sutures are placed through the surrounding areolar fat tissue to further cover the anasto-mosis. The donor and recipient right atria are anastomosed using a con-tinuous suture of 5/0 polypropylene, as in the operation of orthotopic heart transplantation (Figure 21.7). Finally, the two aortae are anastomosed end-to-end, using a continuous suture of 4/0 polypropylene. Myocardial protec-tion is maintained throughout operation by the continuous or intermittent topical application of cold (4 °C) saline.

A vent is introduced into the left ventricle, either through the left atrial appendage, which is to be preferred, or through the ventricular apex. The caval snares are released and a needle introduced into the ascending aorta and pulmonary artery to evacuate air. The venous pressure is raised to facilitate the expulsion of air from the heart and lungs. The aortic cross-clamp is removed, thus reintroducing coronary artery perfusion to the donor heart. It is usually necessary to defibrillate the heart. The patient is rewarmed and, if haemodynamically stable, cardiopulmonary bypass is discontinued, and the various cannulae removed (Figure 21.8). Drains are introduced into the pericardial and pleural cavities, and the chest is closed.

In our experience in the experimental animal, the cardiopulmonary bypass time varies between 1 hour 30 minutes and 1 hour 50 minutes, the total ischaemic time of the graft being $\pm$ 45 minutes.

IMMEDIATE POSTOPERATIVE CARE AND MAINTENANCE IMMUNOSUPPRESSION

The immediate postoperative care is very similar to that of a patient who has undergone heart transplantation alone. The patient is nursed under isolation conditions, and is initially ventilated with a volume ventilator. The central venous pressure is kept low in an effort to prevent reimplantation response (*see below*). If the venous pressure should rise, diuresis is encouraged by drug therapy. Chest physiotherapy is extremely important to prevent atelectasis and clear secretions from the tracheobronchial tree. Suction of the tracheo-bronchial tree is, however, carried out with extreme care to prevent trauma to the tracheal suture line, and also to minimize the risk of introducing infection. In the Stanford experience it is usually possible to extubate the patient within the first 24–48 hours. Chest radiographs are carried out twice daily during the

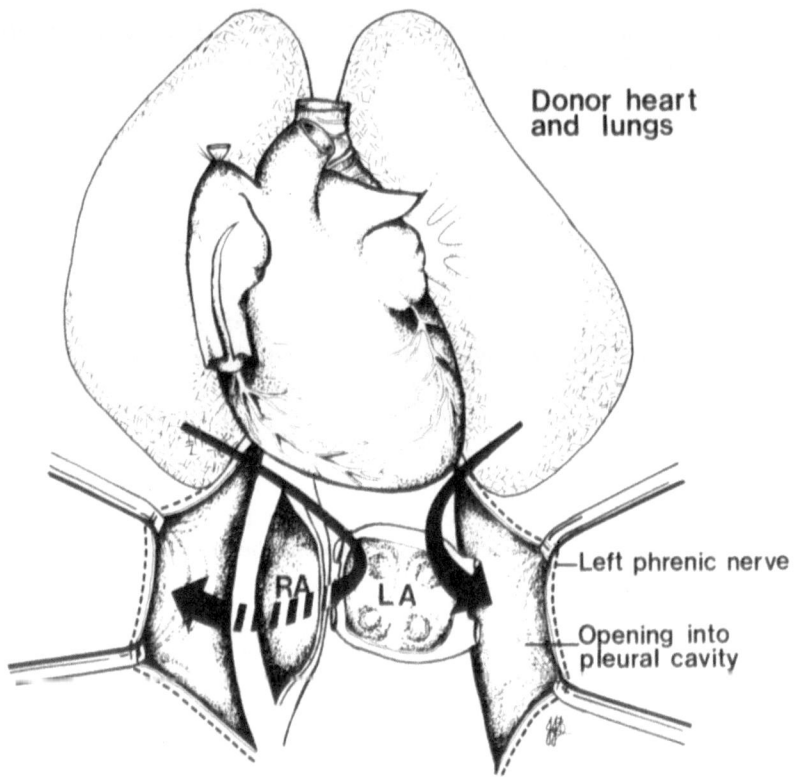

Figure 21.6   Insertion of donor heart and lungs into the recipient thorax. The remnants of the recipient right (RA) and left (LA) atria can be seen. The arrows indicate the route of insertion of the lungs into their respective pleural cavities. Note that both lungs pass posterior to the phrenic nerves and that, in addition, the right lung passes posterior to the recipient right atrium

first few days to detect any possible pneumothorax resulting from a tracheal leak. If no pneumothorax (or haemothorax) is present, it is usually possible to remove the pleural and pericardial drains on the second postoperative day, after which time the patient is actively mobilized.

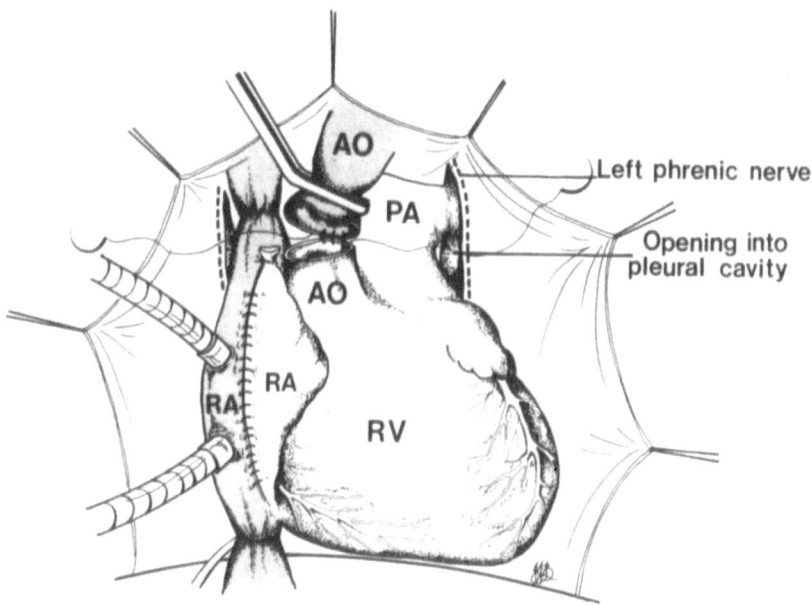

Figure 21.7   View of recipient pericardial cavity during insertion of the donor heart and lungs. The lungs have been positioned in their respective pleural cavities. The shaded area represents the remnants of the recipient's tissue. The right atrial anastomosis has been completed. The aortic anastomosis is in progress. RA = right atrium; RV = right ventricle; PA = pulmonary artery; AO = aorta

A major potential complication of the operation is a failure of the tracheal anastomosis to heal. It is therefore important not to depress fibroplastic activity during the first 2–3 weeks, and for this reason, corticosteroids are avoided unless a definite acute rejection episode has been diagnosed. The major components of the immunosuppressive regimen during this early period therefore consist of cyclosporin A and azathioprine. Methylprednisolone is administered as a single intravenous dose of 500 mg immediately after operation, followed by three further doses of 125 mg during the next 24 h period[27]. No further corticosteroids are administered during the following 2–3-week period, by which time satisfactory healing of the tracheal suture line should have occurred. To compensate partially for this lack of corticosteroid therapy, antithymocyte globulin may be given during the first 2–3 days[28].

Cyclosporin A is begun at 18 mg/kg per day, but reduced with the aim of maintaining a blood trough level of approximately 400 ng/ml, as for patients undergoing heart transplantation alone. Azathioprine dosage is adjusted to maintain a total white blood cell count of 3–5000 cells/mm³, and is usually of the order of 1.5 mg/kg per day. Unless there is evidence suggesting that the tracheal anastomosis has not healed satisfactorily, during the second or third week azathioprine is discontinued and methylprednisolone introduced in a dosage of 0.2–0.3 mg/kg per day[28]. If there is doubt with regard to the healing of the tracheal suture line, it is occasionally necessary to inspect this area by flexible bronchoscopy.

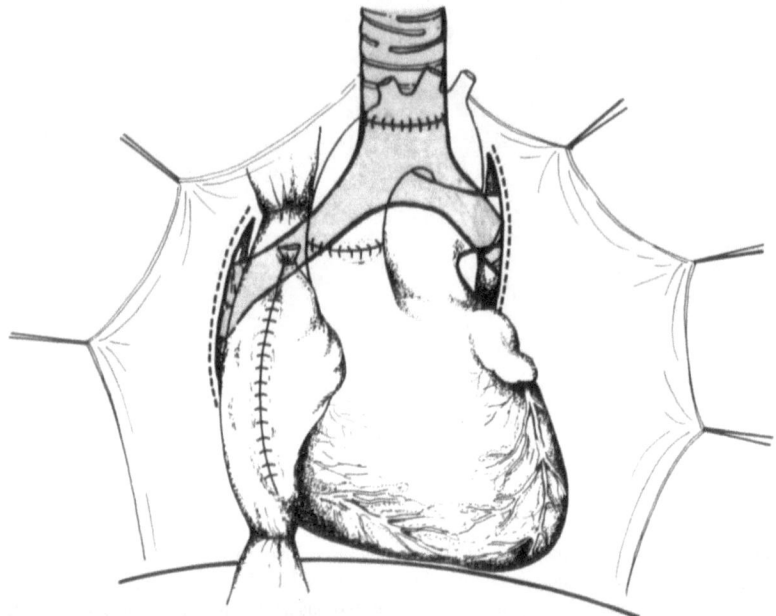

Figure 21.8 The completed operation. The three anastomoses (tracheal, right atrial, and aortic) are shown. The trachea and bronchi, which lie posterior to the other structures and which therefore cannot be seen from the anterior view, have been shaded

COMPLICATIONS

The complications of this operation clearly include those possible following open heart surgery, together with those relating to transplantation of the heart alone. Delayed or imperfect healing of the tracheal suture line has already been discussed. Any air leak with resultant pneumothorax should be treated with intercostal tube drainage; if this fails to correct the situation, further operation is indicated.

Technical

In the initial Stanford series, three of the first six patients required exploration for postoperative bleeding[35]. Haemorrhage may occur from posterior mediastinal dissection in the recipient during excision of the heart and lungs, but also from bleeding points on the donor organs which have been implanted. Retention of the posterior wall of the left atrium has reduced the dissection necessary in the recipient.

Other technical complications in this first Stanford series included three patients who suffered injury to nerves in the mediastinum (Figure 21.9). One required a subsequent pyloroplasty to allow satisfactory gastric emptying following injury to the vagus. A second sustained transient paralysis of the left phrenic nerve, and a third sustained loss of function of the left recurrent laryngeal nerve, requiring Teflon injection into the vocal chord. Subsequent modifications to the surgical technique (incorporated in the section on surgical technique above) have reduced the excessive dissection which was originally carried out and which resulted in these nerve injuries. In particular, retention of the pericardium, the posterior wall of the left atrium, and a small cuff of pulmonary artery attached to the arch of aorta, have reduced the possibility of damaging these mediastinal nerves.

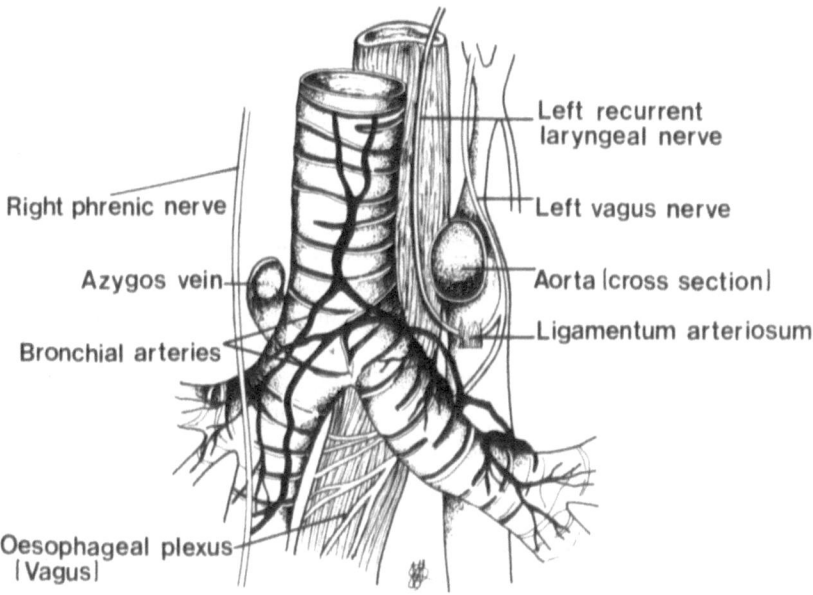

Figure 21.9   Drawing to illustrate the proximity of major thoracic nerves to the trachea, bronchi and aorta. The potential sites of damage of these nerves during the operation of transplantation of the heart and lungs are obvious

Reimplantation response

This complication, which is still poorly understood, has occurred in a large number of the lung transplants performed to date, and may occur whether the transplant involves the heart and both lungs or a single lung[16, 19]. Pulmonary function usually recovers promptly after operation, enabling the patient to be extubated within 24–48 hours. Chest radiographs are normal. During the next few days, however, the radiological appearances change markedly, showing features of a diffuse pulmonary infiltrate. The patient becomes febrile and tachypnoeic, and shows signs of respiratory failure. These are related to a loss of pulmonary compliance, elevation of the pulmonary vascular resistance, a marked fall in arterial PO_2 and an elevation of PCO_2, and pulmonary 'shunting' with ventilation–perfusion imbalance. This syndrome has occurred most commonly between the 4th postoperative day and the end of the 3rd week, after which time it has not been reported[28].

This clinical picture is difficult to differentiate from an acute rejection episode or from infection. The Stanford group has shown evidence that acute rejection in the lungs occurs concomitantly with acute rejection of the myocardium[19], and endomyocardial biopsy may therefore be helpful in differentiating an acute rejection episode from this 'reimplantation oedema'. If the endomyocardial biopsy shows no features of acute rejection, it is unlikely that rejection is occurring in the lungs. Aggressive investigation for a possible pulmonary infection must be carried out; this may involve fibreoptic bronchoscopy. Microscopic examination of fluid collected following bronchial lavage is of little value in differentiating the reimplantation response from acute rejection. It may be helpful, however, in differentiating infection, as micro-organisms may be seen. Microscopic examination of lung affected by this complication shows perivascular cuffs of mononuclear cells, associated with alveolar exudates containing a large quantity of fibrin, pneumocytes and mononuclear cells. If infection is also excluded, then a diagnosis of reimplantation response, as it has become known, can be made with some certainty.

It is likely that many patients with single lung transplants were treated for acute rejection episodes with increased immunosuppression, when in reality they were suffering from this phenomenon of reimplantation oedema. Without the facility for endomyocardial biopsy to distinguish acute rejection in these cases, the diagnosis is particularly difficult. This is clearly one of the great advantages of transplantation of the heart and both lungs over transplantation of a single lung alone.

The aetiology of the reimplantation response is uncertain, but it appears likely that it is related to the ischaemia which the lung has experienced during removal from the donor and reimplantation in the recipient. Though in most reported cases the ischaemic time has ranged between 1 hour 30 minutes and 1 hour 50 minutes, this period is thought to be long enough for the lung to sustain damage; hypothermia alone does not appear to protect the lung completely. Several other factors, however, have been considered as possible aetiological factors in the reimplantation response, though these are probably of less importance than ischaemia[28]. These include the effect of denervation of the lungs, disruption of the lymphatic circulation, and pulmonary trauma from manipulation during the operative procedure.

To a certain extent this complication can be prevented by maintaining a low venous pressure and inducing a diuresis during the early days following transplantation. Should the complication develop, then diuresis is essential, and oxygen should be administered by mask or nasal cannulae. If the pulmonary compliance continues to deteriorate and the arterial PO_2 cannot be maintained above 60 mmHg (8.0 kPa), then continuous positive airway pressure must be introduced. If this should prove inadequate, or if the patient becomes distressed by his respiratory effort, endotracheal intubation and ventilation may be necessary for several days until lung function recovers. Other therapeutic measures which have been found helpful include the infusion of a colloid osmotic agent such as albumin, which helps to draw fluid from the interstitial spaces of the lungs into the circulation.

DIAGNOSIS AND MANAGEMENT OF ACUTE REJECTION

The extreme difficulty of diagnosing acute rejection in the lungs has been discussed above. Fortunately, it would appear that when rejection is occurring in the lungs it is also occurring in the myocardium, and therefore methods of diagnosing acute rejection episodes in the heart can be employed. It is therefore important to perform endomyocardial biopsy at frequent intervals, or to employ other methods of detecting rejection, such as radionuclide scanning (Chapter 11).

Acute rejection of the lungs is associated with an infiltration of mononuclear cells, small lymphocytes, and polymorphonuclear leukocytes; interstitial and intra-alveolar fibrin and erythrocytes may also be present. During infection similar changes can be observed, but significant micro-organisms can also be identified. Bronchial lavage does not usually provide information helpful in making the diagnosis but, on some occasions, can be of value[36].

The treatment of an acute rejection episode is identical to that occurring in a patient with a heart transplant alone. Intravenous boluses of methylprednisolone are administered, together with antithymocyte globulin in severe cases. If a prolonged course of antithymocyte globulin is required, it is essential to regulate the dosage by monitoring the number of circulating T cells.

Though the Stanford experience is that rejection of the heart and lungs occurs simultaneously, our own studies in the Chacma baboon receiving cyclosporin A have shown that the lung may undergo a severe rejection episode whilst the heart shows minimal changes only. It is difficult to obtain satisfactory immunosuppression in the baboon with cyclosporin A, even when administered intravenously twice daily, and this may be a factor in accounting for this observed difference. Our findings would at least suggest, however, that in an inadequately immunosuppressed patient, rejection may occur more rapidly in the lung than in the heart.

RESULTS

The Stanford group has the major experience of patients undergoing transplantation of the heart and both lungs[26, 28, 35]. Of 19 such transplants performed since March 1981, actuarial survival has been 71%, 62% and 62% at 1, 2 and 3 years respectively. The first long-term survivor following this procedure was a 45-year-old woman with primary pulmonary hypertension, operated on at Stanford Medical Center on 9 March 1981. She suffered two documented episodes of acute cardiac allograft rejection at 10 and 25 days respectively, which were reversed using methylprednisolone. Early deaths were from haemorrhage and impaired renal function[28].

In all, approximately 50 heart and lung transplants have been performed by various groups, including those at Stanford, the University of Pittsburgh, the University of Texas Medical Center at Houston, and a small number of European centres. Early results were disappointing and showed a high mortality, but subsequent results have been encouraging.

References

1. Cooper, D. K. C. (1969). Transplantation of the heart and both lungs. I. Historical review. *Thorax*, **24**, 383
2. Cooper, D. K. C. (1968). Experimental development of cardiac transplantation. *Br. Med. J.*, **4**, 171
3. Carrel, A. (1907). The surgery of blood vessels. *Johns Hopkins Hosp. Bull.*, **18**, 18
4. Marcus, E., Wong, S. N. T. and Luisada, A. A. (1951). Homologous heart grafts: transplantation of the heart in dogs. *Surg. Forum*, **2**, 212
5. Demikhov, V. P. (1962). *Experimental Transplantation of Vital Organs*. Authorized translation from the Russian by Haigh, B. (New York: Consultants Bureau)
6. Neptune, W. B., Cookson, B. A., Bailey, C. P., Appler, R. and Rajkowski, F. (1953). Complete homologous heart transplantation. *Arch. Surg.*, **66**, 174
7. Webb, W. R. and Howard, H. S. (1957). Cardiopulmonary transplantation. *Surg. Forum*, **8**, 313
8. Lower, R. R., Stofer, R. C., Hurley, E. J. and Shumway, N. E. (1961). Complete homograft replacement of the heart and both lungs. *Surgery*, **50**, 842
9. Longmore, D. B., Cooper, D. K. C., Hall, R. W., Sekabunga, J. and Welch, W. (1969). Transplantation of the heart and both lungs. II. Experimental cardiopulmonary transplantation. *Thorax*, **24**, 391
10. Nakae, S., Webb, W. R., Theodorides, T. and Sugg, W. L. (1967). Respiratory function following cardiopulmonary denervation in dog, cat and monkey. *Surg. Gynecol. Obstet.*, **125**, 1285
11. Nelems, J. N., Rebuck, A. S., Cooper, J. D., Goldberg, M., Halloran, P. and Velland, H. (1980). Human lung transplantation. *Chest*, **78**, 4
12. Hardy, J. D., Webb, W. R., Dalton, M. L. and Walker, G. R. (1963). Lung homotransplantation in man. *J. Am. Med. Assoc.*, **186**, 1065

13. Pinsker, K. L., Koerner, S. K., Kamolz, S. L., Hagstrom, J. W. C. and Veith, F. J. (1979). Effect of donor bronchial length on healing. A canine model to evaluate bronchial anastomic problems in lung transplantation. *J. Thorac. Cardiovasc. Surg.*, **77**, 669
14. Veith, F. J. (1978). Lung transplantation. *Surg. Clin. N. Am.*, **58**, 357
15. Lima, O., Cooper, J. D. and Peters, W. J. (1981). Effects of methylprednisolone and azathioprine on bronchial healing following lung orthotransplantation. *J. Thorac. Cardiovasc. Surg.*, **82**, 211
16. Siegelman, S., Sinha, S. B. P. and Veith, F. J. (1973). Pulmonary reimplantation response. *Ann. Surg.*, **77**, 30
17. Haglin, J. J., Ruiz, E., Baker, R. C. and Anderson, W. R. (1973). Histologic studies of human lung allotransplantation. In Wildevuur, C. R. H. (ed.) *Morphology in Lung Transplantation.* p. 13. (Basel: Karger)
18. Hudson, C. L., Moritz, A. R. and Wearn, J. T. (1932). The extracardiac anastomoses of the coronary arteries. *J. Exp. Med.*, **56**, 919
19. Reitz, B., Burton, N. A., Jamieson, S., Bieber, C. T., Pennock, J. L., Stinson, E. B. and Shumway, N. E. (1980). Heart and lung transplantation. Orthotransplantation and allotransplantation in primates with extended survival. *J. Thorac. Cardiovasc. Surg.*, **80**, 360
20. Caves, P. K., Stinson, E. B., Billingham, M. E., Rider, A. K. and Shumway, N. E. (1973). Diagnosis of human cardiac allograft rejection by endomyocardial biopsy. *J. Thorac. Cardiovasc. Surg.*, **66**, 461
21. Veith, F. J., Norin, A. J., Montefusco, C. N., Pinsker, K. L., Ramnolz, S. L., Gliedman, N. L. and Emerson, E. (1981). Cyclosporin A in experimental lung transplantation. *Transplantation*, **32**, 474
22. Cooley, D. A., Bloodwell, R. D., Hallman, G. L., Nora, J. J., Harrison, J. M. and Leachman, R. D. (1969). Organ transplantation for advanced cardiopulmonary disease. *Ann. Thorac. Surg.*, **8**, 30
23. Lillehei, C. W. (1970). Discussion of Wildevuur, C. R. H. and Benfield, J. R. A review of 23 human lung transplantations by 20 surgeons. *Ann. Thorac. Surg.*, **9**, 515
24. Barnard, C. N. and Cooper, D. K. C. (1981). Clinical transplantation of the heart: a review of 13 years' personal experience. *J. R. Soc. Med.*, **74**, 670
25. Losman, J. G., Campbell, C. D., Replogle, R. L. and Barnard, C. N. (1982). Joint transplantation of the heart and lungs. Past experience and present potentials. *J. Cardiovasc. Surg.*, **23**, 440
26. Reitz, B. A. (1981). Heart and lung transplantation. *Heart Transplant.*, **1**, 80
27. Borel, J. F., Feurer, C., Gubler, H. U. and Stahelin, H. (1976). Biological effects of cyclosporin A. A new antilymphocytic agent. *Agents Actions*, **6**, 648
28. Reitz, B. A. (1982). Heart–lung transplantation: a review. *Heart Transplant.*, **1**, 292
29. Mancini, M. C., Griffith, B. P., Borovetz, H. S. and Hardesty, R. L. (1983). Static lung preservation in a canine model. *Heart Transplant.*, **2**, 175
30. Veith, F. J., Crane, R., Torres, M., Colon, I., Hagstrom, J. W. C., Pinsker, K. L. and Koerner, S. R. (1976). Effective preservation and transportation of lung transplants. *J. Thorac. Cardiovasc. Surg.*, **72**, 97
31. Modry, D. L., Walpoth, B. W., Cohen, R. G., Seifert, F. C., Bleese, N. M., Warnecke, H., Bieber, C. P., Billingham, M. E., Jamieson, S. W. and Shumway, N. E. (1983). Heart–lung preservation in the dog followed by lung transplantation: a new model for the assessment of lung preservation. *Heart Transplant.*, **2**, 287
32. Grillo, H. C. (1976). Congenital lesions, neoplasms, and injuries of the trachea. In Sabiston, D. C. and Spencer, F. C. (eds.) *Gibbon's Surgery of the Chest.* 3rd Edn., p. 259. (Philadelphia/London: Saunders)
33. Last, R. J. (1978). *Anatomy, Regional and Applied.* 6th Edn., p. 236. (London and Edinburgh: Churchill Livingstone)
34. James, T. N. (1961). *Anatomy of the Coronary Arteries.* p. 205. (New York: Harper & Row)

35. Jamieson, S. W., Reitz, B. A., Oyer, P. E., Billingham, M., Modry, D., Baldwin, J., Stinson, E. B., Hunt, S., Theodore, J., Bieber, C. P. and Shumway, N. E. (1983). Combined heart and lung transplantation. *Lancet*, **1**, 1130

36. Achterrath, U., Blümcke, S., Koerner, S. K., Yipintsoi, T., Siegelman, S. S., Chandler, P., Hagstrom, J. W. C., Torres, M., Cobbah, J. E., Fujii, B. and Veith, F. J. (1975). Alveolar lavage cytology in transplanted lungs. I. Staining methods and findings in dogs with autografts and allografts without immunosuppression. *J. Thorac. Cardiovasc. Surg.*, **69**, 510

22
The Future of
Heart Replacement

INTRODUCTION

The surgical techniques of orthotopic and heterotopic transplantation have been standardized and are unlikely to change appreciably in the foreseeable future. Rejection following the transplant operation can now be reliably detected by endomyocardial biopsy, though this technique may soon be replaced by a non-invasive technique such as radionuclide scanning.

Cyclosporin A (CYA) has certainly increased and improved the therapy available to us in countering acute rejection episodes. It has allowed successful transplantation of the heart and both lungs, a procedure which hitherto had appeared doomed to failure. Even CYA, however, is not entirely effective in this respect, and its action continues to put the patient at risk from infection and malignancy. Its long-term side-effects and its effect on the development of graft arteriosclerosis remain unknown.

Despite these advances, two severely limiting problems remain: (1) prevention of rejection without serious sequelae, and (2) inadequacy of donor heart supply. The relatively non-selective mode of action of current immunosuppressive agents continues to result in much morbidity and mortality. Equally critical to the future development of cardiac transplantation is the worldwide shortage of donor hearts; steps to overcome this shortage are urgently sought.

PREVENTION OF REJECTION

The ultimate goal for which we search is the induction of a stable graft–host relationship without compromising the recipient's immune response to infection or neoplastic mutant cells.

Using the 'conventional' immunosuppressive regimen of maintenance oral *azathioprine* and *corticosteroids*, augmented by intravenous (i.v.) antithymocyte globulin (ATG) during the first 4–6 weeks and i.v. courses of methylprednisolone and ATG during acute rejection episodes, rejection can be prevented or reversed successfully in the majority of cases and most patients brought safely through the critical initial 3-month period. There remains, however, a mortality related to the effects of immunosuppression, namely from infection, not infrequently from unusual or opportunistic micro-organisms, particularly viral or fungal. Furthermore, despite meticulous attention to every detail of patient care, including close control of immunosuppressive therapy, chronic rejection (immunologically-induced accelerated coronary arteriosclerosis) remains the major cause of late donor heart failure, and in some patients significant changes can be seen as early as 2 or 3 months after transplantation. The high incidence of infection, chronic rejection and, to a lesser extent, malignant neoplasia, seen in most series of patients illustrates the point that the immunosuppressive agents used in recent years have been far from perfect.

Recent experimental and clinical studies suggest that cyclosporin A is the most powerful and selective pharmacological immunosuppressive agent yet discovered[1]. Its relatively recent introduction is a major advance in pharmacological immunosuppression, though there remains an associated incidence of infection and other undesirable features, such as depression of renal function, and a continuing risk of malignant tumours, particularly lymphomas[2–5]. The potent immunosuppressive effect of CYA is undisputed and has been well documented in rats, mice, rabbits, pigs, dogs, monkeys and man. The compound may prove to be the first of a whole family of fungal peptides with profound immunosuppressive activity, one of which may ultimately be found to prevent both acute and chronic graft rejection, yet allow the host response to infection to remain unimpaired. CYA has a relatively simple molecular structure (a cyclic peptide consisting of 11 amino acids) that should allow for chemical manipulation to improve its therapeutic index. The quest for the ideal immunosuppressant, however, is by no means over; despite CYA's specificity and potency, it is not without its major side-effects. There is already very preliminary evidence from our own institution that CYA may reduce or eliminate preformed antibodies and therefore permit transplantation even in sensitized patients.

A promising method of manipulating the host's immune system to induce tolerance and prevent rejection is *total lymphoid irradiation* (TLI). Rhesus monkeys receiving as little as 600 rad TLI in 100 rad/daily fractions during the week prior to transplantation, and three doses of rabbit ATG (3 mg/kg i.m.), have consistently demonstrated prolonged cardiac allograft survival greater than 100 days[6]. This prolonged survival suggests that this protocol may have induced tolerance by a brief absolute T cell suppression. Despite these striking results, TLI has not been adapted for clinical use because it does not completely eliminate rejection, and may actually accelerate graft arteriosclerosis[7]. It is also a difficult form of therapy to use, and not without risk. Some form of

TLI may, however, be used as an adjunct to standard immunosuppressive agents in the near future.

Active enhancement, where specific immunosuppression is induced in the recipient after treatment with donor histocompatibility antigens, whether injected as donor whole cells, tissue homogenates, or soluble antigens, offers the possibility of eventually becoming an effective form of immunosuppression[8]. But until the grave risks of sensitization can be safely avoided, active enhancement will remain unsuitable for clinical use.

Although the exact mechanisms responsible for the increased survival observed in kidney transplant recipients with a previous history of blood transfusion are uncertain, they are thought to involve some form of active enhancement, possibly as a result of random sharing of histocompatibility antigens by the blood and organ donors.

Passive enhancement, where specific immunosuppression is attained by treatment with antibodies directed against the donor histocompatibility antigens, is likely to be used as an adjunct to current therapy in the foreseeable future, particularly with the advent of *monoclonal antibodies* produced by B lymphocyte–myeloma clones[9]. The large quantities of pure and highly specific antibodies that can be produced by this method may overcome several of the practical problems of clinical transplantation. Monoclonal antibodies have already been used successfully to combat acute rejection episodes in patients with kidney transplants[10]. The use of monoclonal antiblast antibody to kill only those cells that are reacting against the graft may prove to be a further advance in this field[11].

The selection of recipient donor pairs on the basis of the results of *tissue typing* has been disappointing in cardiac transplantation, and has not led to any significant improvement in patient survival to date. As our knowledge of transplant immunology expands, however, tissue typing may play a more important role.

Recent reports have suggested that *pregnancy is an immunosuppressed state* in which the fetus, despite the presence of paternal antigens, is not recognized as foreign by the mother[12, 13]. Although the mechanisms by which this immunosuppression is established and reversed have not been elucidated, they may reveal newer ways by which the immune system may be modulated.

If any of the methods outlined above are successful in inducing tolerance or achieving an uncomplicated form of immunosuppression, then, of course, the major hurdle to the transplantation of any organ will have been overcome. Similarly, some of the present advantages of heterotopic heart transplantation will be negated or, at least, diminish in importance, and orthotopic transplantation will clearly be the technique of choice in the majority of cases.

DONOR HEART SUPPLY

As the problems of immunosuppression are overcome, and the risks associated with heart transplantation reduced, transplantation will almost certainly be extended to patients with advanced heart disease who would today receive more conservative surgery such as coronary artery bypass grafting or prosthetic valve replacement. If the mortality and morbidity associated with transplantation were reduced to a level comparable with or below that of multiple valve replacement or myocardial revascularization in patients with poor left ventricular function, then transplantation will be clearly preferable. It would result not only in normal valves or coronary arteries, but also in normal left ventricular function. Similarly, there will be increasing utilization of cardiac or cardiopulmonary transplantation in children with uncorrectable congenital malformations, or even in children with complex congenital defects who today are subjected to major surgery that is at best palliative.

The recent encouraging results of transplantation of the heart and both lungs has opened up a wide new field of transplantation in patients not only with advanced cardiac disease, but also with terminal pulmonary disease. There is a large existing untapped pool of patients with advanced lung disease awaiting further advances in this field.

With this great expansion in the number of patients who might benefit from heart and heart–lung transplantation, potential recipients will then far exceed the number of suitable donors which become available. Donor organ shortage will become increasingly critical. In Cape Town this problem has been acute for some time; between one-third and one-half of the patients we currently accept for cardiac transplantation die before a suitable donor becomes available[14].

The shortage of donor hearts may be alleviated or overcome in the future by: (1) improved public and medical awareness and education; (2) improved communications between donor and recipient centres (improved donor procurement organization); improved methods of (3) donor pretreatment and (4) storing donor heart; the use of (5) xenografts and (6) artificial hearts.

1. Public and medical awareness and education

In the Republic of South Africa there are over 10 000 deaths from trauma each year. If only 1% of these patients proved suitable for the purposes of cardiac transplantation, the resulting number of 100 donors would be more than adequate for our purposes in the foreseeable future, as long as all 100 could be utilized. At the present time, however, little more than one tenth of 1% of these actually become available to us for transplantation. This is due to a number of reasons. The relative isolation of Cape Town from the rest of the country greatly reduces the potential donor pool available to us, though this problem will be overcome in part by improved methods of sustaining donor haemodynamic stability and donor heart storage. Large subgroups of the population have religious, superstitious or social beliefs which prohibit them from consenting to donation.

There remains uncertainty on the part of some doctors caring for patients who may become potential donors with regard to the criteria necessary for the diagnosis of brain death, and to the medical, legal and administrative aspects of donation[15]. Continuing education of the medical community as well as of the public in respect to both the problems and possibilities of transplantation is therefore essential.

2. Donor procurement organization

To optimize the number of organs available for transplantation, an efficient organization is necessary to promote and administer the procurement of organs on a regional basis. Such organizations already exist in North America and Europe, but further development of sophisticated methods of communication will eventually be required worldwide. The ability to store hearts for 48 hours or longer will be of little value unless an efficient communications infrastructure exists to facilitate long-distance exchange of such organs.

3. Donor heart pretreatment

The condition of the donor heart prior to transplantation is clearly important. Initial studies in our own experimental laboratory have drawn attention to the myocardial damage that results from sudden brain stem infarction, and to the reduction in circulating levels of various hormones that follows brain death. Donor pretreatment aimed at reducing the myocardial insult to which these hearts are subjected, and to replenishing the rapidly diminishing myocardial energy stores, may contribute to haemodynamic stability. We have also learnt that myocardial damage is minimized if the potential donor is not overloaded with fluid during the period before excision. These and further similar studies should help improve both the pretransplant condition of the donor heart, and its condition after long periods of storage, enable more hearts to be used for transplantation, and result in better initial and long-term function.

4. Donor heart storage

Donor heart supply would obviously be increased if such organs could be obtained at distant centres and transported over long distances to the recipient hospital. This necessitates the need for a method of storing donor hearts for several hours or even days. In most centres involved with heart transplantation at the present time, the method of myocardial protection used is simple flush cooling with a cold cardioplegic agent, bringing about cessation of myocardial contractions within 2 or 3 minutes. The heart is then transported in ice as quickly as possible, usually by air, to the recipient centre, the total ischaemic period not exceeding approximately 4 hours[16]. Under ideal conditions, using private chartered jet aircraft, donor hearts can be procured up to approximately 1500 km (940 miles) from the recipient centre.

In Cape Town we have been interested in trying to prolong donor heart ischaemic time further, both to enable transportation by less expensive methods and to allow time for tests such as tissue typing and lymphocytotoxic cross-matching, and ultimately to allow the transplant operation to be performed as a semi-elective rather than as an emergency procedure. During the past 3 years a team in our experimental laboratory has developed a perfusion system for storage of the donor heart for periods of up to 48 hours. This system has been extensively tested in the experimental laboratory[17-20] and, since 1981, has been used in a small number of clinical cases, with total ischaemic periods extending from approximately 7 to 17 hours.

Further developments in this field are, however, closely linked with a basic understanding of the effect of brain death on the myocardium, as it would appear that neurogenic injury and long periods of ischaemic storage may have an additive effect on the reduction of myocardial energy stores.

The method of long-term storage (weeks or months) that may ultimately prove most successful is freezing or supercooling of the organ. Progress in this field, however, has been slow, and at the present time such techniques lead to irreversible damage of the myocardium.

5. The use of xenografts

Possibly the ultimate way of overcoming the problem of donor supply, which remains the critical limiting factor to the number of transplants being performed in our own and many other units each year, will be by the use of xenografts. Though a non-human primate heart might be immunologically ideal, other animals, such as the pig or sheep, might be anatomically more suitable and certainly more readily available.

In 1977, heterotopic xenografts were used clinically on two emergency occasions at our institution[21]. From this experience with baboon and chimpanzee cardiac xenografts we found that a suitable xenograft could support a failing circulation for at least 2–3 days. Although severe acute rejection destroyed the chimpanzee xenograft completely within 4 days, this experience demonstrated that even using conventional immunosuppression, hyperacute rejection did not necessarily occur between closely related species.

The greater understanding of immunological mechanisms gained recently, and the encouraging results being obtained with new forms of immunosuppression of allografts, has renewed the hope that a solution to the problem of the immune response, even in relation to xenografts, may be found in the not-too-distant future.

6. The use of the artificial heart

Temporary

The successful development of a left ventricular assist pump and/or artificial heart, which can be used routinely to maintain the systemic circulation for periods of weeks and months, would be invaluable in supporting the potential recipient until a suitable donor heart became available. Although forms of temporary mechanical support have been used to support the circulation in patients prior to heart transplantation, long-term survival has not yet been attained following such transplantation[22]. It seems likely, however, that, in the near future, these devices will be used successfully when it is necessary to support a desperately sick patient until a suitable donor becomes available.

Permanent

It seems inevitable that a completely implantable artificial heart will be developed that will enable a recipient to lead an unrestricted, normal life, as do patients with successful heart allografts. But how long it will take to develop such an artificial heart remains uncertain.

In 1969, and again in 1981, a total artificial heart (TAH) was implanted in the chest of a patient at the Texas Heart Institute[23]. Although both patients survived only a few days, this initial experience demonstrated the feasibility of using a mechanical device for the—at least temporary—maintenance of the circulation. More recently, a group at the University of Utah received much publicity for successfully implanting an air-driven artificial heart in a patient (Barney Clark) for 112 days[24].

Most artificial heart devices require large percutaneous tubes connecting the patient to a bulky driving unit and control console. Smaller, more compact, devices, which permit more mobility and freedom, are currently under investigation, though to date the batteries of such portable devices can supply power for several hours only[25].

This problem of an implantable energy source, which will function for months or years, is one of the major factors limiting the more frequent clinical application of TAHs today. Not only do the present large external supplies and control consoles prevent the patient from leading any form of normal mobile life, but the tube or tubes connecting the implanted heart with this external apparatus constitute a risk of infection.

Many of the other problems which face those working in this field, such as the prevention of thrombus formation in the implanted prosthesis itself, appear to have been overcome with varying degrees of success, though material durability continues to present a significant challenge. At present, the major difficulty relates to minute holes in the polymer used to manufacture the heart, which enlarge under the continuous stress of the driving system[26].

For the next few years, therefore, the clinical application of the TAH must surely be considered as a temporary measure to provide circulatory support to the desperate potential recipient awaiting cardiac transplantation.

CONCLUSION

At the present time heart transplantation remains a major undertaking on the part of both the patient and surgical team, but offers carefully selected patients with advanced myocardial disease the possibility of a good quality of life for a number of years. While the cost of a heart transplant in the USA presently ranges from $57 000 to $110 000 for the first year's treatment[27], this formidable financial burden will almost certainly decrease in the near future as more transplants are performed and the management of these patients becomes more routine. With continuing developments in the field of immunosuppression and donor heart supply, it would appear that, during the next decade, the results of transplantation can only improve, and the procedure steadily become available to an increasing number of patients for whom no other therapy is available.

References

1. Green, C. F. (1981). Cyclosporin A. In Salaman, J. R. (ed.) *Immunosuppressive Therapy*. p. 75. (Lancaster: MTP Press)
2. Oyer, P. E., Stinson, E. B., Jamieson, S. W., Hunt, S., Reitz, B. A., Bieber, C. P., Schroeder, J. S., Billingham, M. and Shumway, N. E. (1982). One-year experience with cyclosporin A in clinical heart transplantation. *Heart Transplant.*, 1, 285
3. Thiru, S., Calne, R. Y. and Nagington, J. (1981). Lymphoma in renal allograft patients treated with cyclosporin A as one of the immunosuppressive agents. *Transplant Proc.*, 13, 359
4. Morris, P. J. (1981). Cyclosporin A. *Transplantation*, 32, 349
5. Calne, R. Y., Rolles, K., White, D. J. G., Thiru, S., Evans, D. B., Henderson, R., Hamilton, D. C., Boone, W., McMaster, P., Gibby, O. and Williams, R. (1981). Cyclosporin A in clinical organ grafting. *Transplant Proc.*, 13, 349
6. Bieber, C. P., Jamieson, S., Raney, A., Burton, N., Bogarty, S., Moppe, R., Kaplan, H. S., Strobber, S. and Stinson, E. B. (1979). Cardiac allograft survival in rhesus primates treated with combined TLI and RATG. *Transplantation*, 28, 347
7. Jamieson, S. W., Bieber, C. P. and Oyer, P. E. (1981). Suppression of immunity for cardiac transplantation. In Salaman, J. R. (ed.) *Immunosuppressive Therapy*. p. 177. (Lancaster: MTP Press)
8. Fabre, J. W. (1981). Specific immunosuppression. In Salaman, J. R. (ed.) *Immunosuppressive Therapy*. p. 129. (Lancaster: MTP Press)
9. Kohler, G. and Milstein, C. (1976). Derivation of specific antibody producing tissue culture and tumour lines by cell fusion. *Eur. J. Immunol.*, 6, 511
10. Cosimi, A. B., Burton, R. C., Colvin, R. B., Goldstein, G., Delmonico, F. L., La Quaglia, M. P., Tolkoff-Rubin, N., Rubin, R. H., Herrin, J. T. and Russell, P. S. (1981). Treatment of acute renal allograft rejection with OKT3 monoclonal antibody. *Transplantation*, 32, 535
11. Takahashi, H., Terasaki, P. I., Kinukawa, T., Chia, D., Miura, K., Okazaki, H., Iwaki, Y., Taguchi, Y., Hardiwidjaja, S., Ishikazi, M. and Billing, R. (1983). Reversal of transplant rejection by monoclonal antiblast antibody. *Lancet*, 2, 1155

12. Scott, J. S. and Jenkins, D. M. (1973). The immunology of human reproduction. In Parker, C. W. (ed.) *Clinical Immunology*. Vol. 2, p. 20. (New York: Wiley)

13. Cotton, D. J., Seligmann, B., O'Brien, W. F. and Gallin, J. I. (1983). Selective defect in human neutrophil superoxide anion generation elucidated by the chemoattractant *n*-formyl methionyl-leucylalanine in pregnancy. *J. Infect. Dis.*, **148**, 194

14. Cooper, D. K. C., Charles, R. G., Beck, W. and Barnard, C. N. (1982). The assessment and selection of patients for heterotopic heart transplantation. *S. Afr. Med. J.*, **61**, 575

15. Cooper, D. K. C., De Villiers, J. C., Smith, L. S., Crombie, Y., Boyd, S. T., Jacobson, J. E. and Barnard, C. N. (1982). Medical, legal and administrative aspects of cadaveric organ donation in the Republic of South Africa. *S. Afr. Med. J.*, **62**, 933

16. Mendez-Picon, G. J., Goldman, M. H., Wolfgang, T. C., Szentpetery, S. S., Ducey, K. F., Hess, M. L., Hastillo, A., Guerraty, A. J. and Lower, R. R. (1981). Long-distance procurement and transportation of human hearts for transplantation. *Heart Transplant.*, **1**, 63

17. Wicomb, W. N., Boyd, S. T., Cooper, D. K. C., Rose, A. G. and Barnard, C. N. (1981). Ex vivo functional evaluation of pig hearts subjected to 24 hours' preservation of hypothermic perfusion. *S. Afr. Med. J.*, **60**, 245

18. Wicomb, W. N., Cooper, D. K. C., Hassoulas, J., Rose, A. G. and Barnard, C. N. (1982). Orthotopic transplantation of the baboon heart after 20–24 hours' preservation by continuous hypothermic perfusion with an oxygenated hyperosmolar solution. *J. Thorac. Cardiovasc. Surg.*, **83**, 133

19. Wicomb, W. N., Cooper, D. K. C. and Barnard, C. N. (1982). Twenty-four-hour preservation of the pig heart by a portable hypothermic perfusion system. *Transplantation*, **34**, 246

20. Cooper, D. K. C., Wicomb, W. N., Rose, A. G. and Barnard, C. N. (1983). Orthotopic allotransplantation and autotransplantation of the baboon heart following 24-hour storage by a portable hypothermic perfusion system. *Cryobiology*, **20**, 385

21. Barnard, C. N., Wolpowitz, A. and Losman, J. G. (1977). Heterotopic cardiac transplantation with a xenograft for assistance of the left heart in cardiogenic shock after cardiopulmonary bypass. *S. Afr. Med. J.*, **52**, 1035

22. Pennock, J. L., Wisman, C. B. and Pierce, W. S. (1982). Mechanical support of the circulation prior to cardiac transplantation. *Heart Transplant.*, **1**, 299

23. Cooley, D. A. (1982). Staged cardiac transplantation: report of three cases. *Heart Transplant.*, **1**, 145

24. De Vries, W. C., Anderson, J. L., Joyce, L. D., Anderson, F. L., Hammond, E. H., Jarvik, R. K. and Kolff, W. J. (1984). Clinical use of the total artificial heart. *N. Engl. J. Med.*, **310**, 273

25. Cortesini, R. (1982). Toward artificial heart: medical and ethical dilemmas. *Heart Transplant.*, **1**, 161

26. Taguchi, K., Fukunaga, S., Hasegawa, T., Murashita, J., Matsumura, M., Hamanaka, Y., Isono, M., Ishikawa, M., Sueda, T., Tagami, S. and Hironaka, T. (1982). Problems in artificial heart systems for clinical application. *Heart Transplant.*, **1**, 172

27. Clark, M., Witherspoon, D., Gosnell, M., Carey, J., Shapiro, D., Abrahamson, P., Resener, M., Buckey, J. and Wallace, A. (1983). The new era of transplants. *Newsweek*, 29 August, p. 38

APPENDIX

Heart Transplantation at the University of Cape Town— An Overview

INTRODUCTION

In this volume we have reviewed progress in the field of heart transplantation, with emphasis on our own experience in Cape Town. Though our unit is possibly best-known for its work in transplantation this, in fact, forms only a small part of our activities. Approximately 700 heart operations are performed each year at our institution, one-third of them in children[1]. Only once has the number of transplants exceeded ten in any one year (Figure 1).

ORTHOTOPIC HEART TRANSPLANTATION

Human-to-human heart transplantation was first carried out in Groote Schuur Hospital, Cape Town (Figure 2), on 2 December 1967[2]. Between December 1967 and December 1973 orthotopic heart transplantation was performed in ten patients, using a modification of the technique developed in the experimental animal by Lower and Shumway[3]. This modification, introduced by Barnard, reduced the risk of damage to the sinoatrial node, thus avoiding conduction abnormalities[4].

The recipients were nine men and one woman with an age range of 36–63 years. Six of the ten patients were 50 years or older, with two being more than 60 years. Seven had ischaemic heart disease, two cardiomyopathy, and one rheumatic heart disease. With experience gained since that time, many of these patients would have been considered too old or otherwise unsuitable to undergo the rigours of transplantation, with its accompanying prolonged immunosuppressive therapy[5].

351

Nevertheless, four patients (40%) survived for more than 1 year, enjoying an excellent quality of life. One died from chronic rejection after 12½ years, and one patient remains alive and fully employed approximately 13 years after operation. Ten years' survival has, therefore, been 20%. These two long-term survivors were aged 38 and 44 years respectively at the time of operation. Survival times in this group as a whole might well have been longer if, as would be the case today, younger patients had been selected for transplantation.

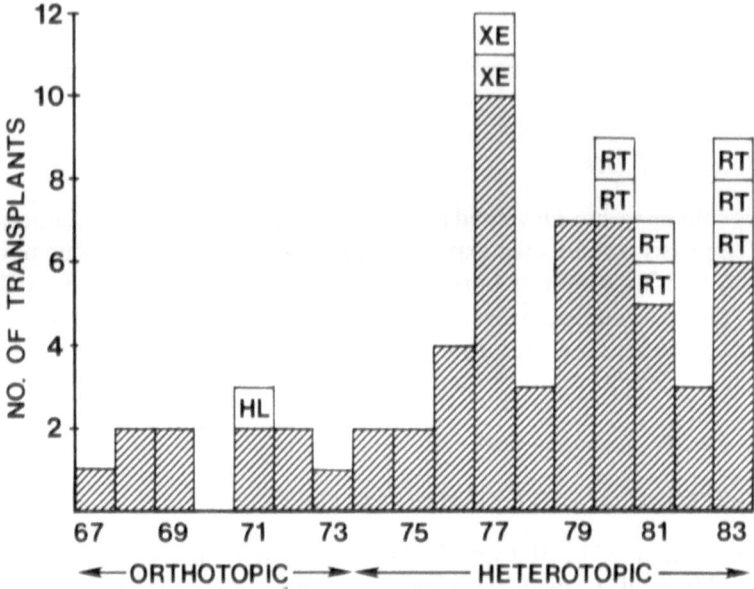

Figure 1 Histogram showing the number of heart transplantation operations performed at Groote Schuur Hospital each year (1967–1983). HL = transplantation of the heart and both lungs; XE = xenografts; RT = retransplant procedure

The first patient to undergo heart transplantation at Groote Schuur Hospital was Louis Washkansky (Figure 3), a 57-year-old man with ischaemic heart disease[2]. He received a heart from an 18-year-old girl who suffered brain death following a road traffic accident. He made a good initial recovery from the procedure and his transplanted heart functioned well. Like many subsequent immunosuppressed patients, however, he developed a chest infection and died of pneumonia on the 18th postoperative day[6].

The second patient, a 60-year-old dental surgeon, Philip Blaiberg (Figure 4), who underwent transplantation on 2 January 1968, could claim to be the world's first 'long-term' survivor, living an active and full life until he succumbed to chronic rejection after 20 months[7].

A 53-year-old man was the third patient, and he also did well, leading an active life until he developed carcinoma of the stomach (possibly related to prolonged immunosuppressive therapy), from which he died after 20 months; his transplanted heart showed no signs of either acute or chronic rejection.

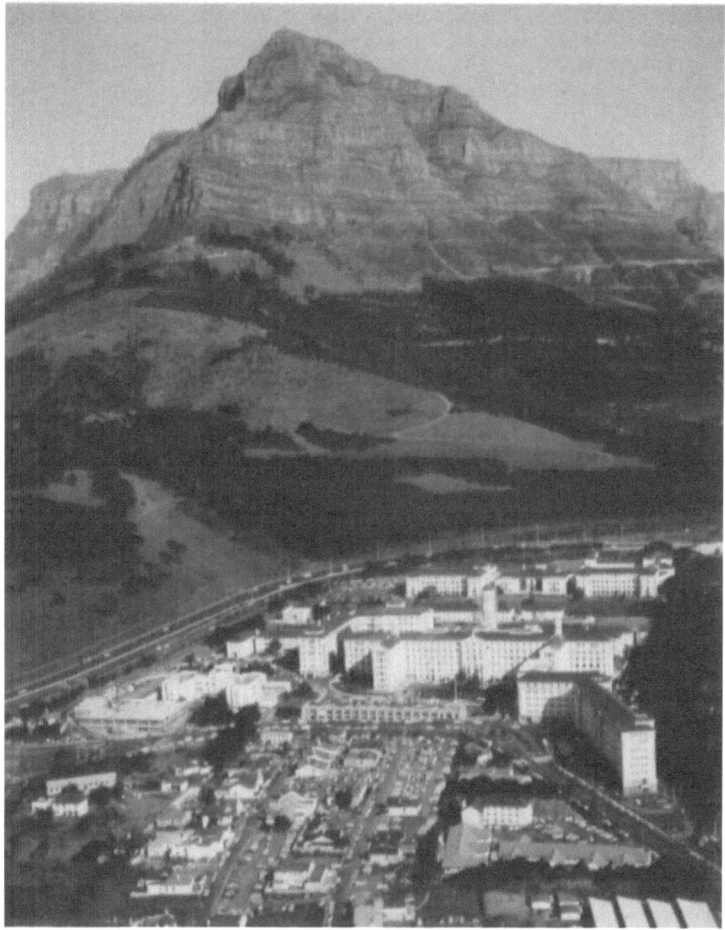

Figure 2   Groote Schuur Hospital, Cape Town

Of the remaining seven patients who received orthotopic grafts during this first phase of the development of heart transplantation at Cape Town, two warrant further comment. The first woman transplanted in our series remained well and active until her death from chronic rejection at $12\frac{1}{2}$ years[8]. The one patient who remains alive today returned to his former work after 3 months and is fully employed almost 13 years later.

The major cause of death in this group was infection, which occurred in five of the patients. There was one operative death related to failure of the donor heart to support the circulation. The death of this patient encouraged the

Cape Town team to initiate an experimental programme to develop a technique of inserting the donor heart as an accessory or auxiliary pump, leaving the recipient's own heart *in situ*.

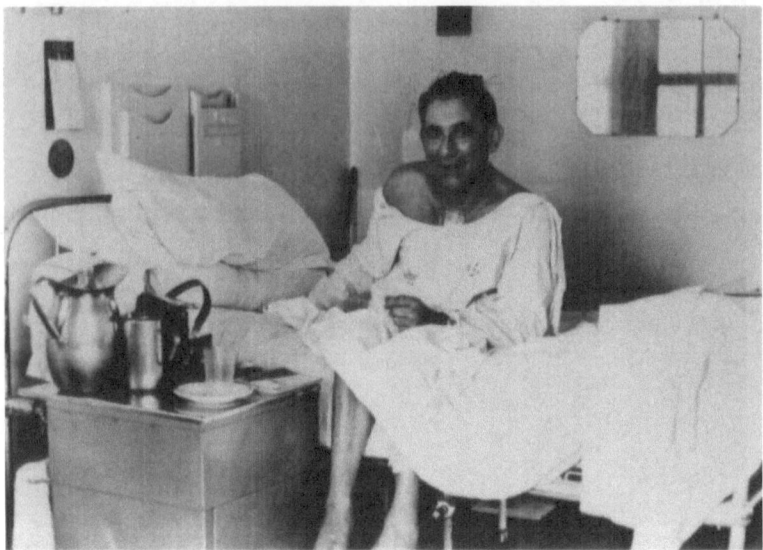

Figure 3 Louis Washkansky, the first patient to undergo orthotopic heart transplantation at Groote Schuur Hospital

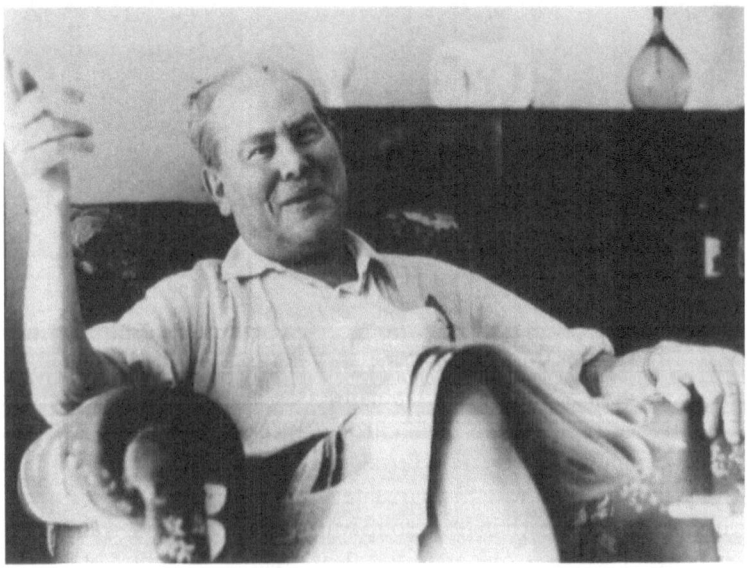

Figure 4 Philip Blaiberg

TRANSPLANTATION OF THE HEART AND BOTH LUNGS

On 25 July 1971 a 49-year-old man with chronic obstructive airways disease and bilateral basal bronchiectasis underwent orthotopic transplantation of the heart and both lungs[9]. He had been ill since 1958 with dyspnoea on exertion and a productive cough, and was diagnosed at that time as having emphysema. He had steadily deteriorated over several years until, 2 months before operation, he had become bedridden and reliant on continuous oxygen therapy, together with antibiotics, steroids, and antifailure medication. The patient had severely deranged respiratory function tests and blood gas analysis.

Transplantation of the heart and both lungs was performed by anastomosing the donor and recipient right atria, aortae, and both bronchi. The patient initially did well, but developed an air leak at the site of the right bronchial anastomosis. An intercostal muscle flap procedure at a subsequent thoracotomy failed to control the leak and a right pneumonectomy was ultimately necessary on the 19th postoperative day. Pneumonia, including a lung abscess, developed in the left lung, and the patient died on the 23rd postoperative day. Autopsy revealed an infected haematoma surrounding the heart and bronchopneumonia of the left lung; there was no significant rejection of the transplanted heart or lungs. The cause of death was considered to be klebsiella pneumonia and septicaemia.

The experience gained from this patient suggested that early acute rejection of the lungs, the organ considered most likely to undergo rapid rejection, could be delayed by suitable immunosuppression. Pneumonia may not have been inevitable if a bronchopleural fistula had not developed.

Successful transplantation of the lungs, however, had to wait another decade until the introduction of a more sophisticated means of immunosuppression (i.e. cyclosporin A). The experimental and early clinical experience at Stanford University using this drug in patients with heart–lung transplants has been encouraging.

HETEROTOPIC HEART TRANSPLANTATION

In November 1974 the Groote Schuur team embarked on a clinical programme of heterotopic heart transplantation using two techniques developed in our experimental laboratory[10–12]. The haemodynamics of the circulation following these procedures were described in Chapter 10. The advantages and disadvantages of heterotopic heart transplantation versus orthotopic transplantation were discussed in Chapter 20. The relative indications for both heterotopic and orthotopic transplantation continue to be modified in the light of other developments, but we believe that the advantages of heterotopic transplantation outweighed its disadvantages in our own particular setting during the past 10 years.

Left ventricular bypass

The technique of left ventricular bypass involves anastomoses of the donor and recipient left atria and aortae. Donor coronary venous blood returns to the recipient right atrium via the donor pulmonary artery (Figure 5).

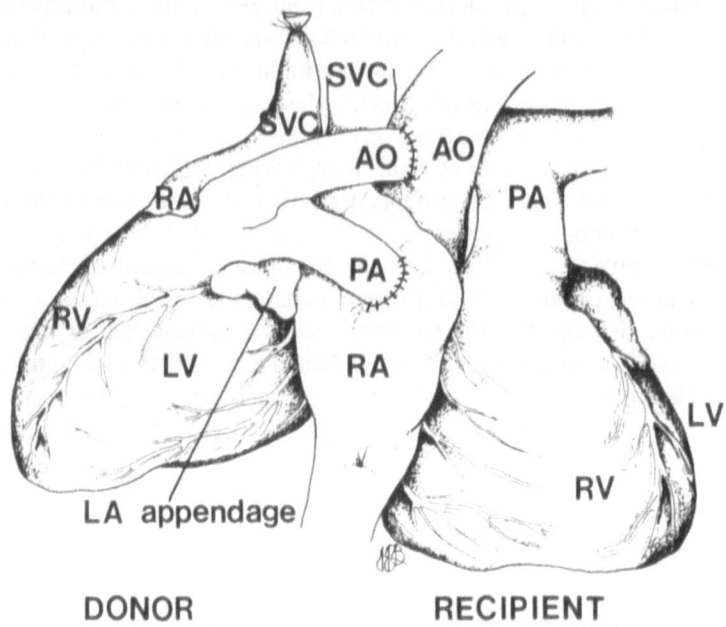

Figure 5   The completed operation of left ventricular bypass. SVC = superior vena cava; RA = right atrium; RV = right ventricle; PA = pulmonary artery; LA = left atrium; LV = left ventricle

Only two patients (both men, aged 59 and 47 years respectively) underwent this procedure. Although the first patient, who underwent operation on 25 November 1974, succumbed to a pulmonary embolus 111 days after transplantation[11,13], the second patient remains alive and well 9 years later[14].

Since both patients suffered from recurrent attacks of recipient heart dysrhythmias, including ventricular fibrillation[15] (although during the attacks the donor heart satisfactorily supported the circulation alone), the technique of left ventricular bypass was superseded by biventricular bypass.

Biventricular bypass

Biventricular bypass is performed by anastomosing the right atria, left atria, aortae and pulmonary arteries, allowing blood to flow through either donor or recipient right heart and either left heart (Chapter 8).

Between April 1975 and December 1983, 47 such transplants were performed in 43 patients, all receiving azathioprine, methylprednisolone, and either antilymphocyte or antithymocyte globulin as the standard immunosuppressive therapy. Seven of these patients subsequently underwent retransplantation for acute or chronic rejection. Patient mean age was 37 years, with a range of 14–52 years. All but three of the patients were men. Fifty-eight per cent of the patients survived over a year, two of whom remain alive 8 years after transplantation.

INTRODUCTION OF CYCLOSPORIN A

Since March 1983, patients undergoing heart transplantation at our institution have been immunosuppressed with cyclosporin A (CYA) and low-dose methylprednisolone. This programme is continuing. In two further patients receiving azathioprine and methylprednisolone, a severe prolonged acute rejection episode, during which donor heart function was lost completely in one case, was successfully reversed after immunosuppression had been changed to CYA[16]. Our short experience with CYA supports the good results that have been obtained by other transplant centres using it as the primary immunosuppressant.

Two patients with sensitization following heart transplantation have shown loss of circulating lymphocytotoxic antibodies following short courses of CYA therapy[17]. If CYA does, in fact, reverse sensitization, then many patients for whom, hitherto, there would be difficulty in finding a suitable donor, may be able to undergo transplantation or retransplantation.

HETEROTOPIC HEART TRANSPLANTATION USING A XENOGRAFT

One of the indications for heterotopic cardiac transplantation is to provide temporary circulatory support to a failing heart when all other measures have been unsuccessful.

Because human donors are often not available when required, xenografts have been used at our institute on two emergency occasions[18]. On both occasions the patient's left ventricle failed to support the circulation when attempts were made to discontinue cardiopulmonary bypass after surgical procedures. Intraaortic balloon pump support was unsuccessful in the first case and not available in the second.

The first patient, operated on in June 1977, received a heterotopic graft from a 30 kg baboon which proved insufficient to support the entire circulation in the presence of repeated attacks of ventricular fibrillation which affected the patient's own heart, the patient dying some 6 hours after transplantation.

The second patient, operated on in October 1977, was supported success-fully by a chimpanzee heart until rejection occurred 4 days later; the recipi-ent's own heart failed to recover sufficiently to support the circulation alone. Higher doses of immunosuppression were used than would be the case with a human donor.

This experience suggested that a heterotopic transplant using a suitable xenograft and heavy immunosuppression could support a patient's circu-lation for at least 2–3 days, and might be indicated where there was evidence that the patient's own cardiac function would recover during this period.

DONOR HEART STORAGE

When the donor heart is excised at a distant location, most groups transport the organ in ice as quickly as possible (usually by air) to the recipient centre; the total ischaemic period normally does not exceed approximately 4 hours. Under ideal conditions, using private chartered jet aircraft, donor hearts can be transported over 1500 km (940 miles) from the donor to the recipient centre.

In Cape Town we have been interested in prolonging myocardial ischaemic time further, both to enable transportation by less expensive methods and to allow time for tests such as lymphocytotoxic cross-matching and tissue typing. Our ultimate goal, however, is to allow the transplant operation to be per-formed as a semielective rather than as an emergency procedure. During the past 4 years, a team in our experimental laboratory has developed a portable perfusion system for storage of the donor heart for periods up to 48 hours[19]. The heart is arrested with cardioplegic solution at 4°C, rapidly excised, and then suspended from a portable perfusion apparatus, where it is continuously supplied with oxygen bubbled into a clear perfusate. The perfusate is con-tinuously circulated by the air-lift pump principle, whereby the flow of oxy-genated gas itself leads to circulation of the fluid.

Consistent survival until rejection has been obtained in immunosuppressed baboons following the orthotopic transplantation of hearts stored for 24 hours; post-transplantation cardiac catheterization has revealed normal pressures and cardiac output. Autotransplantation was carried out in order to assess the long-term effects of donor heart storage uncomplicated by the development of acute rejection[20]. Following excision of the heart and its transfer to the perfusion apparatus, the baboon was supported for 24 hours by an orthotopic transplant from a second baboon. After having undergone continuous hypothermic perfusion for 24 hours, the baboon's own heart was reimplanted. One animal was studied and sacrificed over 2 years later; haemodynamic and histological studies of the myocardium were basically normal (Cooper, D. K. C., Wicomb, W. N. and Novitzky, D., unpublished data).

This perfusion system was first used in clinical practice in September 1981[19]. Total periods of ischaemia have ranged from 6 hours 55 minutes to 16 hours 50 minutes.

THE DIAGNOSIS OF ACUTE REJECTION BY RADIONUCLIDE SCANNING

Though the technique of endomyocardial biopsy, introduced by Caves at Stanford in 1973[21], has proved invaluable in the diagnosis of acute rejection episodes, it is, nevertheless, an invasive technique associated with a small but significant number of complications. Investigators have long been searching for a reliable non-invasive technique which can be performed in the patient's isolation room.

We believe this has recently been achieved at our own institution by the measurement of volume changes of the donor left ventricle by radionuclide scanning using technetium 99M labelled red cells[22, 23]. Experimental and clinical studies have shown excellent correlation between changes in left ventricular volume and histopathological evidence of acute rejection obtained from endomyocardial biopsy. We believe that this technique might well supersede that of endomyocardial biopsy in monitoring for acute rejection in patients with heart transplants, whether they be heterotopic or orthotopic.

Present laboratory and clinical research in our institution continues in the areas of donor heart storage, the diagnosis and management of acute rejection, and the problems of transplantation of the heart and both lungs. We are also applying much attention to the important subject of the effects of brain death on myocardial function, particularly with regard to improving that function before excision and storage of the donor heart.

References

1. Parry, M. W., Cooper, D. K. C. and Barnard, C. N. (1983). Trends in cardiac surgery at the University of Cape Town: an 11-year survey, 1971–1981. *S. Afr. Med. J.*, **63**, 189
2. Barnard, C. N. (1967). A human cardiac transplant: an interim report of a successful operation performed at Groote Schuur Hospital, Cape Town. *S. Afr. Med. J.*, **41**, 1271
3. Lower, R. R. and Shumway, N. E. (1960). Studies on orthotopic homotransplantation of the canine heart. *Surg. Forum*, **11**, 18
4. Barnard, C. N. (1968). What we have learnt about heart transplants. *J. Thorac. Cardiovasc. Surg.*, **56**, 457
5. Losman, J. G., Levine, H., Campbell, C. D., Replogle, R. L., Hassoulas, J., Novitzky, D., Cooper, D. K. C. and Barnard, C. N. (1982). Changes in indications for heart transplantation: an additional argument for preservation of the recipient's own heart. *J. Thorac. Cardiovasc. Surg.*, **84**, 716
6. Thomson, J. G. (1968). Heart transplantation in man—necropsy findings. *Br. Med. J.*, **2**, 511
7. Thomson, J. G. (1969). Production of severe atheroma in a transplanted human heart. *Lancet*, **2**, 1088

8. Rose, A. G., Uys, C. J., Cooper, D. K. C. and Barnard, C. N. (1982). Donor heart morphology 12½ years after orthotopic transplantation. *Heart Transplant.*, **1**, 329

9. Losman, J. G., Campbell, C. D., Replogle, R. L. and Barnard, C. N. (1982). Joint transplantation of the heart and lungs. *J. Cardiovasc. Surg.*, **23**, 440

10. Losman, J. G. and Barnard, C. N. (1977). Haemodynamic evaluation of left ventricular bypass with a homologous cardiac graft. *J. Thorac. Cardiovasc. Surg.*, **74**, 695

11. Barnard, C. N. and Losman, J. G. (1975). Left ventricular bypass. *S. Afr. Med. J.*, **49**, 303

12. Novitzky, D., Cooper, D. K. C. and Barnard, C. N. (1983). The surgical technique of heterotopic heart transplantation. *Ann. Thorac. Surg.*, **36**, 476

13. Uys, C. J., Rose, A. G. and Barnard, C. N. (1975). The autopsy findings in a case of heterotopic cardiac transplantation with left ventricular bypass for ischaemic heart failure. *S. Afr. Med. J.*, **49**, 2029

14. Losman, J. G., Curcio, A. and Barnard, C. N. (1978). Normal cardiac function with a hybrid heart. *Ann. Thorac. Surg.*, **26**, 177

15. Kennelly, B. M., Corte, P., Losman, J. G. and Barnard, C. N. (1976). Arrhythmias in two patients with left ventricular bypass transplants. *Br. Heart J.*, **38**, 725

16. Novitzky, D., Cooper, D. K. C. and Barnard, C. N. (1984). Reversal of acute rejection by cyclosporin in a heterotopic heart transplant. *Heart Transplant.*, **3**, 117

17. Novitzky, D., Cooper, D. K. C., Du Toit, E., Oudshoorn, M., Campbell, E. and Barnard, C. N. (19—). Disappearance of preformed lymphocytotoxic antibodies following cyclosporin A administration in two patients with previous heart transplants. (Submitted for publication)

18. Barnard, C. N., Wolpowitz, A. and Losman, J. G. (1977). Heterotopic cardiac transplantation with a xenograft for assistance of the left heart in cardiogenic shock after cardiopulmonary bypass. *S. Afr. Med. J.*, **52**, 1035

19. Wicomb, W. N., Cooper, D. K. C., Novitzky, D. and Barnard, C. N. (1984). Cardiac transplantation following storage of the donor heart by a portable hypothermic perfusion system. *Ann. Thorac. Surg.*, **37**, 243

20. Cooper, D. K. C., Wicomb, W. N., Rose, A. G. and Barnard, C. N. (1983). Orthotopic allotransplantation and autotransplantation of the baboon heart following 24-hour storage by a portable hypothermic perfusion system. *Cryobiology*, **20**, 385

21. Caves, P. K., Stinson, E. B., Graham, A. F., Billingham, M. E., Grehl, T. M. and Shumway, N. E. (1973). Percutaneous transvenous endomyocardial biopsy. *J. Am. Med. Assoc.*, **225**, 228

22. Novitzky, D., Boniaszczuk, J., Cooper, D. K. C., Isaacs, S., Rose, A. G., Smith, J. A., Uys, C. J., Barnard, C. N. and Fraser, R. C. (1984). Prediction of acute cardiac rejection using radionuclide techniques. *S. Afr. Med. J.*, **65**, 5

23. Novitzky, D., Cooper, D. K. C., Boniaszczuk, J., Isaacs, S., Fraser, R. C., Commerford, P., Uys, C. J., Rose, A. G., Smith, J. A. and Barnard, C. N. (1984). The significance of left ventricular volume measurement in cardiac transplants using radionuclide techniques. *Heart Transplant.* (In press)

Index